ENGINEERING MATERIALS FOR BIOMEDICAL APPLICATIONS

Biomaterials Engineering and Processing Series

Series Editors: **Swee Hin TEOH** (*Department of Mechanical Engineering, National University of Singapore*), **Mauli AGRAWAL** (*Center for Clinical Bioengineering, The University of Texas Health Center, USA*), **Joost D. de Bruijn** (*IsoTis NV, The Netherlands*) & **Yasuhiko TABATA** (*Institute for Frontier Medical Sciences, Kyoto University*, Japan)

Forthcoming

Vol. 2: Principles of Organ Printing
eds. A. Atala (*Harvard University, USA*) & T. Boland (*Clemson University, USA*), R. Markwald (*Medical University of South Carolina, USA*), S. H. Teoh (*National University of Singapore, Singapore*) & V. Mironov (*Medical University of South Carolina, USA*)

Biomaterials Engineering and Processing Series – Vol. 1

ENGINEERING MATERIALS FOR BIOMEDICAL APPLICATIONS

Teoh Swee Hin

National University of Singapore, Singapore

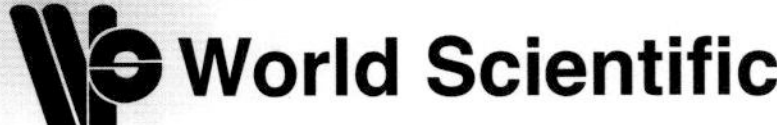

World Scientific

NEW JERSEY · LONDON · SINGAPORE · BEIJING · SHANGHAI · HONG KONG · TAIPEI · CHENNAI

Published by

World Scientific Publishing Co. Pte. Ltd.

5 Toh Tuck Link, Singapore 596224

USA office: 27 Warren Street, Suite 401–402, Hackensack, NJ 07601

UK office: 57 Shelton Street, Covent Garden, London WC2H 9HE

British Library Cataloguing-in-Publication Data
A catalogue record for this book is available from the British Library.

First published 2004
Reprinted 2007

ENGINEERING MATERIALS FOR BIOMEDICAL APPLICATIONS

ISBN-13 978-981-256-061-2
ISBN-10 981-256-061-0

Printed in Singapore by Mainland Press

CONTENTS

3   Corrosion of metallic implants
(D. J. Blackwood, K. H. W. Seah and S. H. Teoh)   **3-1**

4 Surface modification of metallic biomaterials
(T. Hanawa)   **4-1**

5 Biorestorative materials in dentistry *(A. U. J. Yap)* **5-1**

6 Bioceramics: an introduction *(B. Ben-Nissan and G. Pezzotti)* **6-1**

7 Polymeric hydrogels *(J. Li)*   7-1

8 Bioactive ceramic-polymer composites for tissue replacement *(M. Wang)*   8-1

9 Composites in biomedical applications
(Z. M. Huang and S. Ramakrishna) **9-1**

Contents

FOREWORD

This new text on *Engineering Materials for Biomedical Applications*, edited by Prof. Swee Hin Teoh, will be an especially useful reference book for those working with metals and ceramics for hard tissue applications. After a general introductory chapter, the emphasis of most of the remaining chapters is on the compositions, processing techniques, and physical properties of the metallic and ceramic biomaterials and their composites that are commonly used in orthopedic and dental implants. Metal and ceramic processing techniques are not often covered well in other texts, so this will be a valuable contribution of this book. There is detailed coverage of corrosion and surface treatments of metals in two chapters, another chapter on polymer-ceramic composites, and a special chapter on prosthetic appliances for the disabled — an important application area that is also often overlooked in other biomaterials texts. And to "add icing to this rich cake", there are additional chapters on polymeric hydrogels — an important class of synthetic polymers, and chitin — one of the most abundant natural polymers that has great potential in the biomaterials field. This text should provide a valuable addition to the library of the biomaterials scientist and engineer.

Allan S. Hoffman
University of Washington
Seattle, WA 98125 USA
29 July 2004

PREFACE

The success of any implant or medical device depends very much on the biomaterial used. Synthetic materials (such as metals, polymers, ceramics, and composites) have made significant contributions to many established medical devices. The aim of this publication, Volume 1: Engineering biomaterials for medical applications, is to provide a basic understanding on the engineering and processing aspects of biomaterials used in medical applications. Of paramount importance is the tripartite relationship between material properties, processing methods, and design. As the target audiences cover a wide interdisciplinary field of professions ranging from engineers, scientists, clinicians, and technologists to graduate students, the content of each chapter is written with a detailed background so that audience of another discipline will be able to understand. For the more knowledgeable reader, a detailed list of references is included.

Chapter 1 gives a broad overview of biomaterials engineering and processing. Here the requirements of biomaterials and the effects such as grain size, composite layering, molding conditions on mechanical properties are discussed. It also endeavors to give a foretaste of the new emerging field of tissue engineering and the challenges ahead.

Chapter 2 deals with the durability of common metallic implant materials such as stainless steel and titanium. The host-tissue response to metallic debris, the effect of micro motion that leads to fretting fatigue, and the forecast of metallic biomaterials for the future are discussed here.

The main disadvantage of metallic implant materials is that they corrode. This is an important topic which many students without chemistry background will have difficulty in understanding. Chapter 3 therefore deals with the fundamentals of metallic corrosion, giving the audience a strong basic understanding on the thermodynamics and kinetics aspects of corrosion. The case examples cited will be useful to help the audience appreciate how these principles are applied.

Chapter 4 talks about an important aspect in surface modification of metallic implants: it attempts to describe the interactions of cells and proteins on metallic surfaces. This is an interesting chapter which helps the reader to develop a greater appreciation of the basic science of surface chemistry and the adhesion mechanics of cells and proteins.

Chapter 5 gives a good application chapter on dental restorative biomaterials and the technology advancements in this field. Here one can see how ceramics, metals, and polymers have all been used in the early trials of biomaterials.

Chapter 6 introduces a significant topic — bioceramics, which has been a subject of intense research in the biomaterials field. Not only the inert but also the bioresorbable types are important nowadays.

Chapter 7 describes the polymeric hydrogels which have now earned a place in many useful applications — ranging from contact lenses to control of drug release devices. The structure of polymers is an important topic, especially in the quest to engineer and use polymers as biomaterials.

Chapters 8 and 9 are on composites: the former on polymer-bioceramic composites especially the Hapex material, while the latter describes the textile composite which has found some useful applications such as in vascular grafts.

Chapter 10 may seem out of place. But with the latest prosthetic materials and the new technologies that have gone into this traditional field, this chapter sheds new light into what materials engineers have accomplished in the field of prosthetics: lightweight and intelligent lower limb prostheses. The use of computers has indeed revolutionized the way we design materials.

The last chapter, Chapter 11, describes a natural biomaterial — chitin. Chitin is fast becoming a useful material not only in wound dressings, but also in tissue engineering's scaffolds because of its special cell mediation properties.

It is hoped that all the 11 chapters written by many distinguished experts will provide a good start to better understanding in engineering materials for biomedical applications.

SH Teoh
Chair, NUS Graduate Programme in Bioengineering
Professor, Department of Mechanical Engineering
National University of Singapore
18 May 2004

ACKNOWLEDGEMENTS

This book would not have come about without the dedication and active participation of all the authors who over time have become friends and collaborators. They are: Adrian, U. J. Yap, B. Ben-Nissan, D. J. Blackwood, T. Hanawa, Z. M. Huang, E. Khor, J. Li, Peter, V. S. Lee, G. Pezzotti, S. Ramakrishna, K. H. W. Seah, M. Sumita, and M. Wang. I thank them for their patience and for bearing with me.

To all my students in my Biomaterials Engineering and Advanced Biomaterials class, Mechanical Engineering Department, National University of Singapore, over the last 10 years, it has been a joy learning from your criticisms in pointing out the mistakes in my lectures. If not for your feedback, this book would not be able to address some of your concerns. I thank you.

The pictures on the cover were generously provided by Prof E. H. Lee who at the last minute entertained an urgent request from me. I thank him for his kind gesture of friendship over these years.

Last but not least, I thank Ms Rhoda Lim, for her help in editing this volume with surgical accuracy and assisting me in technical matters.

CHAPTER 1

INTRODUCTION TO BIOMATERIALS ENGINEERING AND PROCESSING — AN OVERVIEW

S. H. Teoh

Department of Mechanical Engineering
National University of Singapore
9 Engineering Drive 1, Singapore 117576
E-mail: mpetsh@nus.edu.sg

The success of a material to be used as a biomaterial in medical devices, apart from biocompatibility, is often related to the ability and ease of the material to be formed into complicated shapes. This chapter provides an overview of biomaterials engineering, paying particular attention on the effect of processing methods on the mechanical properties of biomaterials. The effects of grain refinement in metals and ceramics, molding conditions on polymeric wear, and composite lamination are discussed with the aim of introducing the many interesting materials engineering techniques that have been used to enhance the mechanical properties of biomaterials. The chapter concludes by introducing the concept of tissue engineering as the new wave in biomaterials engineering of tissues and organs.

1.1   Introduction

Biomaterials engineering is concerned with the application of biomaterials science in the design and engineering aspects of medical devices' fabrication. Traditionally the study of biomaterials focuses on issues such as biocompatibility, host-tissue reaction to implants, cytotoxicity, and basic structure-property relationships [1–8]. These issues are important. They provide a strong scientific basis for a clear understanding of many successful medical devices such as the mechanical heart valve. However in biomaterials engineering, the manufacturing and processing aspects emerge as a primary concern. While it may be easy to make a one-off laboratory prototype, it is extremely challenging to produce a thousand units of identical devices with good quality control, consistent properties and having to be packed in a sterile manner for storage and easy transportation. Topics such as durability, corrosion, and surface modification are some essential elements in engineering biomaterials for medical applications.

As an example, Figure 1−1 shows the intricate engineering mold design involved in forming a polyurethane (PU) tri-leaflet valve using a thermoforming process. The tri-leaflet heart valve is an interesting design which mimics the natural aortic valve with a central flow. First, a biocompatible PU sheet is thermoformed over the leaflet mold to yield the three-leaflet shape with a central flow. Next, the outer three sinus lobes need to be formed over the leaflet. The valve must be made without any parting lines which are often seen in two-part injection molds. The parting lines can be detrimental as they are lines of weakness and subject to thrombus formation. An engineer developed a three-part mold that allows the PU sheet to be thermoformed over the assembled tool. The latter consists of three detachable lobes which can be unscrewed after the three-sinus-lobe mold is set.

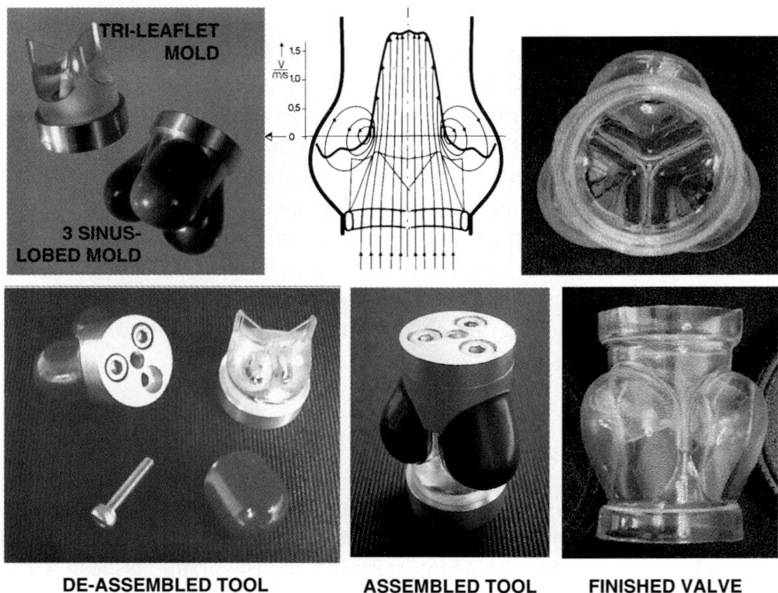

Figure 1−1 Manufacturing steps in making a tri-leaflet polyurethane valve. Note the complex die assembly needed to produce a seamless polyurethane valve by thermoforming.

1.2 Requirements of Biomaterials

Biomaterials must have special properties that can be tailored to meet the needs of a particular application — this is an important concept to bear in mind. For example, a biomaterial must be biocompatible, non-carcinogenic, corrosion-resistant, and has low toxicity and wear [1,2]. However, depending on the application, differing requirements may arise. Sometimes these requirements can be completely opposite. In tissue engineering of the bone, for instance, the polymeric scaffold needs to be biodegradable so that as the cells generate their own extracellular matrices, the polymeric biomaterial will be completely replaced over time with the patient's own tissue. In the case of mechanical heart valves, on the other hand, we need materials that are biostable, wear-resistant, and which do not degrade with time. Materials such as pyrolytic carbon leaflet and titanium housing are used because they can last at least 20 years or more.

Generally, the requirements of biomaterials can be grouped into four broad categories:

1. Biocompatibility: The material must not disturb or induce un-welcoming response from the host, but rather promote harmony and good tissue-implant integration. An initial burst of inflammatory response is expected and is sometimes considered essential in the healing process. However, prolonged inflammation is not desirable as it may indicate tissue necrosis or incompatibility.

2. Sterilizability: The material must be able to undergo sterilization. Sterilization techniques include gamma, gas (ethylene oxide (ETO)) and steam autoclaving. Some polymers such as polyacetal will depolymerize and give off the toxic gas formaldehyde when subjected under high energy radiation by gamma. These polymers are thus best sterilized by ETO.

3. Functionability: The functionability of a medical device depends on the ability of the material to be shaped to suit a particular function. The material must therefore be able to be shaped economically using engineering fabrication processes. The success of the coronary artery stent — which has been considered the most widely used medical device — can be attributed to the efficient fabrication process of stainless steel from heat treatment to cold working to improve its durability.

4. Manufacturability: It is often said that there are many candidate materials that are biocompatible. However it is often the last step, the manufacturability of the material, that hinders the actual production of the medical device. It is in this last step that engineers can contribute significantly.

1.3 Classification of Biomaterials

Biomaterials can broadly be classified as: i) Biological biomaterials; and ii) Synthetic biomaterials. Table 1–1 shows the various classifications and some examples. Biological materials [3,4] can be further classified into soft and hard tissue types. In the case of synthetic materials, it is further classified into: a) Metallic; b) Polymeric; c) Ceramic; and d) Composite biomaterials.

Table 1–1 Classification of biomaterials

I. Biological Materials	II. Synthetic Biomedical Materials
1. Soft Tissue *Skin, Tendon, Pericardium, Cornea*	1. Polymeric *Ultra High Molecular Weight Polyethylene (UHMWPE), Polymethylmethacarylate (PMMA), Polyethyletherketone (PEEK), Silicone, Polyurethane (PU), Polytetrafluoroethylene (PTFE)*
2. Hard Tissue *Bone, Dentine, Cuticle*	2. Metallic *Stainless Steel, Cobalt-based Alloy (Co–Cr–Mo), Titanium Alloy (Ti–Al–V), Gold, Platinum*
	3. Ceramic *Alumina (Al_2O_3), Zirconia (ZrO_2), Carbon, Hydroxylapatite [$Ca_{10}(PO_4)_6(OH)_2$], Tricalcium Phosphate [$Ca_3(PO_4)_2$], Bioglass [$Na_2O(CaO)(P_2O_3)(SiO_2)$], Calcium Aluminate [$Ca(Al_2O_4)$]*
	4. Composite *Carbon Fiber (CF)/PEEK, CF/UHMWPE, CF/PMMA, Zirconia/Silica/BIS–GMA*

1.4 Mechanical Properties of Biomaterials

The mechanical properties of a biomaterial can best be described by its modulus of elasticity, ultimate tensile strength, elongation to failure, and fracture toughness.

- Modulus of elasticity describes the stiffness of the material and is usually obtained from the slope of a stress-strain diagram.
- Ultimate tensile strength describes the ability of the material to withstand a load before it fails.
- Elongation to failure describes how much strain the material can bear before it fails.
- Fracture toughness is an important measurement of the material's resistance to crack propagation.

Figures 1-2(a) to (d) show the comparisons amongst different classes of biomaterial with respect to the four properties mentioned above. It can be seen that metals are generally very stiff and have high fracture toughness. In sharp contrast to the metals are the polymers, which have low stiffness and fracture toughness. However the polymers have high elongation to failure. The high stiffness of metals, on the other hand, can be a disadvantage since this can give rise to "stress shielding" in bone fracture repair. Stress shielding is a phenomenon where bone loss occurs when a stiffer material is placed over the bone. Bone responds to stresses during the healing process. Since the stress is practically shielded from the bone, the density of the bone underneath the stiffer material decreases as a result.

1.5   Effects of Processing on Properties of Biomaterials

1.5.1 Effect of Post Processing and Grain Size

Numerous properties of biomaterials can be improved by processing techniques. Figure 1–3 shows the fatigue strengths of some commonly used metals. It can be seen that the fatigue strengths of forged 316L stainless steel and cobalt–chromium are significantly higher than in their cast state. The increase in fatigue strength can be attributed to the large compressive force applied on the surface of the metal during the forging process, as well as due to grain refinement. How grain refinement leads to an increase in fatigue strength can be understood from the Hall–Petch equation. The equation states that the yield strength of a material (σ_{YD}) is inversely proportional to the square root of the grain size (d):

$$\sigma_{YD} = k \sqrt{d} \tag{1}$$

where k is a constant.

For many years in the steel industry, the subject of grain refinement has been intensely pursued to help improve the yield strength of steel. Nanograin structures have been produced via severe plastic deformation with remarkable success [9]. The other common route is to use powder metallurgy where ultra-fine particles are consolidated, compacted, and sintered at elevated temperature. Figure 1–3 shows that after cobalt–chromium alloy is subjected to hot isostatic pressing (H.I.P.), its fatigue strength is almost double than that in the cast state [10]. The use of isostatic pressure also helps to reduce defects — such as voids — in the alloy.

Brittle materials — such as bioceramics — are sensitive to stress concentrations which exist around pre-existing defects, such as pores, scratches, or cracks. Under an applied tensile stress, σ, the stresses at the tip of a crack can be described by the stress intensity factor K, which is given as follows:

$$K = Y\sigma\sqrt{a} \tag{2}$$

where a is the defect size and Y a geometry factor related to the crack.

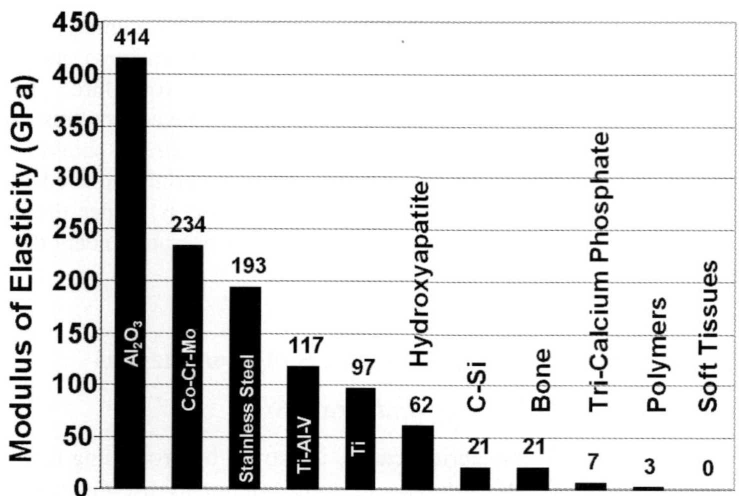

Figure 1–2(a) Comparison of moduli of elasticity of biomaterials. Note the very high values for ceramics and metals.

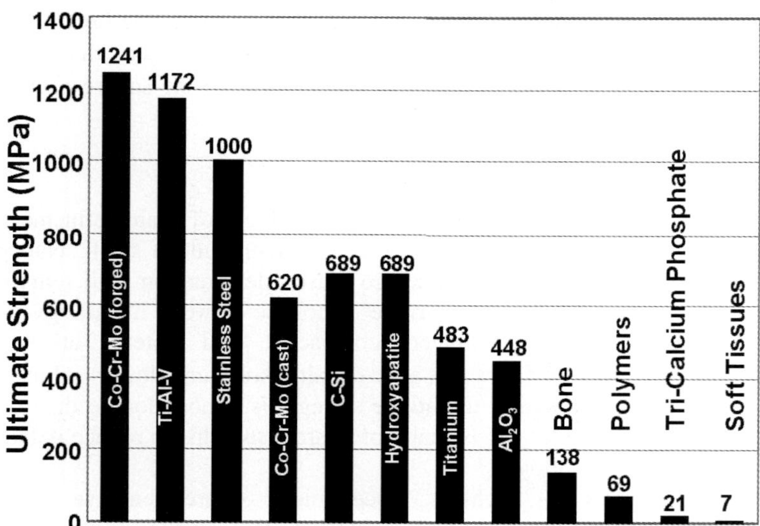

Figure 1–2(b) Comparison of ultimate tensile strengths of biomaterials. Note the exceptionally high values for metals which make the metals an ideal choice for load bearing applications.

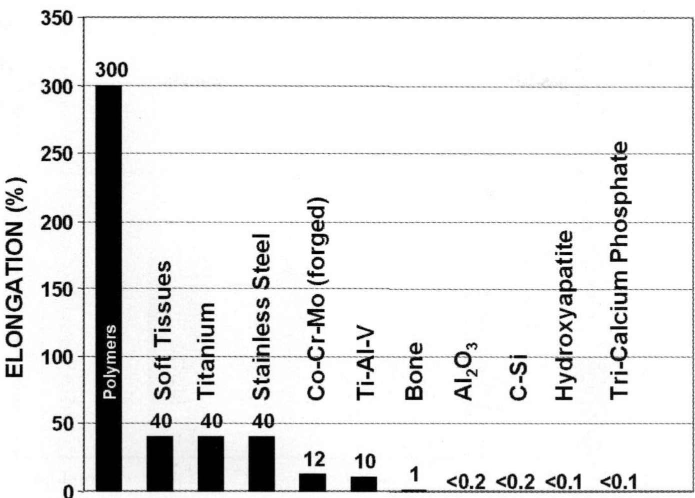

Figure 1–2(c) Comparison of elongation at failure of biomaterials. Note that polymers have exceptional elongation as compared to other materials. This is a measure of their high ductility.

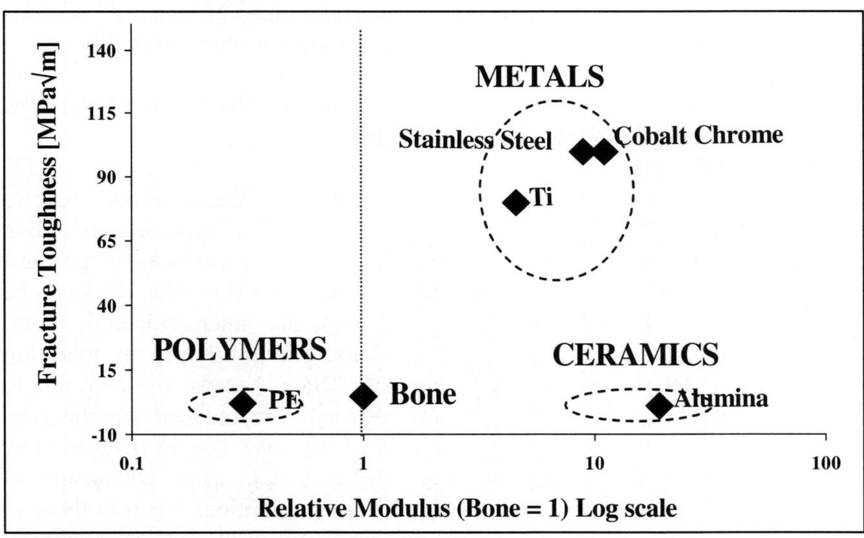

Figure 1–2(d) Comparison of fracture toughness of biomaterials relative to the log (Young's modulus) with bone as the reference. Note that the fracture toughness values of metals are generally several orders of magnitude higher than those of the other materials. The Young's modulus is also much higher than that of bone, giving rise to stress shielding.

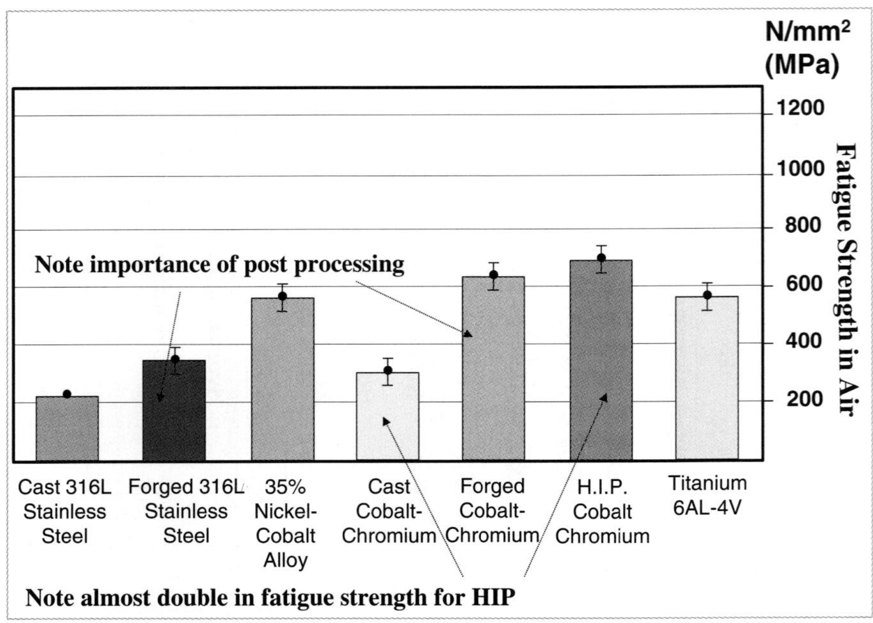

Figure 1–3 Fatigue strengths (in air) of common alloys used as implants. Note the effect of post processing conditions to improve fatigue strength (after Teoh [12]).

Fast fracture occurs when K becomes larger than the fracture toughness, K_{IC}. Fracture strength, σ_S, can then be given by:

$$\sigma_S = K_{IC}/\{Y\sigma\sqrt{a}\} \tag{3}$$

Composite processing by combining two or more phases is one route to produce enhanced properties of biomaterials. Another approach to obtain improved strength and reliability is to refine ceramic processing to produce homogeneous components with a defect size as small as possible. This can be done by refining powder processing to eliminate microstructural flaws. Ceramics such as alumina has been used for femoral heads in total hip replacements (THR) as an alternative to metal. This is because the wear rate in a ceramic-polyethylene combination was shown to be reduced significantly. However, reports of *in vivo* brittle fractures of ceramics due to delayed slow crack growth had brought about a new development in using composites of alumina and zirconia. The influence of processing conditions (such as those in colloidal processing) on the microstructures development of zirconia-toughened alumina composites, and the effect of these microstructures on the mechanical properties of alumina–zirconia composites, are discussed by De Aza *et al.* [11]. They have demonstrated that by using colloidal processing, microstructure refinement has brought about a significant improvement in the fracture toughness of ceramics (see Table 1–2).

Table 1–2 Fracture threshold, toughness and hardness of alumina, zirconia, and alumina–zirconia composites (after De Aza *et al.* [11]

Ceramic	Fracture Threshold, K_{I0} (MPa$\sqrt{m}$)	Fracture Toughness, K_{IC} (MPa$\sqrt{m}$)	Hardness (Vickers)
Alumina (Al_2O_3)	2.5±0.2	4.2±0.2	1600±50
Zirconia (ZrO_2)	3.1±0.2	5.5±0.2	1290±50
Al_2O_3–10vol% ZrO_2	4.0±0.2	5.9±0.2	1530±50

1.5.2 *Effect of Molding Conditions and Irradiation on Polymeric Wear*

Wear of polymeric materials used in implants is perhaps the most difficult to understand [7]. As a result, numerous reports on polymeric wear have emerged over the years [12,13]. In biomedical applications such as occluders in mechanical heart valves and joint prostheses, fatigue fracture and wear of the polymers have been considered to be an important factor in determining the durability of the prostheses. In the case of UHMWPE, many factors influence its wear properties. For example, when UHMWPE was molded between 190 and 200°C and some antioxidants were added during processing, its wear resistance appeared to improve. Molding at higher pressures and increasing the molecular weight, on the other hand, were reported to be detrimental. Nonetheless, there is a possibility that there could be an optimum processing condition and molecular weight distribution that could give the best wear characteristics. More recent work has shown that processing conditions play a vital role on the cyclic fatigue of UHMWPE. In particular, γ-radiation and oxidative aging are very detrimental to the fatigue threshold and crack propagation resistance (Table 1–3). Moreover, compression molding appears to render a better fatigue resistance when compared to extrusion.

1.5.3 *Effect of Composite Lamination*

Nanolaminates' layer of interpenetrating-networked composites such as those found in nature have unique fracture resistance. Examples are seashells which have been shown to yield improved fracture resistance with unique wear characteristics [15] (see Figure 1–4). The microstructure is made of nano brick-type arrangement of ceramic phase sandwiched by ultra-thin polymeric protein layers. Presumably, the small brick-like ceramic components (often biodegradable) allow easy removal/dissolution, a concept which needs to be mimicked in engineering a biomaterial that has wear debris which is eco-compatible. By using the laminate concept, fracture toughness reaching values as high as 16 MPa$\sqrt{m}$ can be achieved — as in the case of boron carbide/aluminum laminates. These laminates also have high flexural strength.

Microlaminates of interpenetrating-networked composites (Figure 1–5) can be produced by bi-axial stretching of one crystalline phase (UHMWPE) or by infiltrating with elastomeric polyurethane (PU) [16]. These microlaminates show significant improvement in strength and fracture toughness, and are used for elastomeric composite membrane (less than 40 μm) in biomedical application.

Table 1–3 Effect of processing conditions on the fatigue threshold (ΔK_{th}) of UHMWPE (after Pruiit and Bailey [14])

Condition	ΔK_{th}
Compression molded	1.8
Compression molded γ-air	1.2
Extruded 90°	1.7
Extruded 0° non-sterilized	1.3
Extruded 0° γ-air	1.0
Extruded 0° γ-peroxide	1.1

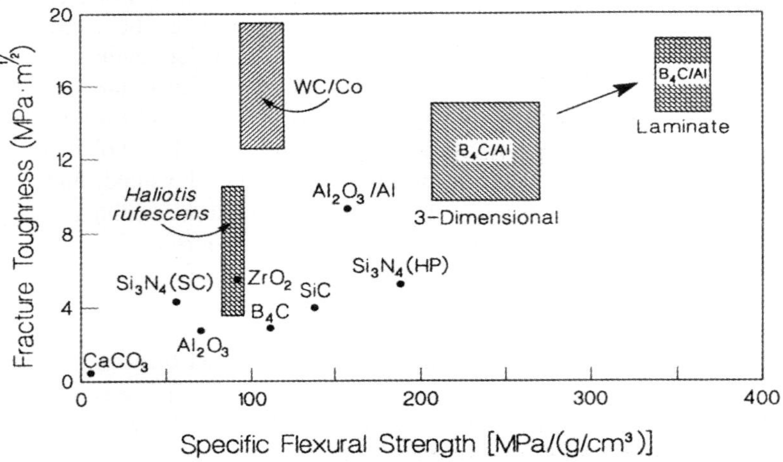

Figure 1–4 Fracture toughness versus specific flexural strength of some bioceramics and nanolaminates of metal matrix-ceramics composites. Note the effect of laminates in improving both fracture toughness and flexural strength (after Saikaya and Aksay [15]; reprinted with permission from Springer–Verlag, Berlin).

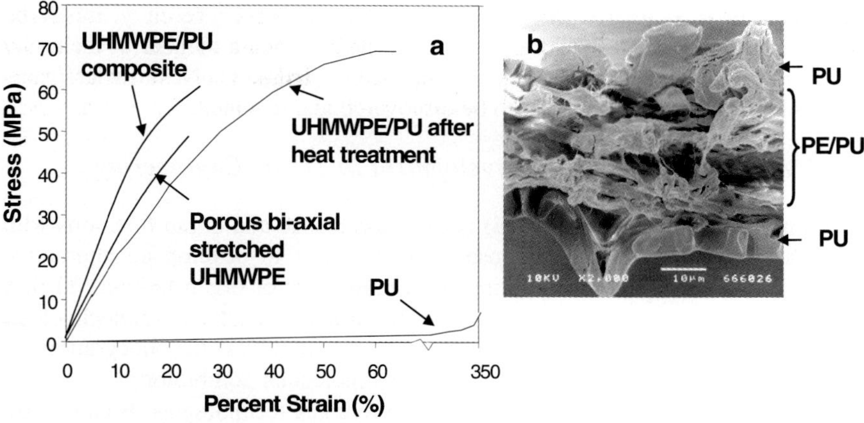

Figure 1–5 (a) Bi-axial stretching of UHMWPE and infiltrating with elastomeric polyurethane (PU) to produce microlaminates with significantly improved mechanical properties; (b) cross-sectional view of internal microstructure (after Teoh *et al.* [16])

1.6 Tissue Engineering — New Wave in Biomaterials Engineering

1.6.1 Need for Organ and Tissue Replacement

Loss of human tissues or organs is a devastating problem for the individual patient. Each year in United States alone, it is estimated that organs failure and tissue loss cost an estimated US$400b. Incidentally, patients waiting for organ transplants are also on the rise. Despite technological advances in biomaterials engineering, the figure significantly — for example from 27,883 in 1988 to 65,677 in 1995. Moreover, as life span increases in developed countries, coupled with rising number of calamities ranging from earthquakes to diseases outbreak and war tragedies, the need for organ and tissue replacement is expected to reach astronomical numbers by late 2010 [17].

1.6.2 Limitation of Current Technologies

Current technology for organ and tissue replacement has limitations. These include donor scarcity, adverse immunological response from the host tissue, biocompatibility, infection, pathogen transfer, and high cost to patient. Then, there is the perennial deficiency of synthetic material to provide the multifunctional requirement of organ. For example, bone is not just a structural element but also a "factory to produce bone marrow". These limitations prompt scientists worldwide to consider alternative technologies, amongst which tissue engineering has been heralded as the promising answer. As a result more than 20 companies were founded, according to an 1998 issue in Business Week

("The Era of Regenerative Medicine", July 27). However, recently, this hype soon met up with the reality of business enterprises when a number of them had to close, merge, or be bought up by large conglomerates. Nevertheless, new technologies and processes need to be discovered and invented.

1.6.3 Platform Technology Development in Tissue Engineering

The aim of tissue engineering (TE) is to restore tissue and organ functions with minimal host rejection. This arose from the need to develop an alternative method of treating patients suffering from tissue loss or organ failure. TE has been heralded as the new wave to revolutionize the healthcare-biotechnology industry. It is a multidisciplinary field and involves the integration of engineering principles, basic life sciences, and molecular cell biology.

The success of tissue engineering lies in five key technologies (Figure 1–6). They are namely: 1) Biomaterials; 2) Cells; 3) Scaffolds; 4) Bioreactors; and 5) Medical Imaging technology. It may seem simple to produce a one-off, tissue-engineered product in the laboratory, but it is a completely different matter to produce hundreds of products of consistent quality for clinical use.

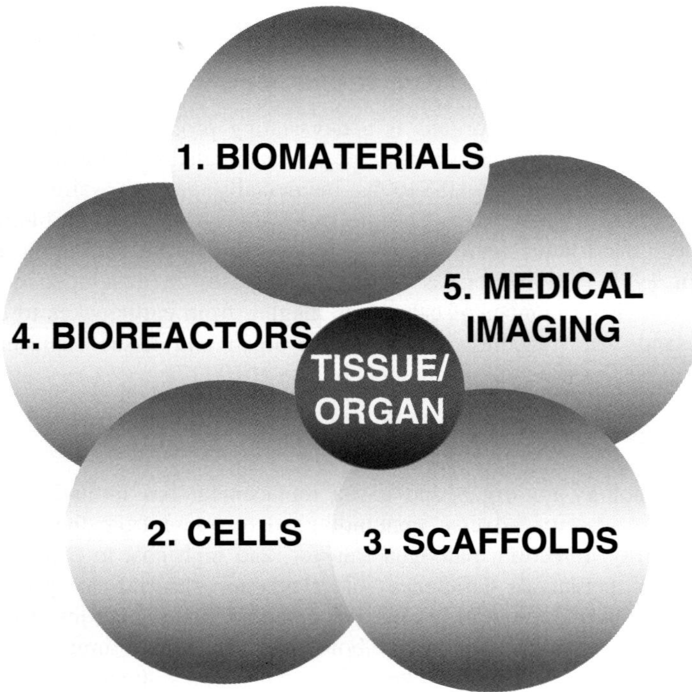

Figure 1–6 Five core technologies (biomaterials, cells, scaffolds, bioreactors, and medical imaging) required for tissue engineering

TE involves a scaffold which acts as a temporary extracellular matrix for the cells to adhere to, differentiate, and grow. Breakthrough has been made in the development of a platform technology which integrates medical imaging, computational mechanics, biomaterials, and advanced manufacturing to produce three-dimensional, porous load bearing scaffolds for tissue engineering of bone [18]. The technology makes use of polycaprolactone (PCL) bioresorbable polymer and Fused Deposition Modeling's (FDM) rapid prototyping advanced manufacturing fabrication process to produce the scaffolds without a mold [19] (Figure 1–7). Controlled three-dimensional architecture with interconnected pores enables good cells entrapment, facilitates easy flow path for nutrients and waste removal, and demonstrates long-term cell viability. Patient-specific scaffolds can now be made using this technology. Already more than 10 patients in Singapore have received scaffolds of this nature for cranioplastic surgery. This biomaterial processing technology has paved the way for patient-specific tissue engineering concepts not dreamed of a few years ago.

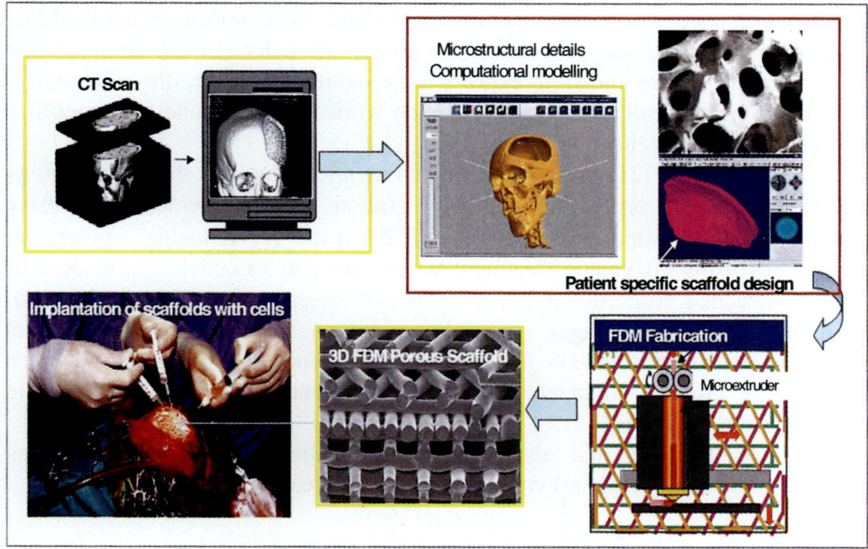

Figure 1–7 Platform technology for patient-specific scaffolds for bone tissue engineering

1.6.4 Tissue Engineering Issues and Challenges

In tissue engineering, there are certainly issues and challenges which are yet to be resolved. These issues range from cell-biomaterial interactions, stem cells technology to know-how in scaffolds manufacturing. For example, in the case of cell-biomaterial interactions, though we can grow single cell sheets such as cartilage, we hardly understand how the cells in composite tissues (such as the heart valve leaflets) recognize their own territories and hence do not cross and violate each other. They seem to know how to live in harmony. Although we no longer need to focus on biochemical effects such as growth factors, we need to study the mechano-induction effects. This is because the manner in which cells differentiate, proliferate, and express their extracellular matrix (ECM) is also a function of the stress fields they experience.

Stem cells and scaffolds technologies also pose some challenges. Recently, some work on human blood vessels was done by Auger's group [20] in Canada. They showed that by growing the cells in sheets and then rolling them into a tube helps to eliminate immunological mismatch. This is because smooth muscles cells (SMCs) re-expressed desmin, a differentiation marker known to be lost under culture conditions. As a result, large amounts of ECM were produced and the structural integrity maintained. However, the handling of the sheets is delicate and it is not clear if the material would survive the viscoelastic compliance mismatch in long-term *in vivo* physiological environment. Other major obstacles exist. One of them is over SMCs proliferation. This could be related to the presence of endothelial progenitor cells (EPCs) in inhibiting SMCs, and EPCs are known to express nitric oxide. However, dipyridalmole is also a strong inhibitor of SMCs, and much work has been done to immobilize this chemical on porous scaffolds.

Okano's group [21] in Japan developed an interesting cell sheets technology where cells grew on culture surfaces grafted with temperature-responsive polymer, poly(N−isopropylacrylamide) (PIPAAm). By reducing temperature (instead of using enzymatic treatment which traumatizes cells), confluent cells simply detached from the polymer as a cell sheet. Layered cell sheets of cardiomyocytes then began to pulse simultaneously and morphological communication via connexin 43 was established between the sheets. When sheets were layered, engineered constructs were macroscopically observed to pulse spontaneously too.

The examples quoted above point to the fact that tissue engineering breakthroughs will further gravitate towards even greater challenges ahead.

1.7   Conclusions

For a material to be used as a biomaterial, it must possess the mandatory properties of biocompatibility and sterilizability. In addition, a biomaterial must be malleable. This is because the ability of a biomaterial to be pulled or pressed into shape often determines its success as a medical device in the long run. When it comes to the manufacturability of a biomaterial, processing techniques often affect the final property of the biomaterial — which means affecting the durability of the device. On this note, engineers need to examine the various processing effects that stem from grain refinement of steel to molding conditions and irradiation on UHMWPE.

Future direction seems to lead us to nanolaminate composites, which give better properties such as fracture toughness and wear enhancement. The era of tissue engineering also paves the way for new biomaterial processes to be developed and invented. The integration of different modalities from cells, biomaterials to medical imaging has opened up new challenges in the healthcare industry.

References

1. B. D. Ratner, A. S. Hoffman, F. J. Schoen, and J. E. Lemons (eds.), Biomaterials science: an introduction to materials in medicine, (Elsevier Sci., New York, 1996).
2. J. B. Park and R. S. Lakes, Biomaterials — an introduction, 2nd Edition, (Plenum Press, New York, 1992).
3. K. C. Dec, D. A. Puleo, and R. Bigirs (eds.), An introduction to tissue-biomaterial interactions, (John Wiley & Sons, NY, 2002).
4. J. Black, Biological performance of materials, 2nd Edition, (Marcel & Dekker, New York, 1992).
5. D. Hill, Design engineering of biomaterials for medical devices, (John Wiley & Sons, New York, 1998).
6. R. S. Greco, Implantation biology: the host response and biomedical devices, (CRC Press, London, 1994).
7. K. R. St. John (ed.), Particulate debris from medical implants, (American Society of Testing and Materials, Philadelphia, USA, 1992) ASTM STP1144.
8. R. D. Jamison and L. N. Gilbertson (eds.), Composite materials for implant applications in the human body, (American Society of Testing and Materials, Philadelphia, USA, 1993) ASTM STP1178.
9. N. Tsuji, Y. Saito, S. H. Lee, and Y. Minamino, ARB (accumulative roll-bonding) and other new techniques to produce bulk ultra-fine grained materials, Adv. Eng. Mat., 2003, 5:338–344.
10. H. A. Luckey and L. J. Barnard, Improved properties of Co–Cr–Mo alloy by hot isostatic pressing of powder, in Mechanical Properties of Biomaterials, eds. G. W. Hastings and D. F. Williams, (John Wiley & Sons, 1980) Ch. 24.
11. A. H. De Aza, J. Chevalier, G. Fantozzi, M. Schehl, and R. Torrecillas, Crack growth resistance of alumina, zirconia and zirconia toughened alumina ceramics for joint prostheses, Biomaterials, 2002, 23:937–945.
12. S. H. Teoh, Fatigue of biomaterials: A review, Int J. Fatigue, (Special Issue on Biomaterials, 2000) 22:825–837.
13. S. H. Teoh, Failure in biomaterials, in Comprehensive Structural Integrity Series, Vol. 9, eds. Y. W. Mai and S. H. Teoh, (Elsevier, London, UK, 2003) Ch. 1.
14. L. Pruitt and L. Bailey, Factors affecting near-threshold fatigue crack propagation behavior of orthopedic grade ultra high molecular weight polyethylene, Polymer, 1998, 39:1545–1553.
15. M. Saikaya and I. A. Aksay, Nacre of abalone shell: A natural multifunctional nanolaminate ceramic-polymer composite material, in Structure, Cellular Synthesis

and Assembly of Biopolymers, ed. S. T. Case, (Springer–Verlag, Berlin 1992), Ch. 1, Fig. 1.

16. S. H. Teoh, Z. G. Tang, and S Ramakrishna, Development of thin composite membranes for biomedical applications, J. Mat Sci: Mat Med, 1999, 10:343–352.

17. S. H. Teoh, Tissue engineering challenges and issues — the Asian perspective, Tissue Engineering, 2003, 9 (Sup 1):S1–S3.

18. D. W. Hutmacher, J. T. Schantz, I. Zein, K. W. Ng, S. H. Teoh, and K. C. Tan, Mechanical properties and cell cultural response of polycaprolactone scaffolds designed and fabricated via fused deposition modeling, J. Biomed. Mat. Res., 2001, 55:203–216.

19. I. Zein, D. W. Hutmacher, K. C. Tan, and S. H. Teoh, Fused deposition modeling of novel scaffold architectures for tissue engineering applications, Biomaterials, 2002, 23:1169–1185.

20. N. L'Heureux, S. Paquet, R. Labbe, L. Germain, and F. A. Auger, A completely biological tissue-engineered human blood vessel, FASEB J., 1998, 12:47–56.

21. T. Shimizu, M. Yamato, Y. Isoi, T. Akutsu, T. Setomaru, K. Abe, A. Kikuchi, M. Umezu, and T. Okano, Fabrication of pulsatile cardiac tissue grafts using a novel 3-dimensional cell sheet manipulation technique and temperature-responsive cell culture surfaces, Circulation Res., 2002, 90:E40–E48.

CHAPTER 2

DURABILITY OF METALLIC IMPLANT MATERIALS

M. Sumita[1] and S. H. Teoh[2]

[1]Biomaterials Center, National Institute for Materials Science
1-2-1, Sengen, Tsukuba, Ibaraki, 305-0032, Japan
E-mail: sumita.masae@nims.go.jp

[2]Department of Mechanical Engineering
National University of Singapore
9 Engineering Drive 1, 117576, Singapore
E-mail: mpetsh@nus.edu.sg

Metallic implant materials such as stainless steel, titanium, and cobalt-based alloys have found many applications as medical devices. This is due to their excellent mechanical properties such as fatigue strength and fracture toughness. Their durability however is dependent on their corrosion and wear resistance. The heat treatment and manufacturing method also affect these properties. The issues of adverse cellular response to wear debris from fretting fatigue and contact motion in artificial joints continue to present many challenges to the design of medical implants. The leaching of metallic ions such as nickel during the corrosion process has caused considerable concerns. This has paved way to development of new nickel-free alloys and amorphous metals that are more biocompatible.

2.1   Introduction

Metallic materials are often used to replace structural components of the human body because they surpass plastic or ceramic materials in terms of tensile strength, fatigue strength, and fracture toughness. As such, they are used in medical devices such as artificial joints, dental implants, artificial hearts, bone plates, staples, wires, and stents. They also possess better electro conductivity qualities, and hence are used for enclosing electronic devices such as pacemaker electrodes and artificial inner ears. Figure 2–1(a) shows typical applications of metallic implant devices, and Figure 2–1(b) shows a stainless steel stent used successfully in a coronary artery.

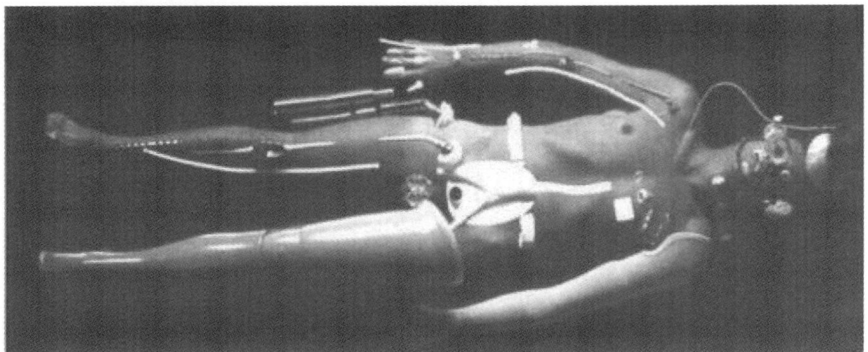

Figure 2–1(a) Some examples of metallic implant devices in the body

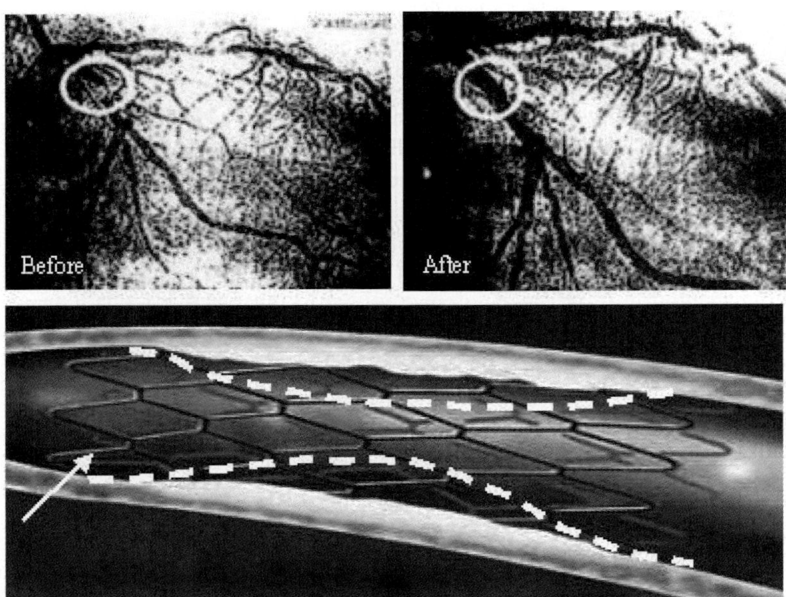

Figure 2–1(b) The first X-ray shows a severe narrowing (circle) of the coronary artery; the second X-ray shows that after the stainless steel stent (arrow) has been put in place, broadening of the artery occurred allowing blood to flow normally

It was in Egypt and Phoenicia that teeth were tied with golden wires as a form of treatment [1]. Golden wires in prosthodontics were used in Egypt 2500 years ago. In Etruria, golden bridges and partial dentures were in use around 700BC. It was during the ancient Greek period that metals were used in orthopedic procedures for the first time. Hippocrates (460–377BC), who is known as the Father of Medicine, is believed to have used golden wires to treat fractures. Records of employing gold, iron, and bronze to suture lacerations in the 17th century were found. As iron and bronze corrode more easily than gold, they have been difficult to verify when they were first used as biomedical materials. The gold and unalloyed metals used then were weak and could not therefore be used for load bearing applications. The unalloyed metals also corroded easily and did not promote osteointegration. They were also not wear resistant.

2.2　Typical Metallic Biomaterials

With the advent of the Iron Age and industrial revolution, steel materials were used in the 19th century as bone plates and screws to fix fractures. Fixing fractures with screws allowed a stronger fixity than the earlier method of fixing with metallic wires. Steel made from nickel-plating steel and vanadium steel later replaced carbon steel materials as steel corrodes easily in the human body. However, these newer materials were not sufficiently corrosion-resistant. It also became clear that they become toxic inside the human body. Consequently stainless steels, cobalt–chromium–molybdenum alloys (Vitallium), titanium, and titanium alloys gradually become the main biomedical materials used presently in orthopedic applications.

Presently the typical metallic biomaterials used for implant devices are:

- 316L stainless steels;
- Cobalt–chromium alloys;
- CP (commercially pure) titanium;
- Ti–6Al–4V alloys; and
- Ni–Ti alloys

These materials were originally developed for industrial uses. They were subsequently used in many implant devices, as a biomaterial, due to their relatively high corrosion resistance. Unfortunately when used as biomaterials, they pose several problems. These include:

- ❖ Toxicity of corrosion products arising from wear and fretting debris;
- ❖ Excessively high rigidity when compared to bone, giving rise to stress shielding and bone loss;
- ❖ High specific gravity, adding extra weight and causes surrounding organs to be subjected to undue stresses;
- ❖ Fracture due to corrosion fatigue and fretting corrosion fatigue;
- ❖ Lack of biocompatibility with surrounding tissue;
- ❖ Inadequate affinity for cells and tissues integration which resulted in the loosening of the metallic devices;
- ❖ Shielding of X-rays which make radiographic examination difficult.

2.2.1 Stainless Steels

Corrosion resistance of various steel types increases with increase in chromium content. Corrosion-resistant steels are made by adding more than 12 percent of chromium, which results in the formation of a thin, chemically stable, and passive oxide film. The oxide film forms and heals itself in the presence of oxygen. Steels containing more than 12 percent of chromium are known as stainless steels. Stainless steel itself does not generally corrode. However, pitting corrosion occurs in saline and chloride environments. Pitting corrosion, resulting from the abnormal progress of internal corrosion, causes deep pits on the metal surfaces. This pitting corrosion is further accelerated when dissolved oxygen reacts with chloride ions [2].

Apart from chromium, nickel and molybdenum are added to stainless steels. Other elements such as carbon, silicone, manganese, and nitrogen are also added. Nickel and molybdenum increase corrosion resistance. Carbon, on the other hand, is detrimental to corrosion resistance in stainless steels. This is because chromium content is decreased when chromium carbides are formed during the manufacturing process like hot working and high temperature heat treatment, and the carbides exist in the matrix as inhomogeneous microstructures.

The microstructures of steel can be classified into three categories based on their crystallographic structures: ferritic (α-body centered cubic, BCC), martensitic (a distorted body-centered cubic, a distorted BCC, obtained by rapid quenching), and austenitic (γ-face centered cubic, FCC) (see Figure 2–2) [3]. Only the austenitic type is non-magnetic. Austenitic stainless steels are more superior to ferritic and martensitic steels in terms of corrosion resistance, toughness, and workability. Nickel is the main alloying element that stabilizes the austenitic form of iron. They are many types of austenitic stainless steels, most of which originate from Type 302 (18Cr–8Ni) stainless steel. Type 316L has its corrosion resistance improved by adding molybdenum and reducing the carbon content.

The use of stainless steels is now confined to temporary devices for load bearing applications because of nickel toxicity to the human body and its susceptibility to stress corrosion cracking and crevice corrosion [4]. However for stents in the coronary artery where there is adequate supply of oxygen in the blood, it has been a successful permanent device for many years. The price of 316L stainless steels is one-tenth to one-fifth of other typical metallic biomaterials' [5]. This is the reason why stainless steels are still used as metallic biomaterials in large quantities, though in terms of quality stainless steels are inferior when compared to cobalt–chromium alloys and titanium alloys. ASTM standards of stainless steels for medical and surgical uses are shown in Table 2–1.

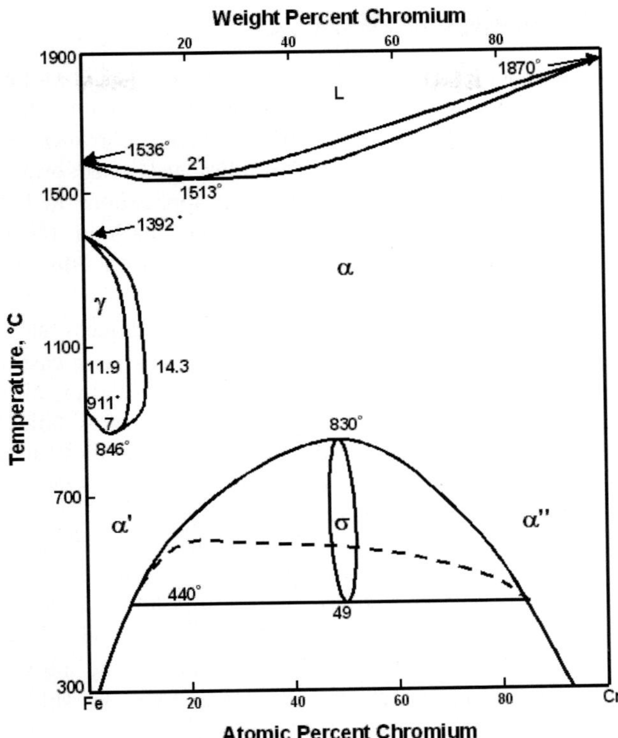

Figure 2–2 Fe–Cr phase diagram

Table 2–1 Standards related to stainless steels for surgical implants (Annual Book of ASTM Standards, Vol. 13.01, 2000)

Specification	Nominal Contents
F 138–97	Wrought 18Cr–14Ni–2.5Mo Stainless Steel Bar and Wire
F 139–96	Wrought 18Cr–14Ni–2.5Mo Stainless Steel Sheet and Strip
F 745–95	18Cr–12.5Ni–2.5Mo Stainless Steel for Cast and Solution-Annealed
F 899–95	Stainless Steel Billet, Bar, and Wire
F 1314–95	Wrought N Strengthened-22Cr–12.5Ni–5Mg–2.5Mo Stainless Steel Bar and Wire
F 1586–95	Wrought N Strengthened-21Cr–10Ni–3Mg–2.5Mo Stainless Steel Bar

2.2.2 Cobalt–Chromium Alloys

At the beginning of 20th century, the cobalt–molybdenum–tungsten alloy — which was called Stellite — was developed by Haynes. It exhibited better strength at high temperature as well as better corrosion resistance when compared to other super alloys. This alloy was used originally in aircraft engines. Then it was used for biomedical applications in the 1930s, during which it was called Vitallium. By modifying Vitallium, the following alloys have been developed: Co–Cr–Mo alloy, Co–Ni–Cr–Mo–W–Fe alloy, and Co–Ni–Cr–Mo alloy [2,6].

Cobalt-based super alloys are superior to stainless steels in corrosion resistance. The Co–Cr–Mo alloy — presently used as a casting alloy — was developed by replacing tungsten with molybdenum. Casting alloys can give rise to course grains, grain boundary segregations, gas blow holes, and shrinkage cavities in the structure. Though inferior to non-cast alloys in terms of fatigue strength and fracture toughness, cast alloys excel in wear resistance, pitting resistance, and crevice corrosion resistance.

Molybdenum is added to refine grain size, enhance solid-solution strengthening as well as increase corrosion resistance. Nickel is added to increase castability and workability; the amount, however, should be limited to less than one percent to ensure low toxicity in the body. Castability is then improved by adding 0.2–0.3 percent of carbon to the alloy to decrease the melting point by about 100°C. Distribution of Cr-rich carbides $M_{23}C_6$ and the work hardenability of this alloy help to increase wear resistance. This alloy allows an artificial hip joint to be made totally of metal due to its excellent tribological properties, though sockets made of plastic materials are generally used presently. The lower the carbon content, the higher the ability to forge the alloy. Forged alloy is inferior to cast alloy in wear resistance, but is superior in fatigue strength and corrosion resistance. ASTM standards of cobalt–chromium alloys for medical and surgical uses are shown in Table 2–2.

2.2.3 Titanium and its Alloys

Compared to stainless steels and cobalt–chromium alloys, titanium is superior in specific strength, corrosion resistance, and biocompatibility, but inferior in tribological properties. Titanium is non-ferrous — its elastic modulus is about half of those of stainless steels and cobalt–chromium alloys. In addition, a very stable passive film is formed at room temperature due to rapid reaction with oxygen [2,7,8]. Titanium has an allotropic transformation temperature at 885°C, where:

- At a lower temperature than this, its structure is hexagonal close-packed (*i.e.*, the alpha form). Elements that stabilize the alpha structure are aluminum, tin, carbon, oxygen, and nitrogen. They elevate the transformation temperature and expand the alpha phase area in the equilibrium diagram (see Figure 2–3).

- At a higher temperature than this, its structure is body-centered cubic (*i.e.*, the beta form). Elements that stabilize the beta structure are molybdenum, niobium, vanadium, chromium, and iron. They decrease the transformation temperature and increase the beta phase area in the equilibrium diagram.

Table 2–2 Standards related to cobalt–chromium alloys for surgical implants (Annual Book of ASTM Standards, Vol. 13.01, 2000)

Specification	Nominal Contents
F 75–98	Co–28Cr–6Mo Casting Alloy and Cast Products
F 90–97	Wrought Co–20Cr–15W-10Ni Alloy
F 562–95	Wrought Co–35Ni–20Cr–10Mo Alloy
F 563–95	Wrought Co–Ni–Cr–Mo–W–Fe Alloy
F 799–99	Co–28Cr–6Mo Alloy Forgings
F 961–96	Co–35Ni–20Cr–10Mo Alloy Forgings
F 1058–97	Wrought Co–Cr–Ni–Mo–Fe Alloys
F 1537–94	Wrought Co–28Cr–6Mo Alloy

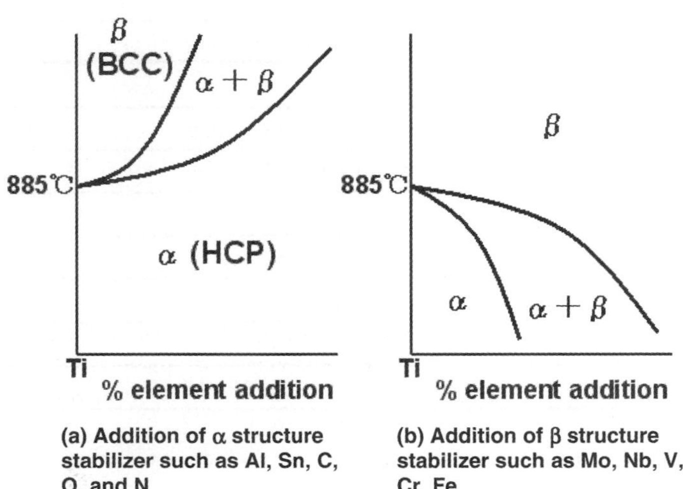

Figure 2–3 Schematic explanation of Ti–X two-phase diagram; 885°C is the allotropic transformation temperature

Addition of beta structure stabilizers makes it possible the existence of a two-phase structure of both alpha and beta structures, or only beta structure at room temperature. Commercially pure titanium (called CP titanium) has an all-alpha structure. Four grades of CP titanium exist, with varying small amounts of iron, nitrogen, oxygen, and other elements. Total amount of other elements increases from Grade 1 to 4 (maximum of 0.7 percent at Grade 4). Tensile strength increases with increase of Grade number. Pure titanium has superior resistance to corrosion, compared to titanium alloys. Compared with beta titanium alloys, alpha titanium alloys are superior in heat resistance and weldability but inferior in strength and workability. Beta titanium alloys are alloys which are solution-strengthened by adding beta structure stabilizers. All-beta structure at room temperature can be obtained by solution treatment (*i.e.*, rapid cooling). Alpha phase precipitates in all-beta structure by aging treatment. Beta structure with precipitated alpha phase has excellent strength.

Two-phase alloys with a dispersion of the beta form in the alpha phase have been developed with excellent properties of each phase. Ti–6Al–4V is a typical two-phase alloy which is used widely. The alloy structure strongly depends on the working and heat treatment. The alloy whose impurities are reduced to improve toughness at low temperature and crack extension resistance is called ELI Ti–6Al–4V alloy (extra low interstitial). ASTM standards of titanium and titanium alloys for medical and surgical uses are shown in Table 2–3.

Table 2–3 Standards related to titanium and titanium alloys for surgical implants (Annual Book of ASTM Standards, Vol. 13.01, 2000)

Specification	Nominal Contents
F 67–95	Unalloyed Titanium
F 136–98	Wrought Ti–6Al–4V ELI Alloy
F 620–97	Ti–6Al–4V ELI Alloy Forgings
F 1108–97a	Ti–6Al–4V Alloy Castings
F 1295–97a	Wrought Ti–6Al–7Nb Alloy
F 1472–96	Wrought Ti–6Al–4V Alloy
F 1713–96	Wrought Ti–13Nb–13Zr Alloy
F 1813–97	Wrought Ti–12Mo–6Zr–2Fe Alloy

2.2.4 Nickel–Titanium Alloys

Nickel–Titanium (Ni–Ti) alloys are shape memory alloys. In terms of application, Ni–Ti alloys are used as metallic biomaterials for stent, catheter, orthodontic wire, the clip for aneurysm repair, as well as guide wire. The chemical composition range for Ni–Ti alloys is 49.5–57.5at%Ni. Shape memory alloys are defined as alloys which possess the function to return to the original shape from a plastically deformed shape due to a small amount of temperature change. The maximum strain is 5–6 percent in terms of shape recovery after plastic deformation. In the family of shape memory alloys, alloys in the Ni–Ti alloy system are the only ones employed as biomaterials — though alloys such as Ag–Cd, Al–Cd, Cu–Al, Cu–Sn, and Cu–Zn have shape memory function too.

In the alloy systems where the shape memory function is present, martensite transformation usually occurs. Shape memory is a phenomenon which is caused by crystallographically reversible phase transformation between the stable phase at high temperature and the stable martensite phase at low temperature. Under martensite transformation, the lattice is deformed by a small shearing-like shift of the atom arrangement while at the same time keeping adjourning relations to each other. Hence martensite transformation is a lattice transformation, not a diffusion transformation. Martensite transformation does not accompany macroscopically plastic deformation.

The transformation starts at martensite transformation starting temperature (Ms) and grows gradually with decrease of temperature. The Ms of Ni–Ti alloys is between −130°C and 60°C. The temperature generally decreases with increase of nickel content. Martensite transformation also grows gradually by applying stress. To return a martensite-transformed structure to its original structure, heat is to be applied or stress be removed as the lattice reverse-shifts against that of martensite transformation.

Ni–Ti alloys exhibit superior ductility, fatigue strength, corrosion resistance, and biocompatibility [9]. For Ni–Ti alloys to be used as metallic biomaterials, there is the ASTM Standard which contains F2063–00 Standard Specification for Wrought Nickel-Titanium Shape Memory Medical Devices and Surgical Implants.

2.3   Body Environment to Metallic Materials

Under normal conditions, human body fluid contains 0.9% saline (NaCl) solution which contains amino acids and proteins. The human body fluid is composed of different fluid types such as tissue fluids, lymph fluids, and blood. It includes cells such as leukocytes, macrophages, and blood corpuscles (e.g., lymphocyte, thrombocytes, erythrocytes). The pH of the fluid is normally 7 but may fall to 4 or 5 when there is inflammation caused by surgery or injury. The normal body temperature is 37°C and 1 atmosphere pressure (where internal partial pressure of oxygen is about one-quarter strength of atmospheric oxygen).

The biological environment of the human body described above is a strongly corrosive one for metallic materials since metals are ionic in nature. Many metallic implants rely on the formation of passive oxide films — such as chromium oxide in stainless steels and titanium dioxide in titanium alloys — for corrosion protection. When the partial pressure of oxygen is reduced inside the body, the corrosion process accelerates. This is because the lower partial pressure of oxygen reduces the recovering speed of the passive oxide film on the surface once it is broken or removed.

Another major concern arises from the adverse host tissue response to wear debris generated by the fatigue and wear process in joint prosthesis. This has been highlighted by Teoh [10] in a recent review on fatigue of biomaterials. This appears to be a natural defense mechanism of the body. The wear debris often invokes an inflammatory and immunological response. This in turn causes blood clotting processes, where leukocytes, macrophages — and for severe cases, giant cells — move in on the foreign wear particles resulting in interfacial problems between the implant and the host tissue. Numerous biochemical activities occur at this stage. These include change of the local environment to a highly acidic one (pH less than 3), and where cells produce superoxides and peroxides such as H_2O_2 [11] to degrade the implant faster. In general, assuming that the wear debris is non-toxic, there are four scenarios:

(i)   The cells will try to digest the foreign debris by releasing chemicals and enzymes to dissolve and later, absorb them so that the by-products can be eliminated through the blood circulation and lymphatic system into various organs such as the kidney and liver;

(ii) If the foreign matter cannot be digested, the body will try to excrete them out of the body system (in the case of fatigue wear in the oral cavity such as wear products from dental biomaterials during the chewing process, the wear products are easily flushed out through the digestive system and are therefore less of a concern compared to other implant materials);

(iii) If the foreign matter cannot be digested or expelled, then cellular fibrous linings will engulf the foreign bodies to keep them away (isolate) from the surrounding host tissue. This scenario is of great concern as the interfacial strength between the implant and the host tissue will drop drastically, giving rise to micro-motion and hence fretting-fatigue-corrosion failure;

(iv) Finally, if the amount of foreign matter keeps increasing in the body and none of the above mechanisms seems to work, the host will send signals to "give up". For example, in the case of a prolonged generation of large amount of wear debris, the host cannot cope and sends osteoclast cells — cells which are involved in the process of bone resorption — to demineralize the surrounding bone, thus causing the prosthesis to loosen.

The majority of tissue-implant activities occur in the surface and subsurface layers (see Figure 2–4), which may lead to the formation of an aqueous sandwich layer of biological components to establish a good bond between the host tissue and the biomaterial. It is here that the host tissue interacts with the implant, and if it is not biocompatible then an avalanche of biochemical reactions occur. However, the molecular absorbed layer is dependent on the underlying passive oxide layer, which protects the base material from corrosion. If the deformed layer has a high compressive stress field (such as in the case of forged stainless steel), the incident of crack initiation is reduced and hence the fatigue strength of the material is increased. One can readily see that the process of removal of these layers (by wear) can greatly affect the fatigue of biomaterials.

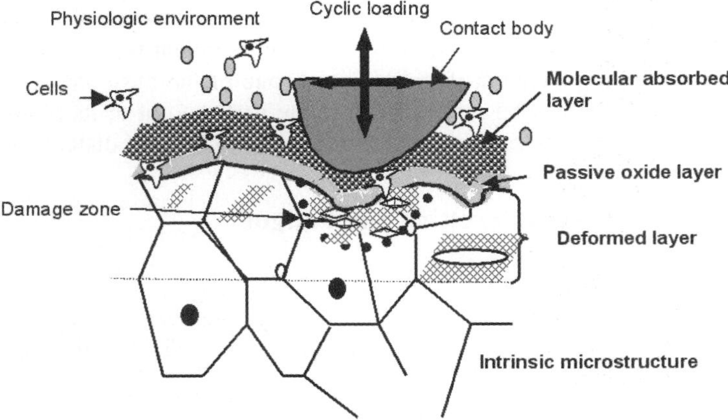

Figure 2–4 Schematic illustration of a cross-section of a deformed metallic biomaterial surface showing the complex interactions between the material's surface and the physiologic environment (after Teoh [10])

2.4　Life of Implanted Metallic Materials

Implanted metallic materials are expected to last the entire lifespan of the patient. Bone plates are an exception. They are implanted to fix failed bones, and in principle, are taken out when the failed bones recover. The life of implanted metallic biomaterials depends on the following two factors:

A. Degree of damages to implanted metallic materials due to the human body environment

This includes concerns for corrosion, corrosion fatigue, and fretting corrosion fatigue. Implanted devices made of metallic materials may fail due to corrosion fatigue and fretting corrosion fatigue [10,12,13], thereby leading to their replacement. They seldom fail due to mere corrosion because higher corrosion-resistant materials are used as metallic biomaterials.

B. Degree of damages to the human body caused by implanted metallic materials

It is inevitable that small amounts of metal ions and debris are released from implanted metallic materials inside the living body during their long-term use [14,15,16]. Metal ions and debris released from the materials may then trigger adverse reactions from cells and tissues, leading to tumor formation, allergy, and teratogenicity [17,2]. In this light, corrosion and fretting/wear of metallic materials and their toxicity are inextricably linked to each other — which means that toxicity may influence the life of implants. As a result, implants may need to be replaced due to inflammation caused by infection, acute pain, necrosis, and complication.

Factors A and B are just two out of the many implant replacement causes. For example, an implanted artificial hip joint, one of the most frequently used biomedical devices, may be replaced due to the wearing out of its plastic-made socket, loosening and stress shielding caused by osteoclasis, or dislocation.

2.5   Corrosion, Wear/Fretting and Fatigue

2.5.1 Fatigue Testing Method

Fatigue failure occurs under conditions of large number of cyclic loading. Fretting fatigue failure occurs under conditions of cyclic loading and cyclic friction loading.

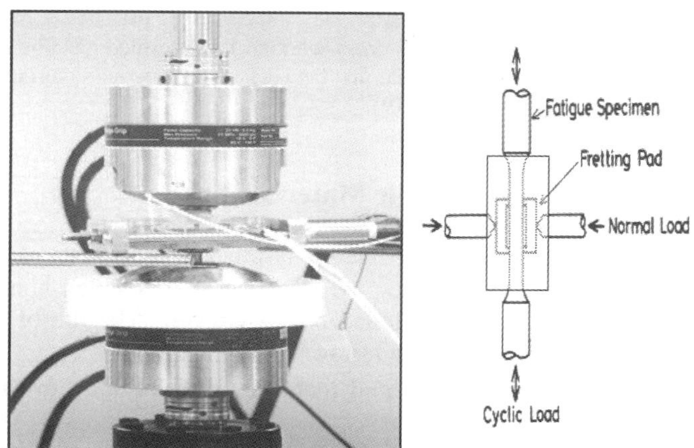

Figure 2–5 Fretting fatigue test in a pseudo-body fluid

A fretting fatigue test is shown in Figure 2–5. A contact normal load is applied to the pads on both flats of the fatigue specimen. When cyclic load is applied to the specimen, a small relative slip occurs between the specimen and the pads, and fretting damage is produced in the contact area. The relative slip between the specimen and the outer edges of the pads is measured using a calibrated extension meter. Frictional force between the fatigue specimen and a pad is measured using gauges bound to the outer edges of the central part of the pad. Fretting fatigue is contributed by friction stress to plain fatigue stress. Cracks can initiate at the contact sites, and one of them may propagate and eventually lead to breakage.

Basic methods of presenting engineering fatigue/fretting fatigue data are by means of the S-N curve and the da/dN-ΔK curve (Figure 2–6), where S is maximum applied stress or stress amplitude, N is number of cycles to failure, da/dN is crack growth rate, and ΔK is stress intensity factor range. It is important to collect data on fatigue strengths and fretting fatigue strengths (*i.e.*, S-N curves) of metallic biomaterials even in pseudo-body fluids. They are useful for material selection, device design, material development, and fracture analysis. On the other hand, da/dN-ΔK curves of materials are used when designing structures such as passenger planes because their designs are carried out based on the fail-safe concept — following the fracture mechanics approach.

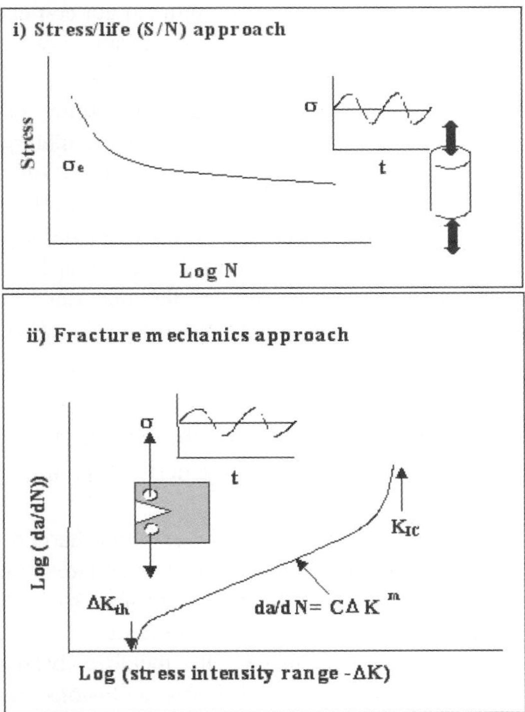

Figure 2–6 Fatigue testing based on (i) stress-life (S/N) approach; and (ii) fracture mechanics approach

For fatigue testing of metallic biomaterials, there is the ASTM standard which contains ASTM designations F1801–97, F1717–96, F1612–95, and F1440–92. For fretting corrosion testing of metallic biomaterials, there is F897–84. However no standards are available for fretting fatigue testing of metallic biomaterials, except for a test procedure described by Nakazawa (1992) [18].

2.5.2 Notes for Fatigue/Fretting Fatigue Tests

(a) Fatigue strength and fretting fatigue strength depend on the following testing conditions:
- Type of cyclic loading (such as uniaxial loading, bending, rotating bending, and reversed torsion);
- Stress ratio (*i.e.*, the ratio of minimum stress to maximum stress in a cyclic stress);
- Testing environment; and
- Stress frequency (under corrosive environment).

Fatigue strength and fretting fatigue strength cannot contend for superiority among specimens if testing conditions described above were not uniformly applied.

(b) Stress raisers such as non-metallic inclusions, blow holes, flaws, and notches should be strictly excluded from the implant material because they decrease fatigue strength. The effect of stress raisers on fatigue strength becomes more pronounced as the work hardening coefficient of metallic material decreases. The effect on fatigue strength is induced using a work hardening model which assumes that when the stress that has been increasing under a given cyclic stress amplitude attains the material's fracture stress, a crack will be initiated at a stress raiser [19]. The fatigue limit with defect, σ_w, can be expressed by the following expression:

$$\sigma_w = 1/10(10/K_s + ((1-K_s)/K_s)1/n)\,\sigma'_y \tag{1}$$

where K_s is stress concentration factor of the defect, n is work hardening coefficient, and σ'_y is yield strength. n is defined by $n = (\varepsilon/\sigma)(d\sigma/d\varepsilon)$, where ε is strain and σ is stress.

Metallic biomaterials have relatively lower work hardening coefficients. This means that their fatigue strengths are sensitive to stress raisers. Flaws on an implant's surface, accidentally scratched by surgical knife during operation, may therefore decrease the fatigue strength substantially. Existence of stress raisers such as non-metallic inclusions in metallic biomaterials is also detrimental to their corrosion resistance because inclusions easily become the starting site of corrosion.

(c) Fretting fatigue strength depends on the contact pressure. The case of a Ti–6Al–4V alloy is shown in Figure 2–7 [18].

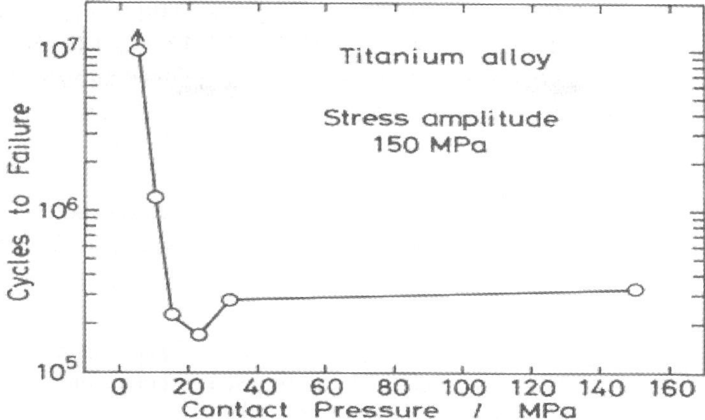

Figure 2–7 Effect of contact pressure on fretting fatigue life in air for a Ti–6Al–4V alloy

The fretting fatigue life exhibits a minimum at low contact pressure, and becomes constant at high contact pressures. The initiation site of the main crack depends on contact pressure (see Figure 2–8):

- When the contact pressure is high and the stick region wide, the main crack initiation occurs near the outer edge of the fretting pad.
- When the contact pressure is low and the stick region narrow, the main crack initiation occurs at the middle portion of the fretted area.

Based on the above observations, the minimum life is probably caused by this high concentration of friction stress amplitude.

(d) Fatigue strength and fretting fatigue strength of metallic materials may depend on the stress frequency in the human body. Fatigue lives decrease as stress frequency decreases in a pseudo-body fluid for CP titanium [20]. It is important to use a stress frequency of roughly 1 Hz for fatigue and fretting fatigue tests of metallic biomaterials, because corrosion is a time-dependent phenomenon and the walking cycle of human beings is about 1 Hz. The use of stress frequency higher than the walking cycle of human beings (such as one higher than 5 Hz) will overestimate the fatigue and fretting fatigue strengths of implant materials.

(e) From the analogy of cyclic stress applied to real hip joints [21], the cyclic stress applied to implants by walking cycle may be a cyclic varying stress composed of various sine waves of different amplitudes. The cyclic varying stress differs between man and woman, and is unique for each person because it is easily influenced by body weight and walking habit. However, the corrosion fatigue strength under cyclic varying stress is almost equivalent to the value obtained under constant cyclic stress for smooth specimens in air and under a corrosive environment [22]. This implies that the Miner's rule (the liner damage addition rule) can be applied. Equivalent stress amplitude, $\sigma_{a,eq}$, and equivalent number of cycles, N_{eq}, are defined respectively by the following expressions (2) and (3):

$$\sigma_{a.eq.} = \alpha \sqrt{} \; \{ \Sigma (\sigma^{\alpha}_{a.i} \cdot n_i) / \Sigma n_i \} \tag{2}$$

$$N_{eq} = \Sigma n_i \tag{3}$$

where $\sigma_{a.i}$ and n_i are stress amplitude and number of cycles for each stage, and α is the exponent of the S-N curve under a constant stress amplitude, which is expressed by:

$$\sigma^{\alpha}_a \cdot N_f = C \tag{4}$$

where σ_a is stress amplitude, N_f is cycles to failure, and C is a constant.

Therefore, constant stress amplitude can be used in corrosion fatigue and fretting corrosion fatigue tests for metallic biomaterials.

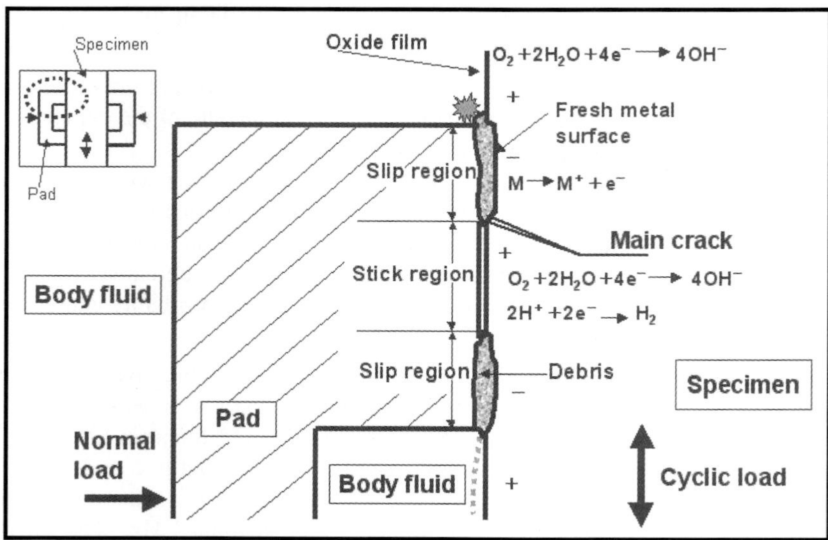

Figure 2–8 Schematic explanation of fretting and corrosion damages on the contacting surfaces of implants in the living body (the part of the circle with broken line in the small figure at the upper left corner is enlarged)

2.5.3 Corrosion Fatigue

In the body, mechanical and chemical effects act simultaneously. Fatigue evaluations of biomaterials use simulated body fluid environment with electrochemical and fretting mechanisms incorporated. When fatigue occurs alongside corrosion, it is known as corrosion fatigue. Metallic materials implanted into human bodies are often damaged by corrosion fatigue or fretting corrosion fatigue [12]. The living body is a chemically and mechanically harsh environment for metallic materials. Moreover flaws on an implant's surface — which can be caused by an accidental scratch of the surgical knife during operation — also decrease fatigue strength. The combined mechanical and chemical processes play a vital role in crack initiation. The inability to repassivate quickly causes the electrochemical breakdown of the surface layers. It is interesting to note the work of Taira and Lautenschlager (1992) — who studied the *in vitro* corrosion fatigue of 316L cold worked stainless steel — which found that the monitoring of corrosion current could give a clear indication of crack initiation which otherwise would have been missed. They have also shown that by applying 200 mV to the metal surface to suppress passivation of the oxide layers, a significant drop in fatigue strength (in the order of 150 MPa) is observed.

Human beings normally walk several thousands of steps a day at a rate of 1 Hz. Artificial hip joints, knee joints, spinal fixations, bone plates, and wires — which have been implanted into a human body — suffer from alternate stresses which correspond to the walking cycle. In the case of artificial hip joints, the stress level is several times higher than that of the body weight. As hip joint is located out of the perpendicular line of the body weight, the balance between body weight and muscular strength pivots on only one leg. As for the pacemaker electrode, the alternate stress corresponds to the myocardium activity. And as for dental implants, the alternate stress corresponds to the chewing cycle.

Inside the living body, surface fretting of metallic materials causes wear — which leads to successive release of metal ions, metallic compounds, and debris. The release of these products into the tissues surrounding an implant may provoke toxicity on local tissue or the affected organ. For example, the black-coloring of the tissue surrounding an implant — a phenomenon called metallosis in clinical orthopedics [23,24] — is due to the release of large amount of debris.

2.5.4 Fretting Corrosion Fatigue

2.5.4.1 Fretting fatigue

Fatigue failure is a mechanical phenomenon where under cyclic load, an initiated crack propagates to failure. If a crack is not initiated by stress raisers such as non-metallic inclusions and notches, it is usually initiated at the root of the intrusion — where shallow channels are formed. The crack initially propagates along the slip line at an angle of about 45° to the tensile stress — because maximum shearing stress lies on a 45° plane, followed by change of the propagation direction to an angle of about 90° to it (as schematically shown in Figure 2–9).

Corrosion usually accelerates crack initiation and its propagation. However as metallic biomaterials in practical uses have higher corrosion resistance, the effect of corrosion on the acceleration of fatigue crack initiation and propagation is very low. Metallic ions release is hardly accelerated by fatigue in PBS(-) (see Table 2–4).

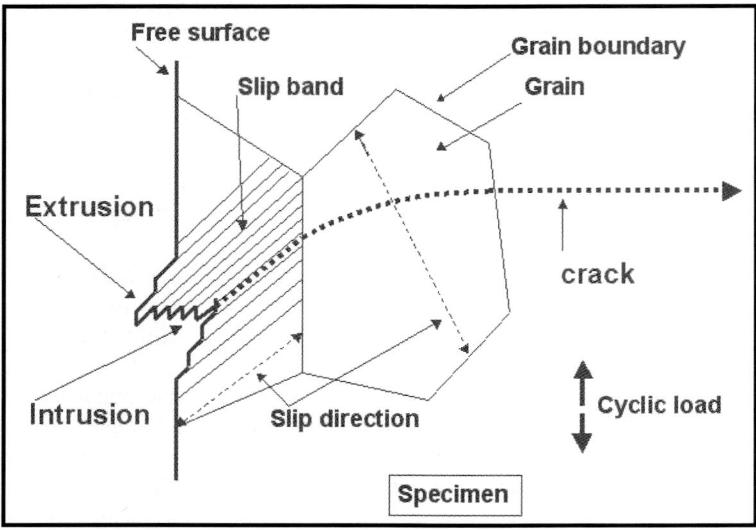

Figure 2–9 Schematic explanation of fatigue crack initiation

Table 2–4 Concentration of metallic elements of a Ti–6Al–4V in test solutions (µg/l)

		Ti	Al	V	Fe	Cr	Ni	Mn
Unused PBS(s)		<5	<2	<5	<2	<2	<1	<1
PBS(-) after	Filtered	<5	2	<5	2	<2	3	<1
Immersion for 30d	Unfiltered	6	3	<5	3	<2	3	<1
Fatigue	Filtered	<5	3	<5	5	<2	<2	1
N_f=3.69x10^6 (21d)	Unfiltered	9	8	<5	12	4	<2	1
Fretting fatigue 1	Filtered	<5	3	11	7	<2	7	3
N_f=1.08x10^5 (0.6d)	Unfiltered	2420	1150	130	42	970	130	110
Fretting fatigue 2	Filtered	<5	3	<5	4	<2	25	2
N_f=4.10x10^6 (24d)	Unfiltered	23	6	8	18	<2	26	4

N_f: Cycles to failure; Stress frequency: 2 Hz

Fretting damage occurs on the contacting surfaces of components which are clamped together and subjected to cyclic loads (see Figure 2–8). Fretting occurs as a result of relative movement with a small amplitude (10–20 micron), which may occur between contacting surfaces of components [25].

From mechanical viewpoint, cyclic shear stress on the surface is a major factor that initiates fretting fatigue cracks. The cyclic shear stress arises from the frictional force induced occasionally by the oscillatory movements. The maximum cyclic stress amplitude, σ_f, at the edge of the fretted area on the surface is calculated as follows:

$$\sigma_f = \sigma_a + 2f_a \tag{5}$$
$$f_a = \mu p \tag{6}$$

where σ_a is plain fatigue stress amplitude, f_a is friction stress amplitude, μ is friction coefficient, and p is contact pressure.

The areas affected by fretting are limited to the shallow surface layers. Fretting fatigue strength is almost mechanically equivalent to the fatigue strength of specimen with short cracks [26]. Fretting fatigue behavior is very much related to notch sensitivity. Non-propagating cracks, which occur easily near the specimen's surface at the fretted areas, are like those that appear easily at the root of shallow notch [12].

The effect of body fluids on fretting fatigue strength is related to friction coefficient change, pits formation on fretted sites, and hydrogen generation due to electro-chemical reaction. Under a certain in-air or in-PBS(-) fretting fatigue testing condition, there exists a stick region at the middle portion of the fretted area and slip regions on either side of it (see Figure 2–8). The relative slip changes — with increase of contact pressure caused by applied normal load — in the following modes: only slip region, narrow stick region plus wide slip region, wide stick region plus narrow slip region.

- In the slip region, the contact surface is heavily damaged and wear debris is produced. Part of the wear debris is displaced out of the fretted area.

  Net contact pressure acting in the slip region is probably lower than the average contact pressure, since the normal load is given through the medium of wear debris.

- On the other hand, in the stick region, the net contact pressure is probably higher than the average contact pressure, since the normal load is increased by a decrease in normal load in the slip region. Hence net contact pressure and net frictional stress amplitude acting in the stick region are higher, while those in the slip region are lower than the average values.

Therefore, stress concentration occurs near the boundaries between the stick and slip regions. The main crack initiation at the boundaries between the slip and stick regions is confirmed by the observation of fracture surfaces using optical microscope [18].

Amount of produced metal debris depends not only on cycles, but also strongly on the relative slip amplitude between the specimen and the pad. The relative slip amplitude is proportional to the stress amplitude. Large relative slip amplitude easily causes a gross slip between the specimen and the pad, producing a large amount of metal debris. The difference in debris amount (concentration of unfiltered metallic elements) between Fretting Fatigue 1 and Fretting Fatigue 2 in Table 2–4 can be explained by the gross slip difference between them.

In the filtered solution recovered after the fretting fatigue test for a Ti–6Al–4V alloy, trace impurities such as nickel, manganese, and iron were detected in relatively high concentrations, compared to the chemical composition of the alloy [27]. Preferential release of certain elements such as chromium and molybdenum were also detected in the fretting fatigue test solutions of a Co–Cr–Mo alloy [28].

2.5.4.2 *Metallic ions release from fretted side*

Metallic ions release is accelerated easily under fretting fatigue tests in PBS(-). This occurred not only for a 316L stainless steel [29] and a nickel-free Co–Cr alloy [28], but also for a Ti–6Al–4V alloy [27] though the metallic materials hardly dissolved due to immersion or fatigue tests in PBS(-) (see Tables 2–4, 2–5).

Table **2–5** Concentration of metallic elements of metallic materials in the immersion test solutions in PBS(-) for 30d at 37°C without load (μg/l)

		Ti	Al	V	Cr	Mn	Fe	Ni
Unused PBS(s)		*	*	*	*	1	2	G
316L	Filtered	*	2	*	*	*	3	3
	Unfiltered	6	5	*	*	*	3	3
CP Ti	Filtered	*	2	*	*	*	3	3
	Unfiltered	6	5	*	*	*	3	3
Ti–6Al–4V	Filtered	*	2	*	*	*	2	3
	Unfiltered	6	3	*	*	*	3	3

* The element analyzed is not detected. The detective limits are shown as follows: 1ppb (μg/l) for Mn; 2ppb for Al, Cr, and Fe; 3ppb for Ni; 5ppb for Ti and V

Under fretting fatigue tests in PBS(-), fresh metal surfaces are produced on the slip region of the fretted site between the specimen and the pads. This production alternates with the formation of very thin oxide films on the fresh metal surfaces during every load cycle. Oxygen near the fresh metal surfaces is consumed to form oxide films. As its supply between the specimen and the pads is delayed due to the crevice, the oxygen concentration under the pads may become lower than that on the area not covered with the pads (see Figure 2–8). Therefore, oxygen concentration cells are formed and electrical potential difference arises between them to accelerate metallic ions release.

However in the case of titanium, the material is insensitive to oxygen concentration. This means that anodic current density seldom changes correspondingly with electrical potential difference. Therefore the metallic ions release mechanism due to oxygen concentration will not be applicable for titanium.

At the same time, passive-active cells are produced at the fretted area [30]. These cells are produced in the presence of a cathode (which is the surface covered with oxide film) and an anode (which is the fresh metal surface). At the anode, metallic ions release can be accelerated according to the following formula:

$$M \rightarrow M^{+} + e^{-} \tag{7}$$

At the cathode, the following takes place:

$$O_2 + 2H_2O + 4e^{-} \rightarrow 4OH^{-} \tag{8}$$

As the supply of consumable oxygen is delayed at the area covered with pads, the generation of OH^{-} decreases. As a result, Cl^{-} invades the crevice to keep the electric balance and metallic salts ($M^{+}Cl^{-}$) are formed as follows:

$$MCl + H_2O \rightarrow MOH + HCl \tag{9}$$

Due to the above hydrolysis, the pH of the fresh metal surface decreases and corrosion accelerates to form a deep pitting.

At the cathode, hydrogen is generated on the stick region by the following formula when oxygen is not supplied:

$$2H^{+} + 2e^{-} \rightarrow H_2 \tag{10}$$

2.5.4.3 *Fatigue and fretting fatigue strengths at high cycle for typical metallic biomaterials in pseudo-body fluid*

Table 2–6 shows fatigue strengths and fretting fatigue strengths at 10^7 cycles in air and in PBS(-) for the following typical metallic biomaterials:

- 316L stainless steel (which contained 12.10%Ni) and 447J1 stainless steel (which contained 0.20%Ni impurity) [31]
- Cobalt–chromium alloy [28]
- Commercially pure titanium [20]
- Annealed Ti–6Al–4V alloy [27]
- STA treated Ti–6Al–4V alloy [27]

                                          M. Sumita & S. H. Teoh

Table 2–6 Fatigue and fretting fatigue strengths at 10^7 cycles

		Stainless steel		Co–Cr	Pure Ti	Ti–6Al–4V	
		316L	447J1			Anneal	STA
UTS (MPa)		602	591	956	440	930	1,104
0.2%P.S. (MPa)		328	525	432	306	861	1,006
Fatigue	Air	205	210	240	150	290	270
Strength (MPa)	PBS	200	200	240	140	290	270
Fretting fatigue	Air	140	150	210	100	120	142
Strength (MPa)	PBS	110	150	210	85	100	105

Fatigue strengths and fretting fatigue strengths are the failure stress amplitudes at 10^7 cycles, respectively

S-N curves for the commercially pure titanium are shown in Figure 2–10 as an example of an S-N curve.

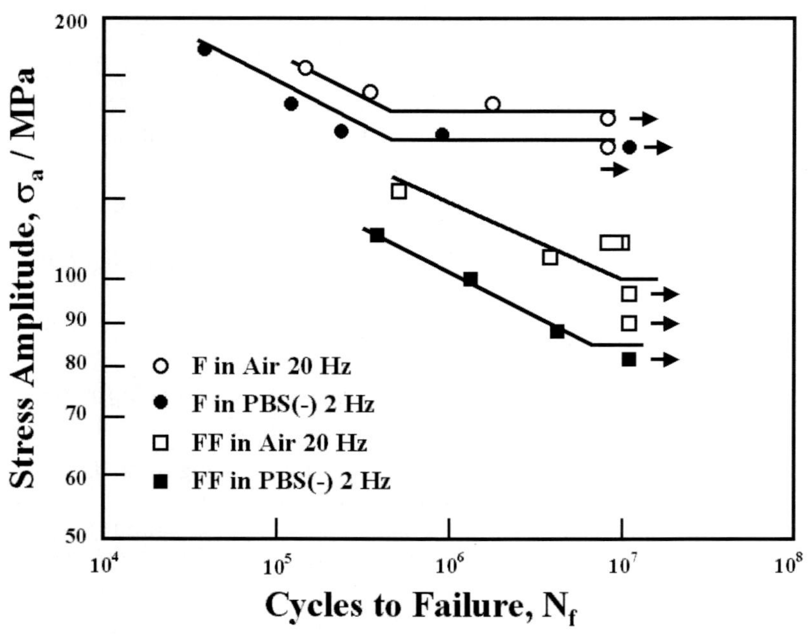

Figure 2–10 S-N curves of CP Ti (JIS grade 3) in air and PBS(-) (F: fatigue and FF: fretting fatigue)

Tests were carried out at tension to tension mode with stress ratio of 0.1 under constant stress amplitude using a sine wave. Stress frequency was 20 Hz in air and 2 Hz in PBS(-) at 37°C.

The following trends are derived from the test results:

(1) Both in air and in PBS(-), the fretting fatigue strength at 10^7 cycles is lower than the fatigue strength at 10^7 cycles for each material tested.

 ❖ The annealed Ti–6Al–4V alloy in PBS(-) presented the largest difference. The fretting fatigue strength at 10^7 cycles was three times lower than plain fatigue strength at 10^7 cycles.

 ❖ The cobalt–chromium alloy in air and PBS(-) presented the smallest difference. The fretting fatigue strength at 10^7 cycles was about 10 percent lower than the plain fatigue strength at 10^7 cycles.

(2) The fatigue strengths at 10^7 cycles increase with increase of ultimate tensile strength; this trend is consistent with the results obtained in air for 15 metallic materials by Waterhouse (1981) [12].

(3) The fretting fatigue strengths at 10^7 cycles do not depend on the ultimate tensile strength; this trend is consistent with the results obtained in air for 15 metallic materials by Waterhouse (1981) [12].

(4) The fatigue strengths at 10^7 cycles in air are almost the same as those in PBS(-).

(5) The fretting fatigue strengths at 10^7 cycles in PBS(-) are lower than those in air for the 316L stainless steel, the commercially pure titanium and the two kinds of Ti–6Al–4V alloy, but are almost the same as those in air for the 447J1 stainless steel and the cobalt–chromium alloy.

The following factors in a quasi-biological environment may influence the fretting fatigue life of metallic biomaterials:

(a) Friction coefficient between the specimen and the pad

The friction coefficient in PBS(-) is about half of that in air at the endurance limit of each material (see Table 2–7). The friction stress amplitude is proportional to the friction coefficient. Therefore, friction stress amplitude applied to a specimen in PBS(-) is about half of that in air.

Table 2–7 Friction coefficient at fretting fatigue limit

	Stainless steel		Co–Cr	Ti–6Al–4V
	316L	447J1		STA
Air	1.0	0.8	0.7	0.6
PBS(-)	0.5	0.5	0.3	0.3

(b) Relative site of the boundary between stick and slip regions at the fretted area of the specimen

It is not clear how the relative site of the boundary is displaced by the existence of PBS(-) (see Figure 2–8).

(c) Corrosion pits formed on the fresh metal surface of the fretted area

Corrosion pits may act as stress raisers to accelerate crack initiation.

(d) Hydrogen generated on the stick regions

If hydrogen is generated on the stick regions, it may accelerate crack initiation and its propagation — which then causes the decrease of fretting fatigue strength. The fretting fatigue strength in PBS(-) is lower than that in air for the 316L stainless steel (Table 2–6). Grain boundary cracking is observed at the crack initiation site as shown in Figure 2–11 [31]. The grain boundary cracking suggests cracking due to hydrogen.

(e) Paring off the micro cracks initiated at the fretted areas

Damages on the fretted surfaces of the cobalt–chromium alloy and the Ti–6Al–4V alloy are shown in Figure 2–12 (a), (b), and (c) [28]. The damage in PBS(-) is more outstanding than that in air. The damage for the cobalt–chromium alloy is greater than that for the Ti–6Al–4V alloy. The large amount of debris produced due to intense paring off may cause delayed crack initiation and crack propagation at its early stage.

(f) Temperature rise on the fretted areas in PBS(-)

The increase of temperature on the surface of a mild steel due to fretting is about 500°C [32]. No experimental findings are available about the increase of temperature on the fretted surface of metallic biomaterials.

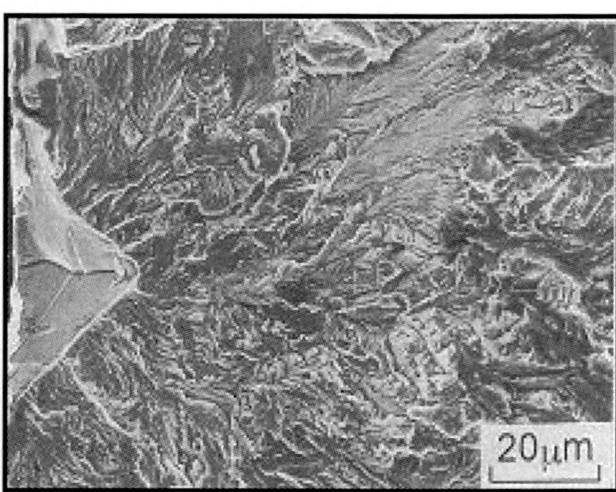

Figure 2–11 Crack initiation site in 316L stainless steel fretting fatigued in PBS(-); σ_a=178 MPa, N_f=2.1x10^5

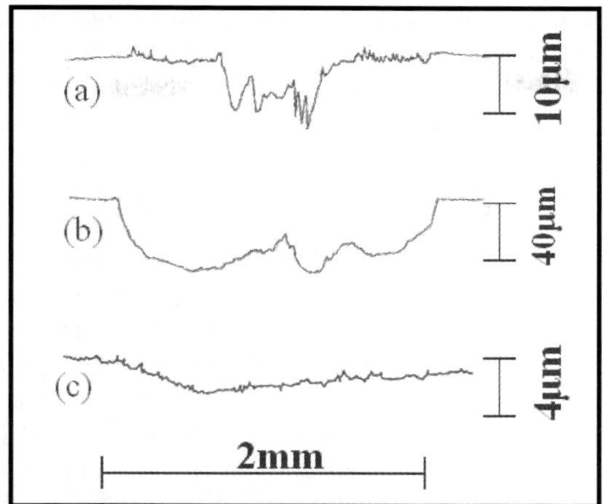

Figure 2–12 Cross-sectional profile on fretted surface: (a) Co–Cr, Air, σ_a=200 MPa, N_f=2.97x10^7; (b) Co–Cr, PBS(-), σ_a=202 MPa, N_f=1.32x10^7; (c) Ti–6Al–4V, PBS(-), σ_a=107 MPa, N_f=4.98x10^6

Among these factors, (a) and (e) may increase the fretting fatigue life of a material in PBS(-). Factors (c) and (d) may decrease the fretting fatigue life in PBS(-), compared to their effects in air. The effects of (b) and (f) on the fretting fatigue life in PBS(-) are not clear. The cancellation and involvement of these factors depend on the stress amplitude, appearing as the difference in the S-N curve under the fretting fatigue load in air and PBS(-).

2.5.4.4 Some failures of implants

For a bone plate made of a pure titanium with the ultimate tensile strength of 450 MPa, the fracture stress after one year of implantation is estimated to be about 50 MPa. For a stem made of a cobalt–chromium alloy with the ultimate tensile strength of 900 MPa, the fracture stress after nine years of implantation is also estimated to be about 50 MPa. These fractures are assumed to be caused by fretting corrosion fatigue [13]. Strengthening methods which can be applied to increase fretting corrosion fatigue strength are not available except addition of compressive residual stress to the surface of metallic materials, while corrosion fatigue strength can be strengthened by heightening material's UTS with high corrosion resistance.

2.6   Toxicity Reaction to Metallic Implants

The most critically indispensable property for biomaterials is low toxicity. Adverse effects of metallic implants on the human body are classified into two categories: chemical and mechanical. When metallic materials are implanted inside the human body they may corrode and wear out, releasing ions and debris which have toxic effects on tissues and organs. From the chemical perspective, toxicity of a metallic biomaterial depends on the kind, amount, and chemical state of metallic elements released from the metallic material [2,33,34,35,36,37]. As for toxicity from the mechanical perspective, mechanical stress is applied upon bones because the Young's moduli of metallic biomaterials are five to 10 times higher than that of the bone. As a result, bone density is decreased due to stress shielding [38].

Metal ions and debris released from implants in the human body not only accumulate in the tissues surrounding the implants, but are also carried to the whole body by the body fluid. Some of them are then discharged out of the body. Toxicity of a chemical to the human body is classified into two types: local and whole. Acute toxicity and chronic toxicity exist for both. Acute toxicity includes inflammation, ocular and skin irritations, clots formation, necrosis, and allergy. Chronic toxicity includes carcinogenicity, calcification, granulation, teratogenicity, and immunotoxicity.

In toxicity, a preceding stage exists prior to the final stage which can be organ disorder or death due to the released metal ions and debris. For example, cancer progresses as follows: metal ions released inside a living body, absorption, distribution, metabolism, molecular initiation, cancerous cells, cancerous organ, and organism response. The abnormal proliferation of cancerous cells exists as the preceding stage of a cancerous property. Cells proliferation is a critical characteristic. This is the reason why cells are used as a significant means to quantitatively estimate metal ions toxicity [39].

Toxicity testing is required for any new biomaterial introduced into the market place. Reactions of animals such as rats, rabbits, and mice to chemicals are the best available predictors of the potential toxicity. However, the use of animals in evaluating chemical safety is costly, time-consuming, and increasingly criticized by animal welfare groups [39]. Toxicity of metallic compounds and chemicals has been evaluated using cultured cells increasingly in detail because of lower cost, shorter term, higher reproducibility, and greater reliability than *in vivo* evaluation. As a result, toxicity evaluation has been carried out *in vitro* using tissue culture techniques on metal plates, metal ions, metal salts, particulate metals, and wear debris [40,33,34,35,36].

Metal ions toxicity is described in terms of the relationship between concentration and biological response such as growth rate or death (see Figure 2–13). The relative cytotoxicity of a metal ion is ranked by its concentration. One that produces 50% RPE (relative plating efficiency) is known as IC_{50} ("IC" stands for inhibitive concentration). ED_{50} ("ED" stands for effective dose) is also shown in the figure. Note that if a poisonous metal ion is administered in small concentration, it renders no toxic effects. Conversely if a nutritious metal ion is administered in excessive amount, it triggers adverse responses.

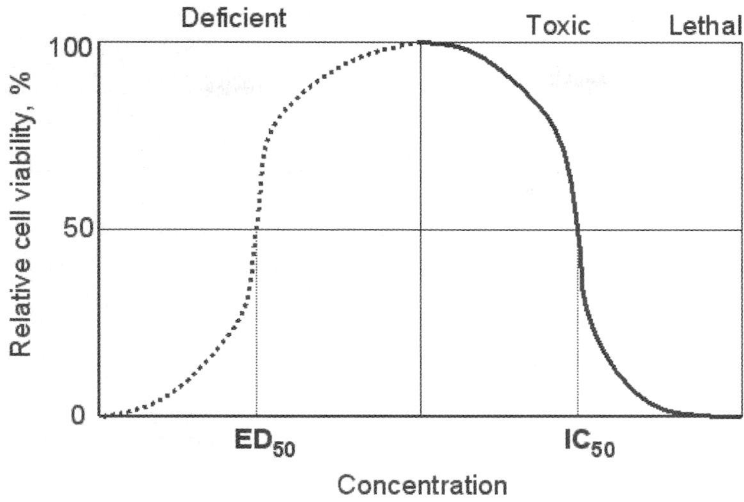

Figure 2–13 Dose-response curve

The C_{50} of metal salts for murine fibroblasts (L929) are shown in Table 2–8. In practical applications, these relatively high-toxic salts such as $K_2Cr_2O_7$, VCl_3, $CuCl_3$, $CoCl_2$, and $NiCl_2$ are included in metallic biomaterials. The toxicity of a metallic compound depends on its chemical species. For example, the IC_{50} of $Cr(NO_3)_3$ is about 500 times larger than that of $K_2Cr_2O_7$ for L929 (see Figure 2–14). This reading indicates that chromium toxicity differs depending on whether it releases hexavalent or trivalent chromium ions (or compounds) in the body. The IC_{50}s of metal salts have a close correlation (correlation coefficient r=0.69–0.94, which are calculated based on metal salts' IC_{50}s in logarithm) among six cell lines (L929, MC3T3–E1, J774.1, HeLa S3, IMR–32, and IMR–90), suggesting the existence of generic tendency in metal salts' cytotoxicity. Note too that cytotoxicity may be correlated to the strength of inflammation, ocular and skin irritations, or acute toxicity [34,35,36].

Mutagenicity is a very fundamental and important toxicity trait related to carcinogenicity and reproductive/developmental toxicity. This is because the damages to genes or DNA can be caused by carcinogenesis and developmental abnormalities. The *umu* test can evaluate the genotoxicity of tested substances by measuring the induction of the bacterial SOS response which is induced by single-strand DNA gaps or DNA fragments produced as a result of damages to DNA. Cu^{2+}, V^{3+}, Cu^+, Rh^{3+}, CrO^{4-}, Ir^{4+}, and Mg^{2+} were tested positive in the *umu* test [37].

Table 2–8 IC_{50} of metal salts for L929

Metal salt	IC_{50} (mol–L^{-1})	Metal salt	IC_{50} (mol–L^{-1})
$K_2Cr_2O_7$	1.58×10^{-6}	$TiCl_4$	1.09×10^{-3}
VCl_3	2.82×10^{-6}	$MoCl_5$	1.19×10^{-3}
$CuCl_2$	4.15×10^{-5}	$ZrCl_4$	1.64×10^{-3}
$CoCl_2$	8.12×10^{-5}	$NbCl_5$	3.63×10^{-3}
$NiCl_2$	1.06×10^{-4}	$Al(NO_3)_3$	4.18×10^{-3}
WCl_6	6.22×10^{-4}	$FeCl_3$	4.42×10^{-3}
$Cr(NO_3)_3$	7.43×10^{-4}	$FeSO_4$	6.95×10^{-3}

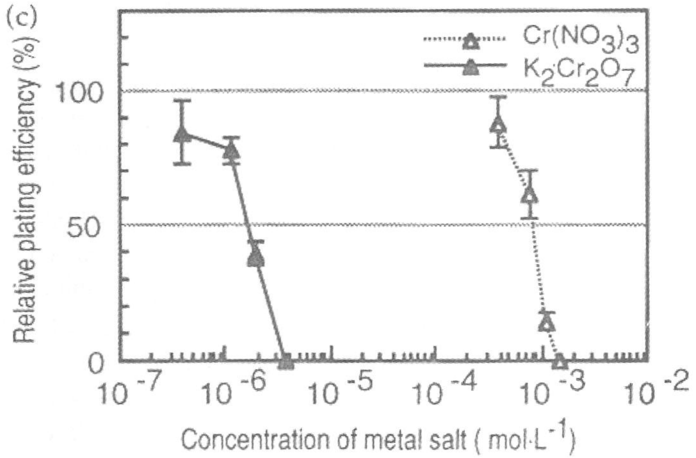

Figure 2–14 Cytotoxicity of the salts of oxo acids of chromium for L929; the error bar in the graph shows the standard deviation

2.7   Metallic Biomaterials for the Future

The safety of metallic biomaterials to the human body has the highest priority among their essential characteristics. It is definitely preferable that metallic biomaterials be constructed without the metallic elements that may produce toxic compounds to the human body. However for a large number of metallic elements and for a wide range of toxicity such as acute toxicity, carcinogenicity, and hyper sensitivity, their toxicity data of metallic ions and compounds are not widely available.

To date, toxicity of metallic elements to the human body is not systematically understood. For example, the International Agency for Research on Cancer (IARC) of World Health Organization (WHO) speculates that Be, Cd, Cr(VI), Ni compounds are carcinogenic, while Co, Pb, Hg compounds, metal Ni, and Ni alloys are probably carcinogenic too [2]. However there are no reported professional literature on the carcinogenicity of metallic materials implanted into the human body [41]. Newly developed metallic biomaterials do not contain metallic elements which have highly suspicious toxicity to the human body, such as nickel and vanadium. Some of these new developments are namely:

- Nickel-free stainless steels [42]
- Nickel-free cobalt–chromium alloys [28]
- Vanadium-free titanium alloys (ASTM F 1813)
- Amorphous alloys [43] — amorphous alloys usually exhibit a higher tensile strength, lower Young's modulus and higher corrosion resistance than crystalline alloys

Devices such as stem, bone plate, artificial knee joint, spinal fixator, sensor, and ventricular assist system need to be downsized as there is no spare space in the human body to accommodate these foreign bodies. Leveraging on this concern, there is a pressing need to develop new materials or new system to break the present impasse on structural biomaterials.

References

1. K. Okuno, The history of metallic biomaterials, Metallic Biomaterials — Fundamentals and Applications, eds. M. Sumita, Y. Ikada, and T. Tateishi, (ICP, Tokyo, 2000) 11–18.
2. IARC Monographs on the Evaluation of Carcinogenic Risks to Humans: Surgical Implants and other Foreign Bodies, Lyon, 1999, 74:65–84.
3. V. Raghavan, Phase diagrams of ternary iron alloys Part 1, Monograph series on alloys phase diagrams, ASM International, 1988, 29.
4. D. H. Kohn and P. Ducheyne, Materials science and technology — a comprehensive treatment, medical and dental materials, Weinheim, 1998, 14:39–41.
5. M. Sumita, Present status and future trend of metallic materials used in orthopedics, Orthopedic Surgery, 1997, 48:927–934.
6. N. S. Stoloff, Metals Handbook, 10th Edition, ASM International, 1996, 1:960–968.
7. J. D. Destefani, Metals Handbook, 10th Edition, ASM International, 1996, 2:586–605.
8. Y. Nakayama, T. Yamamura, Y. Kotoura, and M. Oka, *In vivo* measurement of orthopedic implant alloys: comparative study of *in vivo* and *in vitro* experiments, Biomaterials, 1989, 10:420–424.

9.   H. Hosoda and S. Miyazaki, Shape memory alloys, in Metallic Biomaterials —
      Fundamentals and Applications, eds. M. Sumita, Y. Ikada, and T. Tateishi, (ICP,
      Tokyo, 2000) 133–149.

10.   S. H. Teoh, Fatique of biomaterials: a review, Int. J. Fatigue, 2000, 22:825–837.

11.   S. C. Silverstein, R. M. Steinman, and Z. A. Cohn, Endocytosis, Annu. Rev.
      Biochem., 1977, 46:669–722.

12.   R. B. Waterhouse, Fretting fatigue in aqueous electrolytes, in Fretting Fatigue, ed.
      Waterhouse, (Applied Science Publishers, London, 1981) pp:159–175, 221–240.

13.   M. Sumita, Corrosion fatigue and fretting corrosion fatigue, in Metallic
      Biomaterials — Fundamentals and Applications, eds. M. Sumita, Y. Ikada, and T.
      Tateishi, (ICP, Tokyo, 2000) 233–270.

14.   P. D. Bianco, P. Ducheyne, and J. M. Cuckler, Local accumulation of titanium
      released from a titanium implant in the absence of wear, J. Biomed. Mater. Res.,
      1996, 31:227–234.

15.   Y. Mu, T. Kobayashi, M. Sumita, A. Yamamoto, and T. Hanawa, Metal ion release
      from titanium with active oxygen species generated by rat macrophages *in vitro*, J.
      Biomed. Mater. Res., 2000, 49:238–245.

16.   Y. Mu, T. Kobayashi, K. Tsuji, M. Sumita, and T. Hanawa, Causes of titanium
      release from plate and screws implanted in rabbits, J. Materials Science: Materials
      in Medicine, 2000, 13:583–588.

17.   A. Sato, Biological safety of metallic materials, Zairyo–Kagaku, 1982, 19:193–199.

18.   K. Nakazawa, M. Sumita, and N. Maruyama, Effect of contact pressure on fretting
      fatigue of high strength steel and titanium alloy, in Standardization of Fretting
      Fatigue Test Methods and Equipment, 1992, ASTM STP 1159:115–125.

19.   M. Sumita, I. Uchiyama, and T. Araki, Relationship between effect of inclusions
      on the endurance limits and the work hardening behaviors of carbon steels, Trans.
      ISIJ, 1974, 14:275–284.

20.   N. Maruyama, K. Nakazawa, M. Sumita, and S. Sato, Effect of stress frequency on
      fatigue and fretting fatigue lives for commercially pure Ti and Ti–6Al–4V alloy in
      pseudo-body fluid, J. Jpn. Soc. Biomater., 2000, 18:17–23.

21.   T. Satoh, Biomechanics, The Japan Society of Mechanical Engineers, Ohm–sha,
      1991, p.257.

22.   Maruyama and M. Sumita, Effect of stress amplitude transient on fatigue crack
      initiation and propagation of high strength steel in synthetic sea water under
      cathodic protection, Tetsu-to-hagane, 1992, 78:640–647.

23.   H. F. Hildebrand and J. C. Hornez, Biological response and biocompatibility, in
      Metals as Biomaterials, eds. J. A. Helsen and H. J. Breme, (John Wiley & Sons,
      New York, 1998) 265–290.

24.   R. S. Petrie, A. D. Hanssen, D. R. Osmon, and D. Il Strup, Metal-Blacked Patellar
      Component Failure in Total Knee Arthroplasty: a Possible Risk for Late Infection,
      The American Journal of Orthopedics, 1998, 172–176.

25.   O'Connor, The role of elastic stress analysis in the interpretation of fretting fatigue
      failures, in Fretting Fatigue, ed. R. B. Waterhouse, (Applied Science Publishers,
      London, 1981) 23–66.

26.   I. Nishioka and K. Hirakawa, Fundamental investigations of fretting fatigue, Part 5:
      The effect of relative slip amplitude, Bulletin of JSME, 1969, 52:692–697.

27. A. Yamamoto, T. Kobayashi, N. Maruyama, K. Nakazawa, and M. Sumita, Fretting fatigue properties of Ti–6AL–4V alloy in pseudo-body fluid and evaluation of biocompatibility by cell culture method, J. Japan Inst. Metals, 1995, 59:463–470.

28. N. Maruyama, T. Kobayashi, K. Nakazawa, M. Sumita, and M. Sato, Fatigue and fretting fatigue behavior of Ni-free Co–Cr alloy in a pseudo-body fluid, J. Jpn. Soc. Biomater., 1999, 17:172–179.

29. A. Yamamoto, T. Kobayashi, N. Maruyama, and M. Sumita, Quantitative analysis and cytotoxicity evaluation of metallic elements in pseudo-body fluids used as environment of fretting fatigue test of metallic biomaterials, J. Jpn. Soc. Biomater., 1996, 14:158–166.

30. H. H. Uhlig, Corrosion and corrosion control, 3rd Edition, (John Wiley & Sons, New York, 1989).

31. K. Nakazawa, M. Sumita, and N. Maruyama, Fatigue and fretting fatigue of austenitic and ferritic stainless steels in pseudo-body fluid, J. Japan Inst. Metals, 1999, 63:1600–1608.

32. R. B. Waterhouse, Fretting corrosion, Pergamon Press, Oxford, 1972 (translated into Japanese by J. Satoh, 83, in 1984).

33. J. C. Wataha, C. T. Hanks, and R. G. Craig, The *in vitro* effects of metal cations on eukaryotic cell metabolism, J. Biomed. Mater. Res., 1991, 25:1133–1149.

34. A. Yamamoto, R. Honma, and M. Sumita, Cytotoxicity evaluation of 43 metal salts using murine fibroblasts and osteoblastic cells, J. Biomed. Mater. Res., 1998-a, 39:331–340.

35. A. Yamamoto, Biocompatibility evaluation of metallic biomaterials *in vitro*, Doctoral dissertation at Kyoto University, 1998-b, 59–134.

36. A. Yamamoto, R. Honma, A. Tanaka, and M. Sumita, Genetic tendency of metal salt cytotoxicity for six cell lines, J. Biomed. Mater. Res., 1999, 47:396–403.

37. A. Yamamoto, Y. Kohyama, and T. Hanawa, Mutagenicity evaluation of forty-one metal salts by the *umu* test, J. Biomed. Mater. Res., 2002, 59:176–183.

38. W. H. Harris, The osteolysis phenomena in total hip and total knee replacement surgery, in World Tribology Forum in Arthroplasty, eds. C. Rieker, S. Oberholzer, and U. Wyss, (Hans Huber, Bern, 2001) 17–23.

39. A. M. Goldberg and J. M. Frazier, Alternatives to animals in toxicity testing, Scientific American, 1989, 261:16–22.

40. ISO 10993–5 Biological evaluation of medical devices — Part 5: Test for cytotoxicity – *in vitro* methods.

41. Y. Tabata, Foreign body reaction, in Metallic Biomaterials Fundamentals and Applications, eds. M. Sumita, Y. Ikada, and T. Tateishi, (ICP, Tokyo, 2000) 335–346.

42. J. Menzel, W. Kirschner, and G. Stein, High nitrogen containing Ni-free austenitic steels for medical applications, ISIJ International, 1996, 36:893–900.

43. S. Hiromoto, A. P. Tsai, M. Sumita, and T. Hanawa, Corrosion behavior of zirconium based amorphous alloys for biomedical use, Mater. Trans., 2001, 42:656–659.

CHAPTER 3

CORROSION OF METALLIC IMPLANTS

D. J. Blackwood[1], K. H. W. Seah[2] and S. H. Teoh[2]

[1]Department of Materials Science
[2]Department of Mechanical Engineering
National University of Singapore, Lower Kent Ridge Road, Singapore 119260
E-mail: masdjb@nus.edu.sg

The practice of using metals and alloys to repair or replace human body parts is now well established. Two of the most important parameters in determining a material's suitability for biomedical applications are its biocompatibility and corrosion resistance. This chapter will give a basic introduction to the thermodynamic and electrochemical aspects behind corrosion, focusing on the various forms of localized corrosion that are responsible for most of the *in vivo* failures. This will be followed by a brief review of the successes and, in reality, the remarkably few failures of the traditional materials — which are mainly titanium alloys, cobalt–chromium alloys, amalgams, and stainless steels. The desire to utilize a few advanced materials such as memory-shape alloys, porous materials, and rare earth magnets will then be discussed. Unfortunately nearly all of these materials have inadequate corrosion resistances, such that they cannot be used directly *in vivo* without some form of protection. The chapter ends with some case histories of surgical implant failure.

3.1   Introduction

The practice of using metallic materials to repair or replace bones in the human body is now well established. An important parameter in determining the suitability of a material for use in surgical implants is its corrosion resistance. In many industrial applications, metal corrosion is controlled by these means: altering the local environment, changing the pH, lowering the temperature, or adding chemical inhibitors. Unfortunately, these techniques cannot be used to reduce the corrosion rate of surgical implants since the environment within the human body is fixed. Coatings (e.g., paints) are also widely used to control corrosion. However, these coatings are of limited use to protecting implants. This is because many of these implants (especially orthopedic devices) are subjected to wearing and abrasion processes that will damage most coatings [1]. The only generally successful method of reducing corrosion within the human body is to fabricate the implants from a corrosion-resistant alloy.

This approach has been extremely successful — at least with respect to extending the lifetime of biomedical devices. Up to the late 1970s, corrosion of surgical implants loomed large as a major concern. The development of a range of corrosion-resistant alloys, such as Ti–6Al–4V and high-nitrogen stainless steels, have reduced the number of failures to extremely low levels. Even most of the few failures that still occur are often traced to either poor quality control (for example a 304L screw instead of a 316L screw was used), or to an unexpected and unusually aggressive local environment around the implant (due to pathological changes in the surrounding tissue as it reacts to the surgical procedure). Most of the other earlier implant failures were either due to fatigue or fretting, which might or might not be accelerated by corrosion.

Nevertheless, there remains the concern that extended exposure to even very low levels of corrosion products could result in medical complications. One major problem in this respect is that there is no consensus on what the safe levels are, or even which metals are toxic. For example a few years ago, aluminum was linked with Alzheimer's disease. This has recently been disproved, but iron is now linked to Parkinson's disease [2]. To date, fortunately, titanium — the mainstay of biomaterials — has not been linked to any disease. However, there is no guarantee that it will not be in the future, especially as the average age of patients receiving implants is decreasing due in part to modern popularity of physical sports which place a large strain on joints. Thus the required life expectancy of the implant is increasing, and this obviously increases the risk of a high accumulation of toxic ions as well as increasing the likelihood of failure by fatigue and fretting. As a result, there will be a continued need to develop alloys for surgical use that have lower and lower corrosion rates.

Corrosion problems in dental applications are more common, mainly due to the high acidity and chloride contents of many foodstuffs. Although fixtures in the oral cavity are readily accessible for repair, there is the concern of the toxicity of the metals leaching out. Even more alarming are the potentials that can develop within galvanic cells — they have been linked with oral cancer [3,4].

3.2   Corrosion Theory

3.2.1 *Basic Thermodynamics of Corrosion*

3.2.1.1 *The Nernst equation*

For a typical chemical equation with non-charged species,

$$aA + bB \rightarrow cC + dD \tag{1}$$

the free energy of the reaction is simply the difference between the chemical potentials of the products and reactants (as shown below).

$$\Delta G = \text{(chemical potential of products} - \text{chemical potential of reactants)}$$
$$= (c\mu_C + d\mu_D) - (a\mu_A + b\mu_B) \tag{2}$$

At equilibrium, $\Delta G = 0$ and since the chemical potential of any species can be defined by:

$$\mu = \mu^\theta + RT\ln(M) \tag{3}$$

where μ° is the standard chemical potential, R the gas constant, T the temperature and M either the fugacity or activity of the substance, equation (2) can be expressed as:

$$(c\mu^\theta + d\mu^\theta) - (a\mu^\theta + b\mu^\theta) + RT(c\ln M_C + d\ln M_D) - RT(a\ln M_A + b\ln M_B) = 0$$

which can be rearranged as:

$$\left(c\mu^\theta + d\mu^\theta\right) - \left(a\mu^\theta + b^\theta\right) = RT\ln\left(\frac{[M_C]^c[M_D]^d}{[M_A]^a[M_B]^b}\right)$$

or

$$\Delta G^\theta = -RT\ln K \tag{4}$$

where ΔG^θ is the standard Gibbs free energy of reaction and K is the equilibrium constant.

However, in electrochemical reactions, at least one species will carry a charge. In this case, it is necessary to add an additional term to the chemical potential to represent the electrical free energy (due to the interaction of the charge with its environment). This yields the electrochemical potential which is defined as:

$$\overline{\mu} = \mu + zF\Phi \tag{5}$$

where z is the charge number (including sign, *i.e.*, -1 for an electron), F is Faradays constant (96485 C mol^{-1}), and Φ the Galvani potential.

Now consider a typical electrochemical reaction in which an electron is transferred from a metal electrode into the solution. There it reduces an oxidized species (O) to a reduced species (R) — where one (or both) of which must be charged:

$$O_{sol} + e^-_m \rightarrow R_{sol} \tag{6}$$

Once again, ΔG must be zero at equilibrium. This means that the electrochemical potentials of the products and the reactants must be equal:

$$\overline{\mu}_O + \overline{\mu}_{e,m} = \overline{\mu}_R \tag{7a}$$

In terms of chemical potentials and Galvani potentials, equation (7a) can be expressed as:

$$\mu_O + z_O F\Phi_{sol} + \mu_{e,m} - F\Phi_m = \mu_R + z_R F\Phi_{sol} \tag{7b}$$

Rearranging equations (7a) and (7b) then yields:

$$\Phi_m - \Phi_{sol} = (\mu_O - \mu_R + \mu_{e,m})/nF$$

where n is the number of electrons transferred (*i.e.*, $z_O - z_R$).

Expanding the chemical potential terms as in equation (3) yields:

$$\Delta\Phi_{m,sol} = \Delta\Phi^\theta_{m,sol} + RT/nF \ln (M_O/M_R) \tag{8}$$

Unfortunately, this Galvani potential difference cannot be measured. However, if we place a second electrode into the solution we can measure the cell electromotive force (emf), *i.e.*, the difference between two Galvani potentials (as shown below):

$$E_{emf} = \Delta\Phi_{m2,sol} - \Delta\Phi_{m1,sol} = E^\theta_{emf} + RT/nF \ln (M_O/M_R) \tag{9}$$

This expression is known as the Nernst equation. Fortunately, in practice, most solutions are sufficiently dilute to allow the activities to be replaced by concentrations. As a result, the emf subscript is normally neglected so that the Nernst equation is usually written as:

$$E = E^\theta + RT/nF \ln ([O]/[R]) \tag{10}$$

Furthermore at equilibrium $E = 0$, the concentration terms in equation (10) can also be replaced by the equilibrium constant, hence yielding:

$$E^\theta = -RT/nF \ln K \tag{11}$$

Inserting equation (4) then provides the link between an electrochemical reaction's standard potential and its standard Gibbs free energy change:

$$\Delta G° = -nFE° \tag{12}$$

3.2.1.2 *Standard potentials (E^θ) and the electrochemical series*

As stated earlier, we can measure only the emf potentials between two electrodes (and not the Galvani potential of a single electrode). However, in order to relate this measured potential to any practical energy scale it is necessary to have some reference point. By convention, the standard potential of a reversible hydrogen reaction in a solution — with unit proton activity and hydrogen at a partial pressure of one atmosphere — is taken to be zero at all temperatures (*i.e.*, chemical potentials for proton and hydrogen at unit activity and fugacity are zero).

$$2H^+ + H_2 \Leftrightarrow H_2 + 2H^+ \qquad (E° = 0.000 \text{ V}^*) \tag{13}$$

In other words, the reaction at one electrode is:

$$2H^+ + 2e^- \rightarrow H_2 \tag{14}$$

while that at the other is:

$$H_2 \rightarrow 2H^+ + 2e^- \tag{15}$$

---

* The standard hydrogen electrode potential is in the region of 4.5 eV on the vacuum scale

In practice both reactions (14) and (15) proceed on the same electrode, since they occur at the same potential and no net currents are required.

Reactions that involve the production or consumption of electrons are called "half cell" reactions — they cannot exist independently. The standard potential for any other half cell reaction is defined as the potential that would be measured when the oxidation of molecular hydrogen to solvated protons acts as the second half of the cell with all species being in their standard states (and with activities and fugacities at unity).

For example, the standard potential for a piece of zinc is determined from the following equilibrium reaction:

$$Zn^{2+} + H_2 \leftrightarrow Zn + 2H^+ \tag{16}$$

The conditions required to induce unit activities and fugacities would be a solution that contains 1 mol dm^{-3} of Zn^{2+} ions at pH 1 and subjected to one atmosphere of hydrogen gas. Under such conditions, the measured standard potential is −0.76 V. Note that solids always behave with unit activity and can thus be eliminated from the Nernst equation. It is hence normal to abbreviate reaction (16) to the form below:

$$Zn^{2+} + 2e^- \leftrightarrow Zn \tag{17}$$

Alternatively, if the chemical potentials of all the species involved are already known, the standard potential can be calculated directly from equation (12):

$$E^\theta = -\Delta G \, / \, nF$$
$$E^\theta = - \text{(chemical potential of products} - \text{chemical potential of reactants)} \, / \, nF$$
$$= - \left[(\mu_{Zn} + 2\mu_{H+}) - (\mu_{Zn2+} + \mu_{H2}) \right] \, / \, nF$$
$$= - (-\mu_{Zn2+}) \, / \, nF \quad \text{(all the other terms being zero by convention)}$$
$$= -0.76 \text{ V}$$

The electrochemical series (Table 3–1) lists half cell reactions in the order of their standard potentials. A metal with a high standard potential (e.g., gold) is sometimes referred to as being noble, whereas those with low standard potentials (e.g., magnesium) are termed base.

Placing a base metal in a solution containing more noble ions should cause the noble metal to plate out at the expense of corrosion to the base metal, such as:

$$Fe + Cu^{2+} \rightarrow Fe^{2+} + Cu$$
$$Zn + 2H^+ \rightarrow Zn^{2+} + H_2$$

The second of the above two examples reveals that all metals which have negative standard potentials can be expected to corrode in aqueous (or at least acidic) solutions. However in practice, the presence of oxide films and complex ions can greatly influence the measured potentials. Thus the above series should be used only as a guide.

3.2.1.3 Potential-pH equilibrium diagrams (Pourbaix diagrams)

As shown in Table 3–1, standard potentials for solids in equilibrium with
solutions of their ions can be calculated. In addition, chemical potentials —
when combined with solubility constants — can also be used to calculate the
equilibrium condition of any system that consists of:
- Two solid substances;
- One solid substance and one dissolved species; or
- Two dissolved species.

Pourbaix [5] used this technique to calculate the stable phases at
equilibrium for most of metal/water systems at 25°C. The data are displayed in
the form of a diagram with pH as the X-axis and potential as the Y-axis.

Table 3–1 Electrochemical series of the more common metals

Half cell reaction	Standard potential (volts)
$Au^+ + e^- \leftrightarrow Au$	+1.68
$Pt^{2+} + 2e^- \leftrightarrow Pt$	+1.20
$Hg^{2+} + 2e^- \leftrightarrow Hg$	+0.85
$Ag^+ + e^- \leftrightarrow Ag$	+0.80
$Cu^{2+} + 2e^- \leftrightarrow Cu$	+0.34
$2H^+ + 2e^- \leftrightarrow H_2$	0.00
$Pb^{2+} + 2e^- \leftrightarrow Pb$	−0.13
$Sn^{2+} + 2e^- \leftrightarrow Sn$	−0.14
$Ni^{2+} + 2e^- \leftrightarrow Ni$	−0.25
$Cd^{2+} + 2e^- \leftrightarrow Cd$	−0.40
$Fe^{2+} + 2e^- \leftrightarrow Fe$	−0.44
$Cr^{3+} + 3e^- \leftrightarrow Cr$	−0.71
$Zn^{2+} + 2e^- \leftrightarrow Zn$	−0.76
$Ti^{2+} + 2e^- \leftrightarrow Ti$	−1.63
$Al^{3+} + 3e^- \leftrightarrow Al$	−1.67
$Mg^{2+} + 2e^- \leftrightarrow Mg$	−2.34
$Na^+ + e^- \leftrightarrow Na$	−2.71
$Ca^{2+} + 2e^- \leftrightarrow Ca$	−2.87
$K^+ + e^- \leftrightarrow K$	−2.92

Figures 3–1 and 3–2 show examples of Pourbaix diagram for a number of
important materials. Each diagram is divided into three different domains which
are labeled: Immunity, Corrosion (which has been shaded for ease of reference),

and Passivation. The meanings of these three terms can be explained by considering the following scenario.

When a piece of metal is placed in solution, it will corrode until the activity (effectively concentration) reaches the level required to obtain thermodynamic equilibrium as demanded by the Nernst equation — that is, when the driving force for corrosion is exactly matched by the driving force for electroplating.

- Immunity: the activity of metal ions required to obtain equilibrium is less than 10^{-6} mol dm^{-3}.

- Corrosion: the activity of metal ions required to obtain equilibrium is greater than 10^{-6} mol dm^{-3}.

- Passivity: the activity of metal ions required for an oxide/hydroxide film to form is less than 10^{-6} mol dm^{-3}. In this case, equilibrium is established between the oxide film and the ions in solution.

Note that there is nothing special about the level of 10^{-6} mol dm^{-3} — it was just chosen on the basis that it represents a very dilute solution. Moreover, hinging on the above definitions does not equate immunity to no corrosion. It is only that the amount of corrosion required to raise the concentration of ions to equilibrium levels is very low, and thus one would expect that equilibrium is rapidly established and that the corrosion rate falls to a negligible level. However, at this point, it is worth reiterating that corrosion rates that are considered negligible in most industrial applications may still be significant when applied to a surgical implant, due to the need to prevent high levels of potentially toxic metallic ions building up in the body.

Lines (a) and (b) that are marked on all the Pourbaix diagrams represent the stability zone for water, and thus it is only within this range that equilibrium can be obtained in an aqueous system. Below line (a), water is reduced to hydrogen as follows:

$$H_2 \Leftrightarrow 2H+ + 2e^- \qquad E^\circ = 0.000 - 0.0591pH - 0.0295 \log P(H_2) \qquad (18)$$

Above line (b), water is oxidized to produce oxygen as follows:

$$2H_2O \Leftrightarrow O_2 + 4H^+ + 4e^- \quad E^\circ = 1.228 - 0.0591pH + 0.0147 \log P(O_2) \qquad (19)$$

Naturally line (b) is also the limit below which any oxygen dissolved in the solution can be reduced. However, as we will see later, kinetic and mass transport limitations play an important role in the reduction of dissolved oxygen.

From an industrial perspective, the Pourbaix diagram for iron is the most important — it being the basis of all steels and stainless steels. It can be seen from Figure 3–2(d) that iron is classified as being immune at very negative potentials (*i.e.*, strongly reducing conditions). However, as the potential is increased, there is a tendency for the iron to become oxidized. Under either acidic or highly alkaline conditions, oxidation of iron results in active corrosion. However, in neutral environments passivation results. It can also be seen from the Pourbaix diagram that increasing the potential tends to favor passivation over corrosion.

Examination of Pourbaix diagrams of other metals shown in Figures 3–1 and 3–2 reveals that they have basically the same pattern as that of iron: immunity at very negative potential, corrosion under acidic or basic conditions, and passivity in neutral environments. However, closer examination of the diagrams reveals that for noble metals such as platinum, the immunity domain extends across nearly the entire zone of water stability, hence explaining their excellent corrosion resistance. On the other hand, the immunity domain of active metals — such as zinc and titanium — are located well below the water stability zone, which means that they can be expected to be rapidly oxidized in an aqueous solution. In the case of zinc, the Pourbaix diagram shows that active corrosion occurs almost throughout the whole of the water stability zone, except for a small band around pH 12; hence this is clearly not a suitable material for biomedical applications.

Fortunately, the oxides and hydroxides of titanium have extremely low solubilities — so a passive oxide film readily forms over the titanium's surface. Furthermore, this film is continuous and coherent so that it provides excellent protection to the underlying metal. It is the presence of this oxide film that is responsible for titanium's excellent corrosion resistance, which enables it to be used in surgical applications. However, it is important to note that the Pourbaix diagram still shows two sets of conditions where titanium does undergo rapid corrosion. The first is in neutral or acidic conditions — which are extremely reducing conditions (negative potentials) — where titanium fails to form a passive oxide; the second is under extremely oxidizing conditions where solubilities of titanium hydroxides start to increase[*]. Although both of these regions fall outside the water stability zone, it turns out that the kinetics for both the reduction and oxidation of water at titanium electrode are slow. Thus it maybe possible to enter the negative corrosion region in anoxic environments or the positive region in the presence of a strong oxidizing agent, such as hydrogen peroxide.

Although Pourbaix diagrams form a good basis for the study of corrosion reactions, their limitations when applied to practical problems should be appreciated. The lack of kinetic data is best illustrated by the cases of nickel and cobalt. Figures 3–1(a), 3–1(b) and 3–2(e) show that the Pourbaix diagrams for Ni and Co are very similar — both have rather extensive, theoretical domains for corrosion. However, experimentally, it is found that nickel passivates much more readily than predicted from thermodynamics, and that corrosion is restricted to a much smaller range of conditions (Figure 3–1(b)). The explanation for this behavior is thought to be mainly due to the slow kinetics of the nickel dissolution reaction. In the case of cobalt, there is reasonably good agreement between theory and practice except in non-oxidizing acids, which

---

[*] The corrosion region at positive potentials is often marked with "question marks" due to the difficulty in obtaining reliable fundamental thermodynamic data under these conditions.

thermodynamically should be very corrosive towards cobalt. However, in practice, cobalt is one of the metals least attacked by non-oxidizing acids as the kinetics of hydrogen evolution reaction on its surface are very slow [5].

It is important to remember that Pourbaix diagrams are for the simple metal/water systems. The presence of complexing ions (chloride, cyanide, citrate, *etc.*) can greatly expand the corrosion zone. This is particularly true for the case of chromium, for which the size of the passive domain can be severely reduced in the presence of chloride (Figures 3–1(c) and (d)). Given that chromium plays a dominant role in the formation of oxide films that protect stainless steels, the importance of this phenomenon (with respect to the performance of stainless steel implants) is obvious.

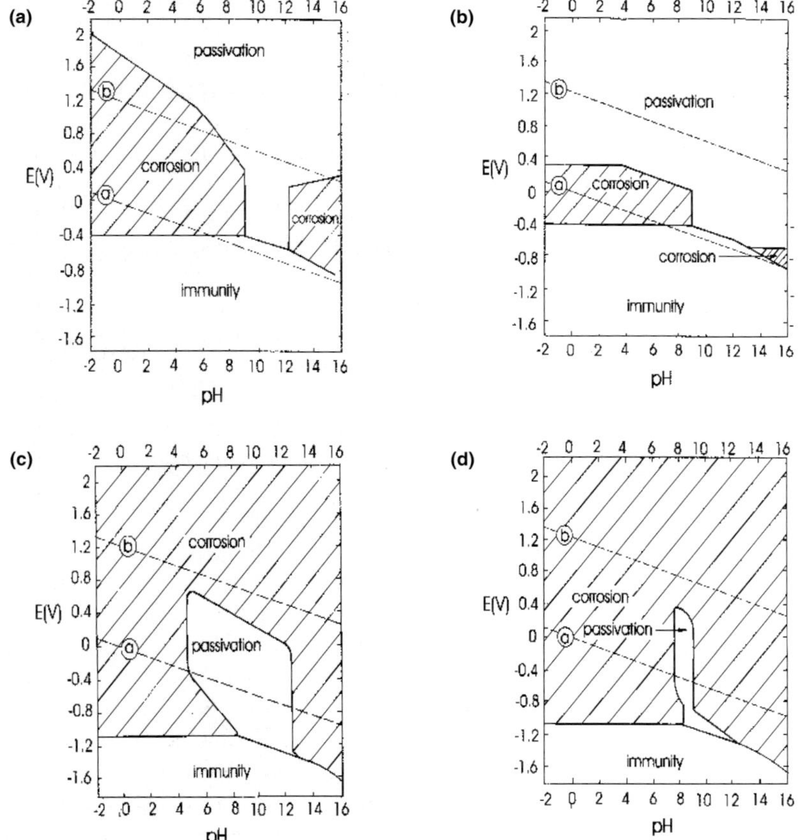

Figure 3–1 Potential against pH Pourbaix diagrams: (a) nickel (theoretical); (b) nickel (experimental); (c) chromium (absence of chloride); (d) chromium (presence of chloride) (Reprinted from reference [5] with permission)

 D. J. Blackwood et al.

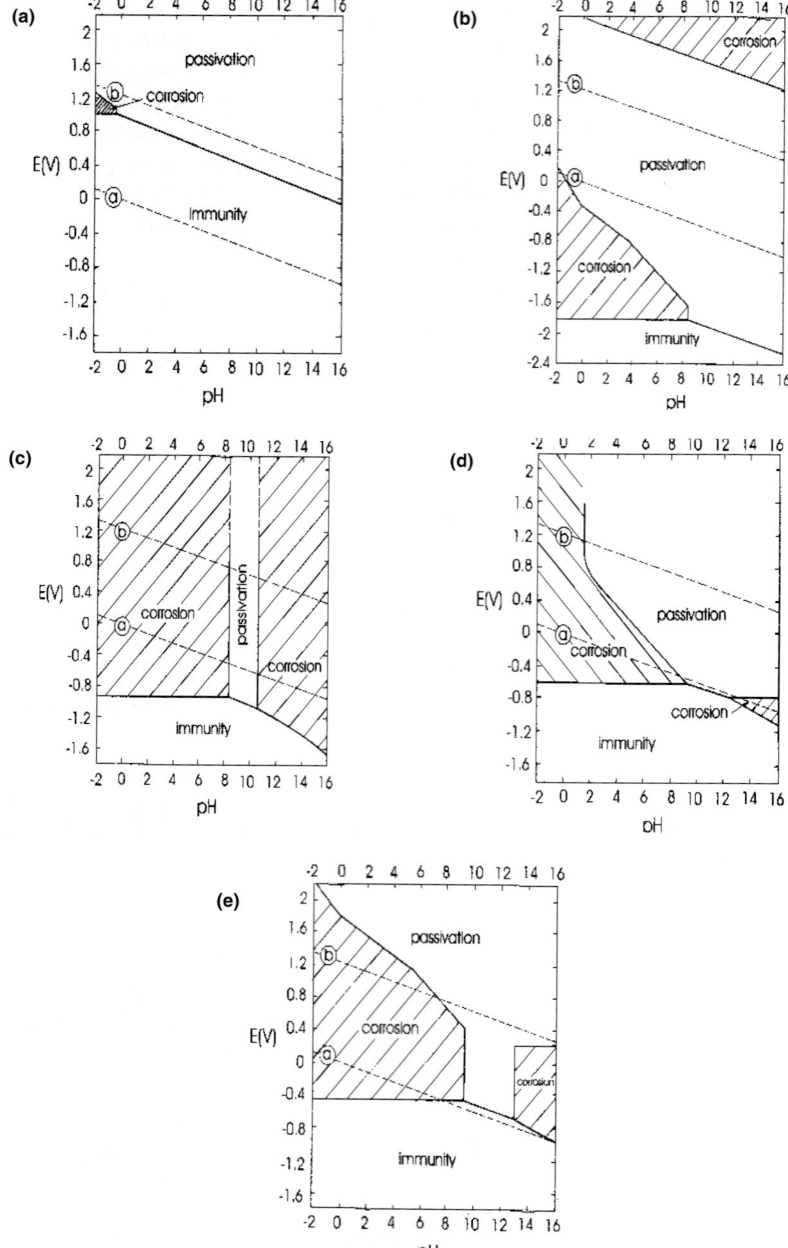

Figure 3–2 Potential against pH Pourbaix diagrams: (a) platinum; (b) titanium; (c) zinc; (d) iron; and (e) cobalt (Reprinted from reference [5] with permission)

3.2.2 Basic Electrochemistry

3.2.2.1 Electrode reactions

An electrode reaction is defined as the transfer of electrons between chemical species and an electrode.

    a)   Chemical species are **oxidized** if electrons are transferred to the electrode (as illustrated below).

$$2H_2O - 4e^- \rightarrow O_2 + 4H^+$$
$$2Al + 3H_2O - 6e^- \rightarrow Al_2O_3 + 6H^+$$

Oxidizing reactions are also referred to as anodic processes, and the electrode at which they occur as the anode. The more positive the applied potential, the faster these oxidizing reactions will proceed. By convention, currents arising due to anodic processes (oxidizing) are considered to be positive.

    b)   Chemical species are **reduced** if electrons are transferred from the electrode (as illustrated below).

$$Fe^{3+} + e^- \rightarrow Fe^{2+}$$
$$2H_2O + 2e^- \rightarrow H_2 + 2OH^-$$

Reducing reactions are also referred to as cathodic processes, and the electrode at which they occur as the cathode.

Overall charge balance must always be maintained. Therefore for every electron transferred at the anode another must be transferred at the cathode. The magnitude of the current flowing is directly proportional to the rate of reaction, and the total charge (q) passed yields the amount of chemical reaction that has taken place via Faraday's law:

$$q = mnF \tag{20}$$

where m is the number of moles of reactant consumed, n is the number of electrons transferred per reactant, and F is Faraday's constant.

3.2.2.2 Electron transfer

Consider an inert electrode (e.g., platinum or gold) placed in a solution containing solution species O and R. A dynamic equilibrium will be established at the surface of this electrode, which can be expressed as:

$$O + e^- \Leftrightarrow R \tag{21}$$

It is very important to understand that equilibriums are dynamic. In other words, both the reduction of O and the oxidation of R are happening continuously — but at an equal rate, no net changes occur. In terms of current flow, this can be expressed as:

$$-\overrightarrow{I} = \overleftarrow{I} = I_0 \tag{22}$$

where $\overrightarrow{I}$ and $\overleftarrow{I}$ are partial current densities of the forward and back reactions, and I_0 is the exchange current density. **No net current flows.**

The potential at which this equilibrium occurs is defined as follows by the Nernst equation:

$$E_e = E_e^{\theta} + \frac{RT}{nF} Ln \frac{c_O^{\sigma}}{c_R^{\sigma}} \tag{23}$$

The superscript σ is used to indicate that it is the concentration at the electrode surface that determines the potential, which may be different from the bulk concentration.

Now make the potential of our inert electrode more negative, *i.e.*, apply an external voltage using a second electrode. Equilibrium can now be re-established only when the ratio between the surface concentrations of O and R has taken up the new value as demanded by the Nernst equation. Therefore a current must flow across the electrode/solution interface to convert O into R. Likewise, if a positive potential is applied a current will flow in the opposite direction to convert R into O. However, the magnitudes of these currents will depend on kinetics rather than thermodynamics.

3.2.2.3 *Kinetics of electron transfer*

At any potential, the net current flowing is given as:

$$I = \overrightarrow{I} + \overleftarrow{I} \text{ (where } \overrightarrow{I} \text{ is negative)} \tag{24}$$

with

$$\overrightarrow{I} = -nF \, \overrightarrow{k} \, c_O^{\sigma} \text{ and } \overleftarrow{I} = nF \, \overleftarrow{k} \, c_R^{\sigma}$$

The k's are rate constants that vary with applied potential (*i.e.*, the potential difference at the electrode's surface during electrons transfer). They usually take the following form:

$$\overrightarrow{k} = \overrightarrow{k}_0 \, Exp\left(\frac{-\alpha_C \, nF}{RT} E\right) \quad \text{and} \quad \overleftarrow{k} = \overleftarrow{k}_0 \, Exp\left(\frac{\alpha_A \, nF}{RT} E\right)$$

where α_A and α_C are constants (usually ≈ 0.5) and for simple electron transfer reaction (as illustrated below):

$$\alpha_A + \alpha_C = 1 \tag{25}$$

Note that overpotential (η) is defined as:

$$\eta = E - E_e \tag{26}$$

and by definition at $\eta = 0$:

$$I_0 = -\overrightarrow{I} = \overleftarrow{I}$$

allows the Butler–Volmer equation to be derived as follows:

$$I = I_0 \left[Exp\left(\frac{\alpha_A\, nF}{RT}\, \eta \right) - Exp\left(\frac{-\alpha_c\, nF}{RT}\, \eta \right) \right] \tag{27}$$

This is the fundamental equation of electrokinetics with three limiting forms:

1. At high positive overpotentials the second term can be ignored, thus yielding:

$$\log I = \log I_0 + \frac{\alpha_A\, nF}{2.3 RT}\, \eta \tag{28}$$

2. At high negative overpotentials the first term can be ignored, thus yielding:

$$\log -I = \log I_0 - \frac{\alpha_C\, nF}{2.3 RT}\, \eta \tag{29}$$

3. At very low overpotentials where $\eta \ll (RT/\alpha_A nF)$ and $\eta \ll (RT/\alpha_C nF)$, and where it is only valid for $|\eta| < 10$ mV the following is obtained:

$$I = I_0 \frac{nF}{RT}\, \eta \tag{30}$$

Equations (28) to (30) are known as Tafel equations and are used to determine the values of both I_0 and α.

3.2.2.4 Mixed potential theory

Corrosion processes differ from the simple case represented by reaction (21) in that the forward and back reactions are not identical. For example, the reactions that occur when a piece of iron is placed into an acidic solution are:

$$Fe \rightarrow Fe^{2+} + 2e^-$$

$$2H^+ + 2e^- \rightarrow H_2$$

However, the iron is at open-circuit, so no net current can flow. Therefore the corrosion potential is defined as the potential at which the forward and back reactions occur at the same rate. Corrosion current density can thus be defined as:

$$-\overrightarrow{I} = \overleftarrow{I} = I_{Corr} \tag{31}$$

As long as both the forward and back reactions adhere to the Butler–Volmer equation, the corrosion current density (I_{corr}) and corrosion potential (E_{corr}) can be obtained by plotting the log of the current density against the applied potential (as shown by the schematic diagram in Figure 3–3). This diagram is sometimes referred to as a Tafel plot or Evans diagram. Note that the slopes of such a plot are often referred to as beta values, and from the Tafel equations (equations (28) and (29)) it can be seen that:

$$\beta = RT / \alpha nF \tag{32}$$

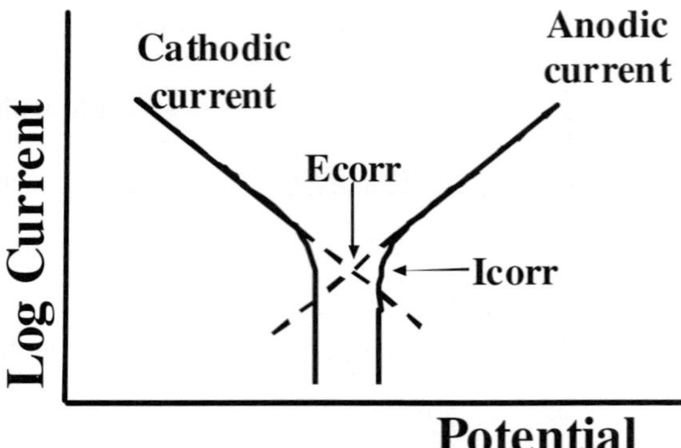

Figure 3–3 Plot of log current versus potential (*i.e.*, polarization curve or Tafel plot) for the case where both the corrosion and cathodic reactions are under electron transfer control. The corrosion current and corrosion potential can be determined from the intercept of the anodic and cathodic regions.

3.2.2.5 *Cathodic reactions*

Under open-circuit conditions (*i.e.*, when the metal is freely corroding), no net current flows. Therefore reducible species are required in the solution to act as a sink for the electrons produced during metal oxidation. It is clear from Figure 3–3 that the rate at which a metal corrodes not only depends on the kinetics of this anodic reaction, but also on the rate at which electrons are consumed by the supporting cathodic reaction. In an aqueous environment, the two most important cathodic reactions are the reduction of dissolved oxygen and the reduction of water (*i.e.*, the hydrogen evolution reaction). It is worth mentioning at this point that equations (18) and (19) reveal that both common cathodic supporting reactions lead to a localized decrease in pH at the metal's surface. In seawater, this can lead to the deposition of protective calcium carbonate scales [6]; in the case of surgical implants, this phenomenon may be helpful in encouraging the formation of hydroxyapatite films [7].

Oxygen Reduction

Under aerobic conditions, the cathodic current is usually supplied from the reduction of dissolved oxygen at the metal's surface (as represented by equation (19)). Unfortunately, the mechanism for reduction of oxygen in aqueous media is complicated with hydrogen peroxide being a possible intermediate reaction product.

$$O_2 + 2H^+ + 2e^- \rightarrow 2H_2O_2 \qquad \text{+0.68V vs. SHE} \qquad (33)$$

Figure 3–4 shows typical polarization curves for the reduction of dissolved oxygen. At very positive potentials, the oxygen reduction reaction is purely under electron transfer control, as illustrated by a straight "Tafel" line.

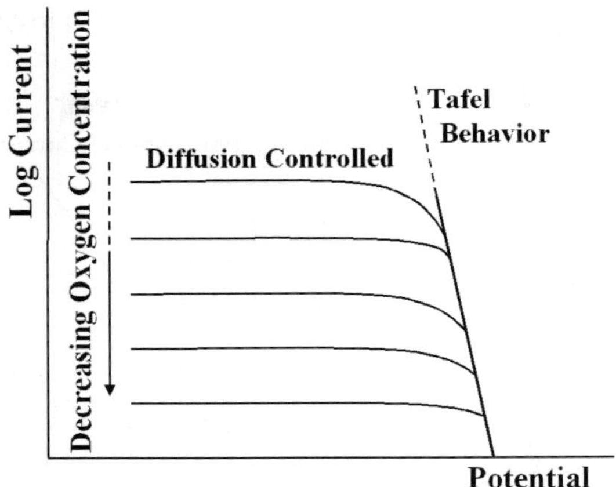

Figure 3–4 Polarization curve for oxygen reduction showing regions under electron transfer and mass transport control

However, solubility of oxygen in aqueous solutions is very low. As a result, the rate of its mass transport — mainly via diffusion — towards the metal's surface is slow. Therefore oxygen reduction can supply only a limited amount of cathodic current before its surface concentration begins to fall and the rate of its reduction partially under mass transport control. This causes the potential dependence of the cathodic current to curve below the Tafel line. At the extreme limit, the dissolved oxygen concentration at the metal's surface drops to zero — at which point the rate of its reduction becomes mass transport limited and therefore independent of potential. In the case where the only available form of mass transport is diffusion, the maximum cathodic current density, I_{lim}, that can be supplied by the reduction of dissolved oxygen is given by [8]:

$$I_{\lim} = \frac{4FDC_O}{\delta} \tag{34}$$

where F is Faraday's constant, D is the diffusion coefficient of the dissolved oxygen ($\sim 10^{-5}$ cm^2 s^{-1}), C_o is concentration of dissolved oxygen in the bulk of the solution, and δ is the diffusion layer thickness ($\sim 10^{-2}$ cm). Clearly, as illustrated in Figure 3–4, the value of the limiting current depends directly on dissolved oxygen concentration. In addition, in the presence of convection (such as fluid flowing through a pipe), the thickness of the diffusion layer reduces such that for a given dissolved oxygen concentration, I_{lim} increases.

Since no net current flows under open-circuit conditions, the corrosion potential adopted by a metal in aerobic conditions is that at which the demand for anodic current from the corrosion reaction is balanced by the available supply of cathodic current from the reduction of dissolved oxygen. Figure 3–5 shows that this decrease in dissolved oxygen concentration will cause the

                              D. J. Blackwood et al.

metal's corrosion potential to shift in the negative direction from intercept (d) to intercept (a).

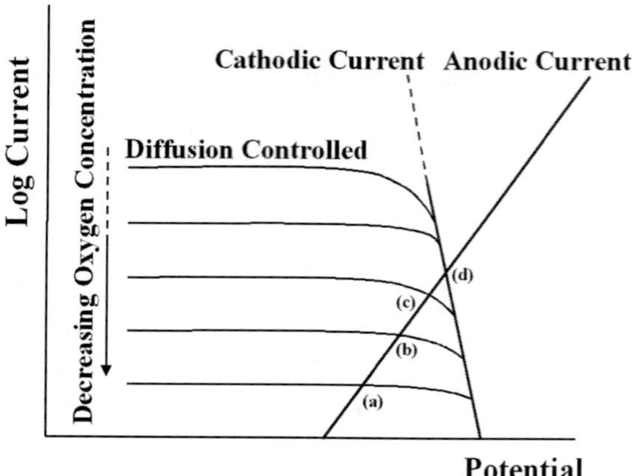

Figure 3–5 Combined polarization curves for active metal and oxygen reduction. The corrosion potential will be at the intercept between the anodic and cathodic currents, that is at (a), (b), (c) or (d), depending on the dissolved oxygen concentration.

Hydrogen Evolution Reaction

If the cathodic current available from dissolved oxygen is insufficient to balance the anodic corrosion current, the system will search for a fresh source of cathodic current. Although there may be a number of reducible species in the body that could potentially supply some of the required additional cathodic current, the only one source in abundance is water — the reduction of which leads to the evolution of hydrogen. However, as indicated by equations (18) and (19), the reduction of water occurs at a much more negative potential than that for the reduction of oxygen. Hence water is only able to support the corrosion of more active metals — which in practice, refer to metals with negative standard potentials (Table 3–1). However, the local chemical environment can reduce the potential at which some of the more noble metals corrode.

Water is nearly always in excess at the electrode interface. Hence its reduction to hydrogen can be expected to be dominated by the kinetics of charge transfer reactions, rather than by mass transport processes. The electrochemistry behind hydrogen evolution reaction has been studied in great detail over the years, and its mechanism is now well understood [8]. The first step is the adsorption of hydrogen atoms:

$$H^+ + e^- + M \rightarrow M\text{–}H \qquad (M = \text{metal surface}) \tag{35}$$

This is followed by either the desorption of hydrogen molecules:

$$2M\text{–}H \rightarrow 2M + H_2 \tag{36}$$

or reaction with a proton:

$$M\text{–}H + H^+ + e^- \rightarrow M + H_2 \tag{37}$$

Note that hydrogen evolution requires both the formation and breaking of a M-H bond. The strength of this bond (free energy of adsorption, ΔG_{ADS}) will depend on the nature of the metal.

- The greater ΔG_{ADS} is, the faster the rate of reaction (35) but the slower the rates of reactions (36) and (37).
- The lower ΔG_{ADS} is, the slower the rate of reaction (35) but the faster the rates of reactions (36) and (37).

This effect is extremely significant as it can lead to reaction rates that vary by as much as ten orders of magnitude on different metals (Table 3–2). Therefore minor alloying elements or impurities can totally control the hydrogen evolution rate, and with it the corrosion behavior of the parent metal. At times, this can be put to good use. For example, hydrogen evolution reaction occurs very slowly on titanium. As a result, there is a danger that the protective passive oxide film does not form in reducing environments. However, this problem can be solved if as little as 0.25% palladium is alloyed to titanium, thereby increasing the hydrogen evolution rate and shifting the corrosion potential into the passive region (see Pourbaix diagram, Figure 3–2(b)).

Table 3–2 Exchange current densities for hydrogen evolution reaction at various metal surfaces (Reprinted from reference [8] with permission)

Metal	$-\log (I_o /A\ cm^{-2})$	Metal	$-\log (I_o /A\ cm^{-2})$
Ag	5.4	Ni	5.2
Au	5.5	Pb	12.2
Cd	11.0	Pd	2.3
Co	5.2	Pt	3.6
Cr	7.4	Ru	2.1
Cu	6.7	Ti	11.3
Fe	6.0	W	7.0
Hg	12.5	Zn	10.5

Definition of Anaerobic Corrosion

From the corrosion perspective, a condition is defined as "anaerobic" if it is necessary for water reduction to occur in order to supply the cathodic current required to support the corrosion reaction. Likewise a condition is defined as "aerobic" when the concentration of dissolved oxygen, plus those of any other reducible species, is sufficiently high to support corrosion process without the need for water reduction. It should be noted that the corrosion behaviors of various implant metals are different. Furthermore, corrosion depends on factors such as local pH and salinity levels. These definitions for anaerobic and aerobic conditions are very metal specific, *i.e.*, a single environment can appear as aerobic to one metal, yet anaerobic to another.

3.2.2.6 *Nature of electrode reactions*

Consider the reaction:

$$2Fe + O_2 + 2H_2O \rightarrow 2Fe^{2+} + 4OH^-$$

In its simplest form, this reaction involves three steps:

(1) Mass Transport: Dissolved oxygen moves from the bulk solution to the surface of the iron (water is in excess so it does not have to travel to the iron's surface).

$$O_{2(bulk)} \rightarrow O_{2(surface)}$$

(2) Electron Transfer: Electrons are transferred from the iron to the dissolved oxygen, which then steals protons from the surrounding water.

$$2Fe \rightarrow 2Fe^{2+}_{(surface)} + 4e^-$$
$$O_{2(surface)} + 4e^- + 2H_2O \rightarrow 4OH^-_{(surface)}$$

(3) Mass Transport: Products created by step (2) move away from the surface of the iron into the bulk solution.

$$Fe^{2+}_{(surface)} \rightarrow Fe^{2+}_{(bulk)}$$
$$OH^-_{(surface)} \rightarrow OH^-_{(bulk)}$$

Any one of these three steps can be rate limiting. Step (3), the removal of products, deserves further consideration. If the hydroxide ions are not efficiently removed, localized pH will increase — which as seen from the Pourbaix diagram may favor passivation (Figure 3–2(d)). If metal cations are not efficiently removed, localized concentration may exceed its solubility limit, thus forming a solid corrosion product — which may or may not take the form of a protective passive film.

In practice, the real situation is likely to be further complicated as follows:

- The four electrons in step (2) are likely to be transferred one at a time with the creation of a number of intermediate species;
- Once the reactants reach the surface, they may have to be adsorbed before electrons transfer can take place. Likewise the products may have to be desorbed after the electrons transfer step;
- Phase formation may occur, such as gas bubbles and oxide films;
- Coupled chemical reactions may take place.

3.2.3 *Passivation*

3.2.3.1 *Electrochemical behavior of active/passive metals*

Corrosion is the term used to describe the oxidation of metals by the surrounding environment. Equation (38) reveals that there is a simple relationship between the corrosion rate and the density of the anodic current flowing through the metal.

$$M \rightarrow M^{n+} + ne^- \tag{38}$$

Once a metal is oxidized, one of these processes will take place: either it forms a soluble ion as in equation (38) or it forms an insoluble compound, usually an oxide, as in equation (39).

$$nM + mH_2O \rightarrow M_nO_m + 2mH^+ + 2me^- \tag{39}$$

Which of these processes occurs simply depends on the solubility of the compound (M_nO_m) in the local environment [5]. In many cases, the compound forms a dense impermeable film on the metal's surface, thereby isolating it from the surrounding environment. The film then prevents, or more accurately, greatly slows down further corrosion. This phenomenon is known as passivation and is central to the corrosion resistance of virtually all metals commonly used in medical applications. Exceptions such as the alloys of noble metals (e.g., Au, Pt, and Pd) are sometimes used in dentistry, because noble metals are inherently corrosion-resistant.

In the absence of any aggressive anion that might induce localized corrosion phenomenon, Figure 3–6 shows a typical relationship between the anodic current density (corrosion rate) and the polarization potential for a passivating metal (e.g., stainless steel in neutral and alkaline environments) [9]. Such plots are referred to as polarization curves. The polarization potential, which in the laboratory is controlled by the application of an external potential, represents the oxidizing power of a given environment. For example, applying a more positive potential can be envisaged as adding an oxidizing agent, such as hydrogen peroxide.

Tracing the curve in Figure 3–6 from the negative potential end towards the positive end, one can see that the corrosion current increases initially — corresponding to a region of active corrosion. Eventually, the corrosion current reaches a peak due to the formation of a passive oxide film. After which, the corrosion current rapidly drops to a small value that is virtually independent of any potential. Beyond this passive region, the corrosion current again rises sharply as the passive film breaks down for a variety of reasons [10], and this is known as transpassive behavior. In the case of the metals and alloys used in biomedical implants, transpassive behavior occurs at potentials positive of that required to oxidize water — thus this phenomenon should not normally be observed within the body. One possible exception is in the presence of hydrogen peroxide, which is a very powerful oxidizing agent. Such a situation may arise during the initial stages of inflammatory response of the surrounding body tissue after an implant is inserted [11].

Since there is a direct relationship between current density and corrosion rate (equation (38)), it is best to maintain the metal within the passive region. However, the potential range of this region depends both on the nature of the metal and that of the surrounding environment. Furthermore, unless subjected to some form of pre-treatment, most passive films in *in vivo* environments are very thin — typically 5–10 nm. Thus small isolated areas of the oxide film are susceptible to breakdown due to a series of processes known as localized corrosion (which will be discussed in more detail in Section 3.3.2). Therefore an awareness of the mechanisms of the formation and destruction of passive oxide films is central to understanding the corrosion behavior of medical implants.

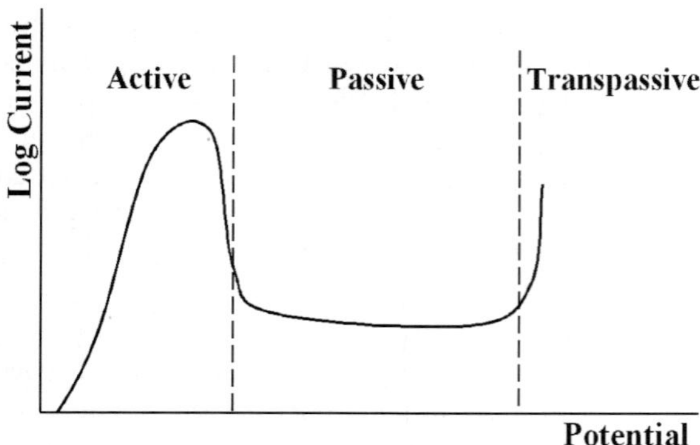

Figure 3–6 Polarization curve for an active-passive metal

3.2.3.2 *Nature of passive film*

A film develops on the surface of a corroding metal if the local concentration of ions exceeds that of the solubility product of the least soluble salt in solution (equation (39)). In practice, under the environments encountered in biomedical applications, the first films to develop are nearly always oxides or hydroxides. One common exception is the black sulfide films that cause tarnishing on dental amalgams. However, the formation of a film does not automatically imply passivation of the underlying metal, as this requires the film to be continuous, non-porous, and well-adhered. The Pilling–Bedworth ratio, which is the ratio of the oxide volume to the volume of the metal it replaces, can be used as a guide to predict whether an oxide film will provide protection [12]. If this ratio is less than 1, the oxide is too porous or discontinuous to protect the underlying metal. If the ratio is greater than 2, the stress resulting from the necessary volume expansion causes the oxide to spall off and so again it provides poor protection. Values that range between 1 and 2 predict an adherent, non-porous protective coating. Although many metals follow the Pilling–Bedworth prediction when the oxide film is formed thermally, *i.e.*, produced by heating a metal in air, it is less useful in aqueous solutions where the film is likely to contain hydrated oxides and hydroxides. Another complicating factor in alloys is that the composition of the oxide film is usually not representative of that of the parent alloy. For example, the passive oxide on stainless steels consists mainly of chromium oxide, although there is typically only 18% chromium in a stainless steel.

The thickness of a passive oxide film results from the balance between its rates of growth and chemical dissolution. On one hand, the rate of growth is governed by the size of the electric field across the metal/solution interface, which controls the migration rates of the charged species through the oxide to the position of growth. This may be either at the metal/oxide interface or the oxide/solution interface. Since the electric field is approximately given by the potential drop across the metal/solution interface divided by the thickness of the oxide itself, it is clear that the rate of growth decreases as the oxide thickens [13]. On the other hand, the rate of chemical dissolution of the passive oxide film is a function of its solubility (which by definition is very small) and the rate at which metal ions are transported away from the oxide/solution interface.

Although a full discussion of the processes controlling the thickness of passive films is beyond the scope of the present chapter, suffice it to say that passive oxide films are very thin — typically only 5–10 nm. Hence the presence of soluble foreign particles within the film, which may have dimensions of the order of microns, can lead to a serious breach of the protective barrier. In the case of metals and alloys used in biomedical applications, the foreign particles are usually either contaminants from the production process, or due to inclusions of sulfides and phosfides (which may be deliberately added to the alloy to obtain the required mechanical properties, or may simply be present as impurities). Acid pickling is usually performed to control the former problem [14], while additional alloying elements, such as molybdenum, can be used to reduce the problems associated with sulfide and phosfide inclusions [15].

Besides adding alloying elements, the degree of protection afforded by passive films can also be increased by increasing their thickness by anodization — that is, the passage of an electric current in a benign solution such as sodium borate [16]. Alternatively, the degree of protection can be increased by sealing — a process that improves the oxide's crystallinity and blocks pores, and can often be achieved by simply heating to about 80°C in distilled water [17].

Once formed, a passive film's main role can be envisaged as providing an impermeable barrier separating the metal from the surrounding environment. However, there are two important differences between passive films and other barrier coatings such as paints: one of which is an advantage while the other a disadvantage. The advantage is that unlike a coating of paint, the oxide has some potential to repair itself if it is mechanically damaged. The disadvantage arises from the fact that passive films are normally n-type semiconductors rather than insulators. As such, electrochemical reactions still occur at their surfaces. In particular, if a damaged film is unable to repair itself, the cathodic reactions necessary to support corrosion can take place on the undamaged parts of the passive film, leading to rapidly accelerated corrosion at the damaged site.

Finally it is also important to remember that a passive film does not reduce the corrosion rate to zero (since all oxides do have some solubility in aqueous media, albeit extremely small). Although the rate is reduced to levels that are considered insignificant for most industrial applications, this may not be the case for biomedical applications. This is because the structural integrity of the metallic implant itself is not the only concern. It is also necessary to consider what happens to the corrosion products once they leave the medical device. Hence extreme care needs to be taken to guard against the build-up of metallic ion concentrations to potentially hazardous levels.

3.2.3.3 *Influence of cathodic supporting reactions*

Figure 3–7 shows that if the dissolved oxygen concentration is very low, the limiting cathodic current it can supply may fall below that which is required to maintain the passive anodic current. At this point, a fresh source of cathodic current is required and is most likely to be from the reduction of water, which leads to the evolution of hydrogen. However, as indicated in Figure 3–7, reduction of water occurs at a much more negative potential than reduction of oxygen. As a result, the corrosion potential of the active-passive metal will shift dramatically negative. In some metals, this negative potential shift can be sufficient to prevent the formation of the passive oxide film such that rapid active corrosion occurs. This is the case for titanium in highly reducing environments (more reducing than expected to be found in biomedical applications), where it is necessary to add a small quantity of palladium (typically 0.25 percent) to catalyze the hydrogen evolution reaction in order to shift the titanium's corrosion potential back into the passive region [18].

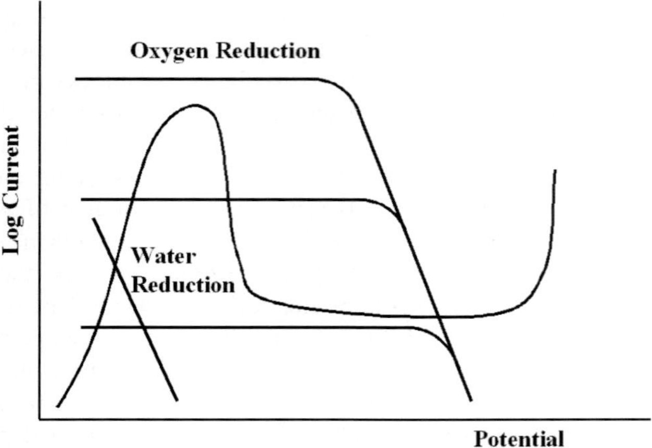

Figure 3–7 Combined polarization curves for an active-passive metal and oxygen/water reduction

3.3 Types of Corrosion

3.3.1 General Corrosion

When metal loss is occurring at a uniform rate across the entire exposed surface, the metal is considered to be undergoing general or uniform corrosion. For metals capable of forming passive films, Figure 3–7 shows that general corrosion can occur in both the active and passive regions of the polarization curve. In other words, the anodic and cathodic currents can cross in either of these regions. However, corrosion rates found within the active region are normally too high for the metal to be of interest in medical applications. In the passive region the general corrosion is sometimes referred to as passive corrosion, and in the long term its rate depends on a balance between the rates of growth and dissolution of the passive film. For a successful implant material, the long-term general corrosion rate should fall to less than 1 µm per year. For almost any other application, such low corrosion rates would be considered insignificant. However, even at these rates it has been reported that after eight years of implantation, the levels of nickel, chromium and cobalt in surrounding tissues can be five times higher than the normal values [19]. It has also been shown that the presence of metal ions suppresses cell growth of human gingival fibroblasts [20].

3.3.2 Localized Corrosion

As mentioned earlier, stable oxide films formed on many metals in neutral and alkaline environments reduce corrosion rates to very low levels. However, in the long term, even these very low corrosion rates could lead to high levels of metallic ions within the body. Of more pressing concern is what happens if these very thin protective passive films are damaged or chemically broken down. This results in small areas of metal at the breakdown points in the oxide film being exposed to a potentially aggressive environment, thus leading to very high corrosion rates. The localized corrosion rate is further aggravated by the fact that the driving cathodic reaction (equation (3)) can occur on the much larger, intact oxide surface. Breakdown of the passive film occurs under different circumstances such as pitting corrosion, crevice corrosion, stress corrosion cracking, *etc.*, as described in detail below.

3.3.2.1 Pitting corrosion

In the presence of aggressive ions, particularly those of chloride, the rate of chemical dissolution of the passive film at flaws (such as sulfide inclusions) can be increased. This leads to the initiation of pitting corrosion. Once formed, a pit is analogous to a tiny crevice, and propagation is thought to proceed via the acidification process described in Section 3.3.2.2. The likelihood of pitting corrosion increases with increased aggressive ion concentration, higher temperature and oxidizing potential, and lower pH. On the other hand, increased solution flow rate and higher dissolved oxygen concentration decrease the probability of pitting. Environments that are not quite aggressive enough to cause active pitting corrosion may still lead to the development of metastable pits. These are pits that initiate, but are unable to obtain the required degree of acidity within their occluded cells to propagate and thus repassivate. A number of papers have been published on this so-called "birth and death" of pits [15,21] — a phenomenon that has important implications for stress corrosion cracking (Section 3.3.2.3).

Pitting corrosion was a common problem with the early stainless steel implants that were mainly of grade 304. However, the addition of Mo (2–3 percent) to form the 316L grade stainless steel has greatly reduced the number of failures due to pitting corrosion, although the mechanism by which Mo reduces the pitting process is still uncertain [15,22]. From a review of failures during 1980–89, Zitter [23] suggested that a pitting resistance equivalent (%Cr + 3x%Mo + 16x%N) greater than 26 is required to prevent *in vivo* pitting corrosion. This is above the pitting resistance equivalent of 316L stainless steels which ranges between 23 and 26. However, if nitrogen additions are included the value should exceed the threshold of 26.

Concerns that pitting corrosion of implants based on cobalt-based alloys could lead to carcinogens being released into the body have resulted in numerous *in vitro* studies [24–29]. All of these reported that under static conditions these alloys were resistant to pitting. However, pitting corrosion of Co–Cr alloys was reported when these alloys were subjected to cyclic loads or had previously been severely cold worked [31,31].

Pure titanium can be considered immune to pitting corrosion in any *in vivo* environment likely to be encountered. Titanium alloys are less resistant, as the alloying elements represent discontinuities in the protective oxide film. However, to date, no *in vivo* pitting related failures have been reported. Nevertheless, *in vitro* experiments have shown that Ti–6Al–4V alloy suffers superficial pitting corrosion at high potentials (>1500 mV vs. SCE) in 1% NaCl solutions [32].

The resistance of nickel–titanium memory-shape alloys has yet to be fully investigated. Results from *in vitro* experiments are pessimistic with the Ni–Ti alloy appearing to be less resistant than 316L stainless steel [33]. However, the results from *in vivo* tests are more encouraging with the Ni–Ti alloy outperforming 316L stainless steel [34].

3.3.2.2 Crevice corrosion

Crevices are formed whenever two surfaces come together trapping a stagnant layer of solution. The width of a crevice needs to be sufficiently small so that natural convection no longer allows the trapped solution to mix with the bulk solution outside, and such that diffusion is the only form of mass transport by which dissolved oxygen can enter the occluded region. Typically this restricts crevices to widths less than 3 mm. In such crevices, the supply of dissolved oxygen within the trapped solution can be depleted. As a result, the location of the anodic and cathodic reactions becomes twain — that is, the anodic corrosion reaction occurs in the crevice and the supporting cathodic reduction reaction on the much larger surface outside the crevice. Inside the crevice, the reaction is of the following type:

$$Fe \rightarrow Fe^{2+} + 2e^- \tag{40}$$

To maintain charge neutrality, anions need to migrate into, and cations out of, the crevice (Figure 3–8). In the event that the salts of the anions moving into the crevice are more soluble than the corresponding oxide/hydroxide, the local pH value will fall. For example, if the incoming cation is chloride, the following reaction may occur:

$$Fe^{2+} + 2Cl^- + 2H_2O \rightarrow Fe(OH)_2\downarrow + 2H^+ + 2Cl^- \tag{41}$$

This increased acidity within the crevice will cause corrosion to accelerate further, thereby increasing the need for yet more anions to migrate into the trapped solution, and eventually resulting in a lower pH value. Hence the crevice corrosion mechanism is autocatalytic in nature. The final pH value within the crevice is restricted only by the solubility of the salt, *i.e.*, in the case of equation (41), final pH value is restricted by the solubility of $FeCl_2$. The environmental factors that influence the likelihood of crevice corrosion are the same as those mentioned for pitting corrosion.

Typical examples of crevices that might be found in biomedical applications are beneath the heads of fixing screws and within the pores of some of the porous materials currently being proposed for use in surgical implants [35].

Crevice corrosion of stainless steel implants is a very serious problem even in the molybdenum-containing 316L grade. In 1959, Scales *et al.* [36] reported that 24 percent of type 316 stainless steel bone plates and screws removed from patients showed evidence of crevice corrosion. Reducing the non-metallic inclusion content by vacuum melting to form 316LVM stainless steel and an austenitic microstructure that is free of delta ferrite [37] have been shown to reduce the extent of, but not eliminate, crevice corrosion.

Syrett *et al.* [26] found no crevice corrosion on Co–Cr–Mo specimens that had been implanted in dogs and rhesus monkeys for two years. Likewise, Galante and Rostoker [38] found no crevice corrosion on implants removed from rabbits after one year. However, these authors did find single pits in the crevice regions. It is possible that if the experiments had been left for a longer period of time, these pits may have developed into crevice corrosion.

Crevice corrosion of titanium in neutral chloride environments has only been reported at temperatures in excess of 70°C [18]. However, Blackwood *et al.* [17] have shown that at a temperature of only 45°C, the protective oxide film on titanium will slowly dissolve if the environment is anaerobic and pH<2. Although such conditions are theoretically possible within a crevice, they would probably take several years to develop *in vivo*. Nevertheless Galante and Rostoker reported single pits in the crevice regions of Ti–6Al–4V specimens, again after implanting in rabbits for one year; but no actual crevice corrosion was detected. As with pitting corrosion, titanium alloys will be less resistant to crevice corrosion than pure titanium. Crevice corrosion has also been proposed as the reason why porous titanium [39] and porous Co–Cr–Mo alloys [40] have much poorer corrosion resistances than their solid counterparts. This is because the porous matrix itself provides ready-made crevices.

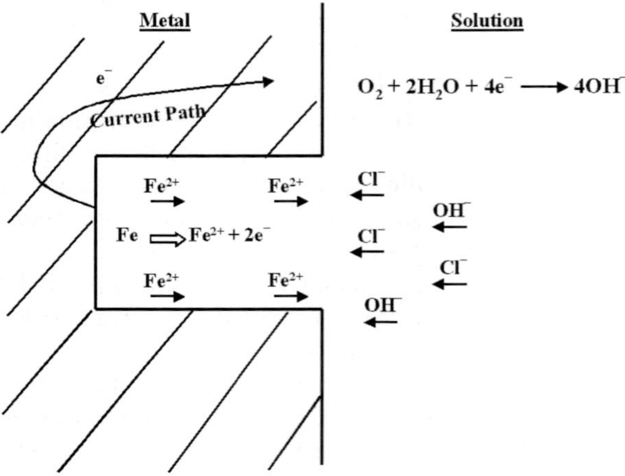

Figure 3–8 Schematic representation of corrosion within a crevice

3.3.2.3 Stress corrosion cracking

Stress corrosion cracking (SCC) is a general term used to describe stressed metals and alloys that fail due to the propagation of cracks in corrosive environments [41]. SCC can initiate and propagate with little external evidence. Failure due to SCC is therefore insidious, and fracture can occur without visible warning. SCC frequently initiates at surface discontinuities which have resulted from fabrication processes or as a consequence of poor design or workmanship. Features such as burrs, groves, laps, and joints provide potential sites for the initiation of crevice corrosion, which likewise favor crack initiation [42]. In solutions containing chloride, SCC is known to initiate from localized corrosion sites such as pits or crevices [43–46]. The transition between localized corrosion and cracking is dependent on the same parameters that control SCC, *i.e.*, the electrochemistry occurring at the base of the pit and the presence of a stress-strain system.

One of the essential requirements for cracks to propagate is a sharp tip at which the stress can be concentrated. Hence, SCC tends not to occur on specimens undergoing either active general corrosion or localized pitting corrosion. This is because these other forms of corrosion tend to blunt the crack tips. In the case of the metals and alloys commonly used in medical devices, this means that SCC usually occurs in conditions slightly less aggressive than those required for active pitting corrosion. In other words, SCC occurs in the "metastable" pitting region mentioned in Section 3.3.2.1. Furthermore, as passive films are essentially ceramic materials, they are not as ductile as the underlying metal. Hence any elongation of the metal by applied tensile stress cannot be matched by the brittle films, which thus will break. Similarly, anything in the local environment that can cause embrittlement of the metal's surface increases the likelihood of SCC occurrence.

Paradoxically, metals and alloys that are highly resistant to general corrosion due to their ability to readily form passive films are at greater risk to SCC failures than nominally less corrosion-resistant materials. This is because rapid reformation of the passive film helps keep the crack tip sharp and thus concentrates the stress — which then leads to rapid crack propagation (Figure 3–9).

Another stress related corrosion phenomenon is hydrogen embrittlement. This is very similar to SCC, except that it occurs at negative rather than positive potentials. If the potential is sufficiently negative for hydrogen to be formed, then hydrogen atoms can enter the metal's lattice and form metal hydrides at the surface. These tend to be brittle and thus crack when subjected to stress.

To the best of the authors' knowledge, SCC has not been observed on recovered surgical implants. Although implants may exhibit cracks, these do not show the physical characteristics associated with SCC and thus are believed to be due to mechanical damage that occurred either during manufacture or the recovery process [47]. Laboratory experiments appear to confirm that the common implant alloys are not susceptible to SCC in *in vivo* environments [48]. However, Edwards *et al.* [49] have shown that Co–Cr–Mo alloys may be susceptible to hydrogen embrittlement in Ringer's solution if polarized at such negative potentials that significant amounts of hydrogen evolution could occur on their surfaces. In practice, such a situation is only likely to occur *in vivo* if the Co–Cr–Mo alloy was galvanically coupled to a more active material, such as stainless steel.

Bundy *et al.* [50] have shown that crack propagation continues in 316L stainless steel that has been pre-cracked in acidic $MgCl_2$ solution before being transferred to Ringer's solution and subjected to an applied positive potential. Although these authors concluded that SCC of 316L stainless steel could occur *in vivo*, it is unlikely that their experimental conditions would ever exist in reality.

An excellent review of the advances in the theory and practice of SCC, including a discussion of the various SCC mechanisms, was published in 1990 by Newman and Procter [51].

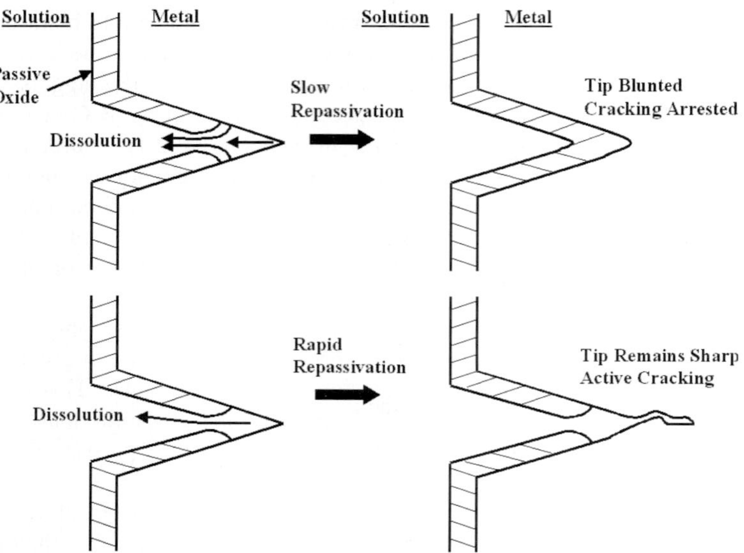

Figure 3–9   Schematic representation of how repassivation rate influences stress corrosion cracking

3.3.2.4 Corrosion fatigue

Corrosion fatigue is very similar to stress corrosion cracking, the difference being that the load is now applied in a cyclic manner. Just as with mechanical failures, cyclic loads tend to cause corrosion failures at lower stresses than static loads. However, unlike normal mechanical fatigue, where there is a fatigue limit and where the number of cycles required for failure to occur is independent of frequency, corrosion fatigue shows no fatigue limit (*i.e.*, no safe loading) and is worse at low frequencies. This makes laboratory testing of corrosion fatigue extremely time-consuming (e.g., it takes almost a year to complete one million cycles at 1 Hz). It is thought that the frequency dependence of corrosion fatigue is due to the stressed metal being in contact with the aggressive solution for longer periods at low frequencies. Unfortunately, many medical devices are subjected to these low frequency loads that are so conducive to causing corrosion fatigue. For instance, simply walking would result in a hip implant being subjected to a cyclic loading at about 1 Hz.

In 1982, Leclerc [52] reviewed the extensive literature related to corrosion fatigue of prosthesis implants. He concluded that as long as the manufacture and metallurgical condition of the device conformed to international standards (e.g., BS 7252, ISO 5832, or ASTM F138), corrosion only made a minor contribution to most fatigue failures. However, Leclerc did note that the longer the prosthesis was implanted in the patient, the more significant was the role of corrosion. A later review by Zitter [23] in 1991 came to similar conclusions as Leclerc. On the other hand, Morita *et al.* [53] reported that the *in vivo* (rabbits) fatigue strengths of 316 stainless steel and a Co–Cr–Ni–Fe alloy were considerably less than their values in air. They proposed that this was due to the corrosive action of body fluids on the materials.

In his review of clinical fatigue related failures, Bechtol [54] claimed that the root cause of the problem was failure of the bone-cement support interface — which eventually led to a widening of the separation between the metal prosthesis and cement, and finally to deformity of the metal stem. This view was recently supported by von Knock *et al.* [55] who found no evidences of corrosion on 11 Co–Cr alloy femoral components retrieved after two to 15 years of service. They speculated that the major component of micromotion between implant and bone occurred between the cement and the bone.

Hughes *et al.* [56] reported that the corrosion fatigue resistance of titanium has been shown to be almost independent of pH over the range 2 to 7, whereas the fatigue strength of stainless steel declines rapidly below pH 4. This is consistent with the findings of Yu *et al.* [57] that pitting corrosion facilitates the initiation of corrosion fatigue in stainless steels. These authors also reported that the corrosion fatigue resistance of Ti–6Al–4V can be enhanced by nitrogen implantation and heat treatments to produce fine prior-β grain sizes.

The importance of materials selection and design were again emphasized by Piehler *et al.* [58] who tested hip nail plates and found that large plates had better corrosion fatigue resistance than small ones, and that Ti–6Al–4V outperformed 316L stainless steel.

3.3.2.5 *Fretting corrosion and mechanical wear*

If the passive oxide film is mechanically worn away, the underlying metal will immediately undergo active corrosion in an attempt to reform it. Since mechanical wearing does not involve the development of aggressive chemical conditions associated with crevice corrosion (Section 3.3.2.2) and as long as the process causing the wear does not occur frequently, only minimal corrosion is required to successfully complete the repassivation process. In other words, the occasional scratch does not significantly cause long-term metal loss. However, with frequent wearing or fretting, the amount of metal loss in periods of active corrosion increases accordingly. In the extreme case of near-continuous wearing, the passive film may never re-form — thus resulting in rapid corrosion.

There are two common causes of wear. The first common cause arises from the rapid flow of solution across the metal surface, leading to a phenomenon termed "erosion corrosion". However, in the case of medical applications, high solution flow rates are only likely to be encountered in a small number of applications such as at valves and pumps where the problem can often be solved by choosing a material that is highly resistant to erosion corrosion, such as titanium. The second common cause of wear arises from the rubbing of two solid surfaces, which leads to fretting corrosion. In fact, fretting corrosion represents the single most important form of attack on load bearing surgical implants. This is because thus far, all the successful metallic implant materials are based on passive metals. Hence any process that wears away the protective oxide film is of major concern [59].

However, in biomedical situations such as the ball-joint of a hip implant, it is likely that a thin film of solution will exist between the two rubbing surfaces. This has led to some debate on whether the corrosion that is observed is really due to fretting or if it is actually a form of crevice corrosion [60] (Section 3.3.2.2). Regardless of the true mechanism, corrosion at joints can be a serious problem as it not only results in metal loss but also increases the dimensions of the joint, thus causing fixation problems. Naturally, mechanical wear at joints can also lead to loss of the surrounding cement or bone, which, apart from being a serious problem in itself, increases the amount of movement of the implant, thereby increasing the likelihood of corrosion fatigue [54]. However, mechanical wear at joints is beyond the scope of the present chapter.

All the three major classes of prosthesis implant materials — namely Ti alloys, Co–Cr alloys, and stainless steels — suffer from fretting corrosion [61]. The situation is made worse by the fact that the corrosion products collect locally as particles. For example, black titanium oxide debris is often found — which causes further abrasion of the implant. The shearing micro-movements that eventually lead to fretting corrosion appear to be due to the large differences between the elastic moduli of the solid metallic implants and the surrounding bone or PMMA cement [61]. For the Ti–6Al–4V alloy, its most serious drawback with regards to use as an implant material is its poor fretting resistance. Thus, considerable effort has been dedicated to finding possible solutions [16,62–64].

3.3.3 Galvanic Corrosion (Bimetallic Corrosion)

When two different metals are electrically coupled together, the anodic corrosion reaction of the more base metal can be supported by cathodic reactions occurring on the more noble metal. Effectively the system forms a battery which leads to an increased corrosion rate on the base anode metal, while the more noble cathode metal is protected from corrosion. Galvanic corrosion, also known as bimetallic corrosion, not only occurs between two different metals, it can also occur internally between different phases of a multiphase alloy. This is a phenomenon common in dental amalgams [65], or between particles of metallic impurities and the parent metal.

Unfortunately, the thermodynamically-derived standard emf series for metals is insufficient to determine which one of any two given metals will be more noble, as the presence of passive films and complexing ions influences the relative corrosion potentials of different metals. Instead, it is necessary to use a galvanic series that has been experimentally determined in the medium of interest. Although there is insufficient data available to construct a full galvanic series for metals in body fluids, the extensive galvanic series that has been produced for seawater can be used as a reasonable substitute [66].

Factors that influence the extent to which the galvanic coupling between two metals accelerates the respective corrosion rate of the anode include [67]:

i)   The difference in the individual, uncoupled corrosion potentials of the two metals. This can be envisaged as the magnitude of an open-circuit voltage across a battery.

ii) The ratio of exposed surface areas of the coupled metals. This is also seen in the case of crevice corrosion where the large cathode area outside the crevice accelerates the corrosion of the small anode within (Section 3.3.2.2).

iii) The nature of the kinetics of cathodic reactions on the coupled metals. As the rates of cathodic reactions can vary by up to 10 orders of magnitude [8], very small impurities or minor alloying additions of an efficient cathode can dominate the corrosion process.

iv) The conductivity of the surrounding medium. A higher conductivity allows the two metals to interact over longer distances.

v)   The polarizability of the two metals in a couple. When two metals are electrically coupled together, they must adopt a common potential — which entails shifting both metals from their individual, uncoupled potentials to the new potential of the couple. The polarizability of a metal is a measure of the amount of current that has to flow in order to shift its corrosion potential.

In the case of most biomedical devices, the last of these factors (*i.e.*, polarizability) requires further consideration. From Figure 3–7, it can be seen that actively corroding metals require large currents to shift their potentials. On the other hand, within the passive region, the currents are very small and virtually independent of potential. This means that for a metal in the passive state, which is the case for most practical biomedical devices, the galvanic couple is not expected to cause any significant change in the corrosion rate so long as the metal remains within the passive region. Unfortunately, such a happy state of affairs is rarely found in practice. Although shifting a passive metal to a more positive potential may not increase its general corrosion rate, reference to Section 3.3.2 reveals that such a shift increases the likelihood of localized corrosion. This increased threat of localized corrosion is the major concern when considering the influence of galvanic corrosion on biomedical devices.

Furthermore, it is worth remembering that the conditions required to initiate localized corrosion are more aggressive than those required for its continued propagation. Therefore if localized corrosion is initiated due to an accidental short-term galvanic coupling event, then breaking that galvanic couple will not stop the localized corrosion from continued propagation.

Rostoker *et al.* [68] found that 316L stainless steel suffered pitting corrosion in 1% NaCl solution at 37°C when it was coupled to either graphite, Ti–6Al–4V, or Co–Cr–Mo alloy. No pitting corrosion was found when any two of the other three materials were coupled together.

In the event that titanium and any cobalt–chromium alloy are coupled together, it is likely that the passive titanium would become the cathode. Thus accelerated corrosion of the Co–Cr alloy may be anticipated. However, titanium is a poor cathode. The kinetics of the oxygen and water reduction reactions are slow on its surface, and since its passive current is virtually independent of potential it is easily polarized. This means that the extent of accelerated corrosion caused to any metal from coupling to titanium should be small. This view has been confirmed in a literature review by Mears [69]. Likewise for titanium–cobalt alloy combinations, this view has been found applicable by the *in vitro* experiments of Lucas *et al.* [30] and by clinical use as reported by Jackson–Burrows *et al.* [70].

Galvanic corrosion in the oral cavity has caused particular concern. The high potential differences that can develop, such as between a gold crown and an amalgam core, not only cause accelerated corrosion but have also been linked to a number of serious oral conditions, including leukoplakia and oral cancer [65].

3.3.4 Selective Leaching

Selective leaching, also referred to as "parting" and "dealloying", is the removal by corrosion of one element from a solid alloy. It differs from internal galvanic coupling in that it can occur within a single-phase alloy. In most cases, the dimensions of the alloy are not reduced. However, there is usually a drastic loss of strength. In terms of medical applications, selective leaching is of concern if it releases toxic elements in the body, e.g., mercury from dental alloys and chromium or nickel from stainless steel implants.

3.3.5 Intergranular Attack

Industrially, the most important form of this corrosion involves alloys that rely on the formation of a chromium oxide layer to maintain their passivity, such as stainless steels. Most of these alloys contain some carbon, which helps provide strength. However, during various forms of heat treatment, most notably under conditions encountered in welding, chromium can react with carbon to form chromium carbide. This leads to grain boundary areas that are depleted of free chromium. Hence the passive film is significantly weaker at these areas, rendering them susceptible to corrosion. In practice, chromium depletion can be avoided through proper post-welding treatment or by choosing one of the specially formulated low carbon alloys (<0.03%) which are denoted by the suffix L, e.g., 316L stainless steel. Hence, although intergranular attack was a problem with the stainless steel implants prior to the 1960s [36], it should not be so in modern biomedical applications.

Dental amalgams are multiphase alloys. As such, they are susceptible to intergranular corrosion between the different phases. In terms of mechanism, this can be considered as a form of localized galvanic corrosion. In conventional amalgams, it is the phases that contain silver which are noble and which cause accelerated corrosion of the non-silver phases. The most vulnerable is the γ_2 phase (Sn_7Hg), which releases mercury when it corrodes [71]. The high-copper amalgams contain no γ_2 phases and are more resistant to corrosion than silver–tin amalgams [72]. The most corrosion-prone phase in high-copper amalgams is the η' phase (Cu_6Sn_5), which does not lead to mercury release [73]. However, it has recently been shown that corrosion of dental amalgams only makes a minor contribution towards the total amount of mercury within the average human body; the vast majority (>90%) enters via the food-chain [74].

3.3.6 Influence of Cold-working

Cold-working, without subsequent annealing, can have two effects on the corrosion of metals and alloys. The first is that cold-working increases the density of dislocations. This effect renders the advantage of increasing the material's strength, but it also causes the worked areas to be slightly more susceptible to corrosion than unworked areas. The second effect is the occurrence of phase changes in the crystal structure. For example, cold-working of the austenitic 304L stainless steel can result in some areas being developed into hard martensite phase, which renders the material more susceptible to stress corrosion cracking. However, this occurs to a much smaller extent in 316L stainless steel used in biomedical applications.

Nevertheless, cold-working followed by short-term tempering has been reported to improve the static and fatigue strengths of high-nitrogen stainless steels without any detrimental effect on their corrosion behaviors in NaCl solutions [75].

3.4   Environments Encountered in Biomedical Applications

3.4.1 Surgical Implants

The compositions of body fluids are complicated. However, from the corrosion perspective, the most important characteristics are the chloride, dissolved oxygen and pH levels. A 0.9% NaCl solution is considered to be isotonic with blood, and under normal conditions most body fluids have a pH of 7.4 and a temperature of 37°C. In these respects, body fluids appear to be slightly less aggressive than seawater. This is reflected by the fact that for stainless steels, a pitting resistance number (PREN) of greater than 26 is recommended for surgical implants as compared to the value of 40 usually required for stagnant seawater [23]. However, the dissolved oxygen levels in blood are lower than those of saline solutions exposed to air atmospheres, by a factor of about 2 for arterial blood and 6 for venous blood. Conversely, bicarbonate levels are about 20 times higher in blood than in seawater [53].

The many other components in body fluids, e.g., phosphates, cholesterols, phospholipids, *etc.* are usually thought to either play no role in the corrosion process or exist at inconsequential levels. As a result most *in vitro* experiments have been conducted in either 0.9% NaCl solution or standard isotonic solutions (such as Ringer's or Hank's solution) in which the presence of bicarbonate and calcium chloride poses as the main difference from the NaCl solution. A review by Solar [76] in 1979 concluded that inorganic solutions based on diluted NaCl were indeed satisfactory substitutes for human body fluids when studying the behavior of passive metals. However, when conducting *in vitro* experiments, no attempts are usually made to lower the dissolved oxygen content of the isotonic solution to that of venous blood. This has been proposed as an explanation for some of the differences observed in the *in vivo* and *in vitro* corrosion behaviors of implant materials [53,56]. Furthermore, the minor components in blood have occasionally been blamed for the accelerated *in vivo* corrosion. For example, it has been postulated that sulfur present in amino acids may enhance crevice corrosion of stainless steels [19].

Figure 3–10 shows the typical environmental conditions expected within a range of different body fluids superimposed on the Pourbaix diagram for chromium in the presence of chloride ions. From this diagram, it can be predicted that stainless steels are likely to suffer corrosion in many of the environments found within the body. However, passivation of stainless steel is likely to occur in those body fluids most likely to be encountered by an implant (e.g., blood which typically has a redox potential in the vicinity of 0 V and pH

7.4). On this note, titanium can be expected to be in a passive state for virtually all the physiological solutions shown in Figure 3–10.

Finally, the surgical operation plus the presence of the implant itself may cause the surrounding tissue to undergo several pathological changes that eventually develop into a more corrosive environment [77]. Laing reported that the pH around a newly inserted surgical implant can drop to as low as 4.0 due to the build-up of haematomas — a condition that could last several weeks [1,78]. Hydrogen peroxide may also be generated during the initial stages of inflammatory response of the surrounding body tissue after an implant is inserted [11,79]. The extents to which these pathological changes occur depend on the biological activity of any corrosion product emanating from the implant, and also on its size and shape. The influences of size and shape mean that the extents of pathological changes will vary across the surface of the implant, which could lead to the development of electrochemical cells [80]. Variations in the local pH on titanium alloys have even been observed during *in vitro* experiments, which could also generate the potential gradients required to drive localized corrosion [81].

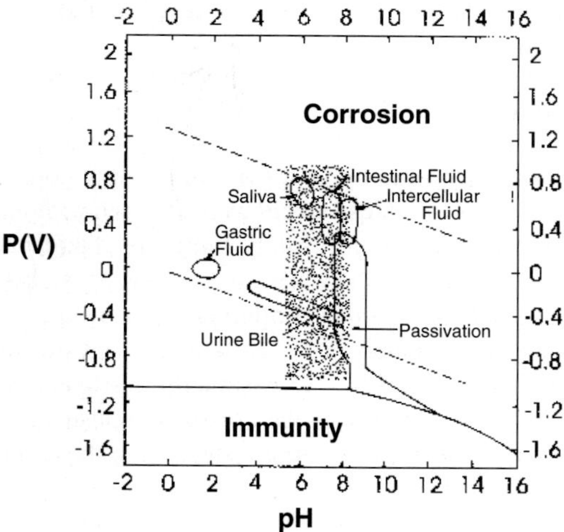

Figure 3–10   Representative environmental conditions for various body fluids superimposed on Pourbaix diagram for chromium in solutions containing chloride; the shaded zone represents the conditions for physiological solutions as suggested by Schenk (Reprinted from reference [82] with permission)

3.4.2 Dental Applications

The environment within the oral cavity is not well defined. Although there are a number of recipes for artificial saliva, the most popular being that of Fusayama's — NaCl, 0.400g dm^{-3}; KCl, 0.400 g dm^{-3}; CaCl$_2$.H2O,

0.795 g dm^{-3}; NaH$_2$PO$_4$.H$_2$O, 0.69 g dm^{-3}; Na$_2$S.9H$_2$O, 0.005 g dm^{-3}; pH 5.5 [83]. In reality, the make-up of human saliva varies considerably between individuals, especially in the sulfide content which can cause tarnishing of both silver- and gold-based amalgams. In any case, many foodstuffs are acidic with high chloride levels and are thus far more corrosive than salvia [84]. Moreover, oral hygiene has a strong affect on the corrosiveness of the oral environment. What rots the teeth is also likely to corrode the amalgams and dental fixtures. Finally, many dental products and solutions contain fluoride, with some of the specialist varnishes used by dentists exceeding 2 wt% fluoride [85].

3.5 Common Metals and Alloys Used in Biomedical Applications

3.5.1 Surgical Implants

All the metals and alloys used for surgical implants rely on the development of a passive oxide film to reduce their corrosion rates to acceptable levels. The actual specifications of modern surgical implant alloys, including chemical compositions and heat treatments, are now covered by the international standard ISO 5832.

3.5.1.1 Stainless steel

Stainless steels are in fact a family of ferrous alloys that contain more than 12% chromium. In the 1930s, stainless steels were the main implant materials [86]. With respect to surgical implants, usually the more ductile austenitic stainless steels containing at least 8% nickel are used — the most important one being grade 316L. 316L stainless steel has a nominal composition of 17Cr, 8Ni, 2Mo, balanced Fe, and an extremely low carbon content to prevent chromium depletion, hence the suffix 'L'. Occasionally nitrogen is added at about one-quarter percent level to improve the corrosion resistance of the alloy. The relative corrosion resistance of stainless steels can be estimated from their pitting resistance number (PREN):

PREN = %Cr + 3.3x%Mo +16x%N

However, 316L stainless steel can corrode within the body — especially in regions where there is insufficient oxygen to maintain the passive film or where crevices are formed (e.g., under the heads of screws). In addition, stainless steel femoral components can fracture. Therefore stainless steel is more suitable for temporary implant devices. Nevertheless, there are cases where 316L fracture plates have been removed from patients after more than 20 years of service, yet show no evidences of corrosion (see case histories in Section 3.8).

One final word of caution on stainless steels is that different grades should not be mixed as this can result in galvanic corrosion. Since it is not possible to visually distinguish one grade of stainless steel from another, careful quality control must be exercised. There have been examples of failure arising simply because one out of a group of screws holding a 316L fracture plate in position was fabricated using the lower 304L grade.

3.5.1.2 Cobalt–chromium alloys

Amongst cobalt–chromium alloys, the main ones used for surgical implants are either Co–Cr–Mo alloys (which have been used extensively in dentistry and more recently for artificial joints), or Co–Ni–Cr–Mo alloys (which are used to make the stems of prostheses for heavily loaded joints). Cobalt–chromium alloys have very good resistance to most forms of corrosion, including crevice corrosion and stress corrosion cracking. However, corrosion fatigue can still cause failures.

A major concern with using these alloys is the potential release of chromium, a known carcinogen, into the body. This worry also applies to stainless steels since they too contain chromium, although at lower levels.

3.5.1.3 Titanium and titanium alloys

Titanium has an excellent strength-to-weight ratio. Coupled with its excellent biocompatibility, titanium has become an attractive material for medical devices. During the 1950s and 1960s, it was the preferred choice of material [87]. Titanium has excellent corrosion resistance to most environments likely to be found *in vivo*, with the possible exception of anoxic regions where the protective passive oxide does not form. If this latter situation is a possibility, then the titanium should be alloyed with a small amount of palladium (Section 3.2.2.5.2). The ability of the passive oxide film to provide corrosion protection can be improved by anodizing (which results in a thicker film), or by "sealing" (which can be achieved by simply heating in distilled water [17]).

Titanium alloys have even better strength-to-weight ratios than pure titanium. For example, the Ti–6Al–4V alloy has now become the most popular implant material. However, titanium alloys do not have quite the same resistance to pitting corrosion as the parent metal and problems arise when the local redox potential is high. Such a condition can result from a situation where hydrogen peroxide is produced during the initial stages of inflammatory response after an implant is inserted. However, on the overall, titanium alloys have better corrosion resistance than cobalt–chromium alloys and stainless steels.

Despite their excellent corrosion resistance and biocompatibility, titanium and its alloys are not the perfect implant material as it has poor shear strength, making it unsuitable for screws *etc*. Titanium also has a high coefficient of friction, which means that wear particles may form if it rubs against bone or another implant surface. The latter case can also lead to fretting corrosion if the passive oxide film is worn off.

3.5.1.4 *Porous titanium*

Although titanium alloys have suitable corrosion characteristics for the construction of surgical implants, their elastic moduli are much higher than that of human bone. This means that stresses are not transferred to the surrounding bone effectively, and this can cause irregular bone growth. To overcome this problem, interest has focused on using porous implant materials, with lower elastic moduli that are closer to that of bone, instead of the traditional solid implants [88]. Porous materials not only encourage more regular bone growth, but also allow the bone to grow into the implant itself, thereby improving the retention. Unfortunately, the corrosion rate of porous titanium in simulated body fluids has been reported to be significantly higher than that of solid titanium [89,90]. Apparent increased corrosion rate is in part due to the much larger surface area that a porous structure exposes to the surrounding environment compared to its solid counterparts. However, it also appears that crevice corrosion occurs within the porous matrix. Furthermore, techniques that improve the properties of the passive film on solid titanium (e.g., anodizing) are less effective on porous titanium [91].

3.5.1.5 *Nickel–titanium alloy*

The Ni–Ti alloy has interesting memory-shape properties [92] which have prompted interest in its potential use in both surgical and dental applications [34]. Although the corrosion resistance of Ni–Ti has not yet been fully assessed, it appears to be slightly more resistant than 316L stainless steel [93]. The most common form of corrosion on Ni–Ti is pitting corrosion, which raises the concern of how much nickel (which is toxic and carcinogenic) might be released into the body. Initial studies suggest that the answer depends on the local environment, with tests in artificial saliva showing similar Ni release rates for Ni–Ti and 316L stainless steel [94]. On the other hand, in physiological simulating fluids the Ni–Ti releases three times as much of nickel [95].

3.5.2 *Dental Materials*

3.5.2.1 *Amalgams*

Modern dental amalgams are prepared mainly from two alloy types. Conventional silver–tin amalgam is prepared from a silver–tin alloy containing small amounts of copper and zinc. High-copper amalgams are prepared from either a mixture of silver–tin and silver–copper alloys (*i.e.*, admixed alloys) or from a ternary silver–copper–tin alloy (*i.e.*, single composition alloy). High-copper amalgams have been reported to have superior clinical properties with a higher resistance to corrosion [72]. However, the corrosion of both types of amalgam is of concern as it leads to the release of toxic mercury into the body.

Dental amalgams are multiphase alloys (as they require high strength), exposing them to localized galvanic or intergranular corrosion between the different phases. In conventional amalgams, it is the phases that contain silver which are noble and which cause accelerated corrosion of the non-silver phases. The most vulnerable is the γ_2 phase (Sn_7Hg), which releases mercury when it corrodes [71]. High-copper amalgams contain no γ_2 phase and are thus more resistant to corrosion than silver–tin amalgams. The most corrosion-prone phase in high-copper amalgams is the η' phase (Cu_6Sn_5). However, preferential corrosion of the η' phase does not release mercury [73].

Amalgams with high percentage of gold and other precious metals appear to be corrosion-resistant in nearly all oral environments. The exception occurs when high fluoride levels are introduced into the mouth, such as during some dental cleaning procedures, which can result in pitting corrosion in gold alloys and titanium [96,97].

Furthermore, in some patients, both silver- and gold-based amalgams can suffer from tarnishing, in which a thin black layer (probably a sulfide) develops across the surface. Although tarnishing does not dramatically affect amalgam performance, nor is it likely to increase mercury release rate, it is unsightly and is thus a matter of concern. The solution to the problem is more likely to be the elimination of the sulfide source, e.g., changing the patient's diet, rather than replacing the amalgam with a more corrosion-resistant material.

3.5.2.2 *Rare earth magnets*

There are a number of ternary alloys that contain rare earth elements (such as those of the NdFeB family) which have remarkably strong magnetic properties. This makes them desirable for a number of specialized medical applications, for example as dental keepers. Unfortunately, these rare earth magnets have very poor corrosion resistances, hence corroding rapidly in a humid atmosphere. One approach to overcome this problem is to completely seal the magnet inside a stainless steel cladding; however, the stainless steel must not reduce the effectiveness of the magnetization. In this respect, austenitic steels are ruled out. Ferritic stainless steels with chromium levels as high as 55 percent have been used, which should be sufficiently corrosion-resistant to survive in the oral cavity. In addition, particular attention must be given to the stainless steel seal, which is normally achieved by laser welding.

3.6 Detection Methods

There are several methods of monitoring and measuring the corrosion rate of a metal in an electrolyte. Detailed explanations of each technique are beyond the scope of the present work, so the interested reader is advised to consult one of a number of specialized corrosion texts [98,99]. Technical standards for corrosion testing include ASTM G1 for metal loss calculation, ASTM G46 for analysis of localized corrosion, and NACE TM–01 for corrosion testing.

The simplest method, which requires just the minimum of equipment with hardly any specialized instrumentation, is the weight-loss method. In this method, the test specimen is weighed after it is thoroughly dried before and after the corrosion test, and the difference in weight is calculated. This gives an indication of the extent of corrosion that the specimen has undergone. In addition, visual inspection of the test sample reveals the type of corrosion that has occurred, e.g., pitting or general corrosion. However, in practice, the formation of oxide films — which give rise to weight gains — impedes the accuracy of this simple technique. Nevertheless this is still the only technique that lends itself well to *in vivo* trails.

The second method, which is more sophisticated, is to construct a Tafel plot. This is obtained by polarizing the specimen over a range of potentials, typically 300 mV on either side of the corrosion potential. Then the resulting current is measured, the log of the current is plotted against applied potential and the linear regions are extrapolated back to the corrosion potential to yield the corrosion current density. However, in practice, the linear regions — which also provide the Tafel slopes — are often ill-defined. This makes extrapolation difficult, leading to large errors because of the log scale. Moreover, steady state currents should also be measured — hence making the technique very time-consuming.

The third method is the linear polarization resistance (LPR) method in which the specimen is perturbed by the application of a small potential (10 mV) and the steady state current recorded after a few minutes. Alternatively, the potential may be applied in the form of a slow ramp with the current being monitored continuously. In both cases, a charge transfer resistance (R_{ct}) can be calculated from the applied potential and the resulting current. Simple equations are then used to convert R_{ct} into a corrosion rate. However, this method neglects effects due to non-Faradaic processes, such as the resistance of the solution and the double-layer capacitance. Moreover, the equations used to convert R_{ct} to a corrosion rate require knowledge of the Tafel slopes, which as mentioned above, may be inaccurate or unavailable.

The fourth — and more modern — technique is electrochemical impedance spectroscopy (EIS), which is somewhat similar to the LPR technique except that the perturbing potential is applied over a range of frequencies (0.01 Hz to 10 kHz). This method takes into account all the non-Faradaic processes, giving a more accurate value of R_{ct}. However, although EIS is a great improvement over earlier techniques, the presence of oxide films and mass transport effects can make data interpretation difficult, and knowledge of the Tafel slopes is still required.

The fifth — and most modern — technique is electrochemical noise, in which two identical specimens are coupled together via a device called a zero resistance ammeter. Small fluctuations in the current flowing between them and in their corrosion potentials are simultaneously recorded. A so-called "noise resistance" can be extracted from the standard deviations in the current and voltage fluctuations, and this is believed to be equivalent to the R_{ct} of the LPR method. The main advantage of the noise technique is that the specimen is not perturbed, so there is no danger of the experiment altering the corrosion rate. However, in practice, this method requires more sophisticated equipment and once again the Tafel slopes are required to calculate the corrosion rate. As a result, electrochemical noise has not yet obtained the status where it can surpass the EIS technique.

A final method is potentiodynamic polarization, in which a slow positive potential ramp (1 mV/s) is applied to a specimen until the measured current exceeds some predetermined value. Unlike the other techniques, this method does not provide a corrosion rate. Instead information obtained is on whether the specimen forms a passive oxide film in a given environment, and if it does, how much resistance this film can provide against localized corrosion, e.g., pitting corrosion. The more positive the potential at which the specified current limit is exceeded, the more corrosion-resistant the specimen is.

3.7   Corrosion Prevention

As mentioned at the beginning of this chapter, most of the traditional methods of controlling corrosion cannot be used for surgical implants as the environment within the human body is fixed. The only methods available are to fabricate the implants from a corrosion-resistant alloy or to use a coating — either of which must be able to withstand any abrasion and wear to which the device may be subjected. Nevertheless, a number of steps must be taken to help reduce the risk of corrosion related failures of surgical implants [100,101].

3.7.1 Coatings and Surface Treatment

Paints and other forms of organic coating have a very limited (if any) role in protecting implants, since they are unable to withstand abrasion. Coatings that may be of use include titanium or titanium nitride films on Ni–Ti memory-shape alloys [102] and very high chromium ferritic stainless steel claddings on rare earth magnets used as dental keepers. The poor fretting resistance of the Ti–6Al–4V alloy represents its most serious drawback with regards to its use as an implant material; thus considerable effort has been dedicated to improving its surface properties. Techniques that have yielded the most encouraging results are anodizing [16] and generating of titanium nitride coatings either by ion implantation [62], magnetron sputtering [103], or nitriding [63,64].

3.7.2 Quality Control

Many corrosion related failures of surgical implants can be traced back to poor quality control. Problems usually stem from one of two points in the supply line. Firstly the manufacturer must follow the appropriate standards (e.g., BS 7252, ISO 5832, or ASTM F138) during fabrication, metallurgical conditioning or application of the surface finishing on the implant. Secondly, since it is impossible to tell the composition of a metallic alloy simply by visible inspection, the alloy type of each component must be clearly labeled and different alloys must be stored separately. This second problem has been particularly associated with screws. For example, type 304L stainless steel screws have been used by mistake instead of the more corrosion-resistant type 316L. The adoption of a quality assurance system, as per the recommendations given in ISO 9000, would eliminate these failures.

3.7.3 Reduce Risk of Galvanic Corrosion

Wherever possible, the coupling of different metals and alloys (including different grades of stainless steel) should be avoided. However, it is recognized that this may not always be possible. For example, titanium alloys do not possess the tensile strength required for use as screws or wires. Therefore, a galvanic couple may be unavoidable if a titanium alloy implant needs to be secured through screwing or wiring. If such a situation should occur, remember that of the common implant materials stainless steels are the most vulnerable to galvanic corrosion. Thus, stainless steel should be used in a couple only as a last resort. For example, to secure a titanium alloy implant, it would be far better to use screws fabricated from a cobalt–chromium alloy than from any grade of stainless steel [68,104,105].

3.7.4 Handling/Sterilization/Assembly

Scratches or small cracks on a surface can act as initiation points for both fatigue and corrosion. Therefore, it is important to handle all implants with great care and to avoid scratching by surgical tools. It would be preferable to keep all implants in protective packaging until the time of use.

Chloride ions are aggressive towards most metallic alloys, particularly at elevated temperatures. Therefore sterilization of implants in saline solutions should be avoided. Although the sterilization procedure may take only a short period of time, it is sufficient for small pits to develop on the implant's surface, which then act as initiation points for corrosion or fatigue.

Contamination of an implant's surface can also lead to corrosion. Such contamination can result from the transfer of metal from surgical tools to the implant. It is thus recommended that drill guides be used to prevent contact between the drill and plates [105]. When assembling implants, care must be taken not to introduce additional crevices. On this note, the importance of stable fixation cannot be over-stressed — it helps to reduce the risks of mechanical fatigue, corrosion fatigue, and fretting. Suggestions on how to improve fixation include the following:

- Plasma-spray a titanium coating with a specific surface roughness on the surface of Ti–6Al–4V alloy [106];
- Engineer the shape, topography, and composition of the implant to facilitate either tissue ingrowth or enhanced on-growth of mineralized bone [107];
- Deposit strongly adhered hydroxyapatite coatings which should fuse with the growing bone [108].

3.7.5 Education

Both surgical teams and dentists need to be aware of the basic causes of corrosion and fatigue. In particular, they should be adequately educated on the importance of avoiding bimetallic couples, of careful handling of implants and of providing stable fixation.

3.8 Case Histories

Case Study A

A housewife born in 1941 had a history of tuberculosis of the left hip. She had a fusion of her hip done in 1947 with limb length corrective surgery. It was done at the level of mid-shaft with a femoral plate, and the implant was secured to the site using screws. The implant was an 8-cm four-hole bone plate, with four 4-mm diameter screws, and 28 mm in length. The plate and screws were not removed until 1997 (50 years later), when the patient complained of thigh and knee pain with an associated swelling on the right side. Histology of the tissue surrounding the implant site showed features consistent with foreign body reaction. The fibrous tissue was observed to have deposits of a black foreign material. No malignancies were seen in the tissue specimens. In removing the plate, the proximal quarter with its two proximal screws had to be broken off to ease the removal of the implant. Figure 3–11(a) shows that one end of the plate was badly corroded, especially under the screw heads, while the screws and the other end of the plate were less affected. The X-ray image in Figure 3–11(b) reveals that the less corroded end of the plate was protected by an overgrown layer of bone; the remains of a drill bit accidentally left in the patient at the time of the original operation can also be seen. Analysis revealed that the plate was constructed from a ferritic stainless steel containing only 12% Cr, while the screws were made from austenitic 304L stainless steel. A level of only 12% Cr is insufficient to prevent pitting corrosion on the plate by body fluids. Moreover, the situation was aggravated by galvanic coupling to 304L stainless steel screws, leading to severe crevice corrosion beneath the screw heads.

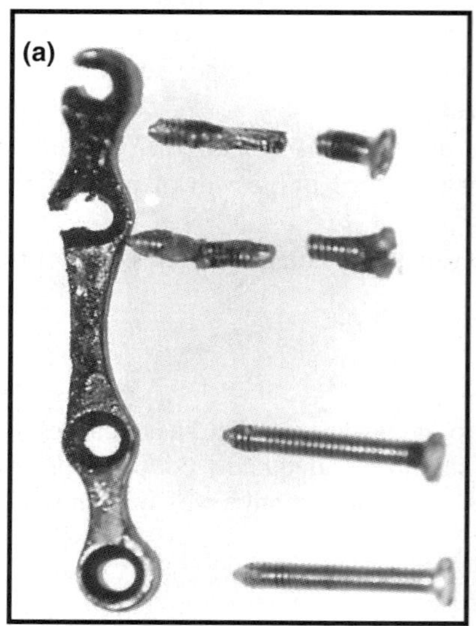

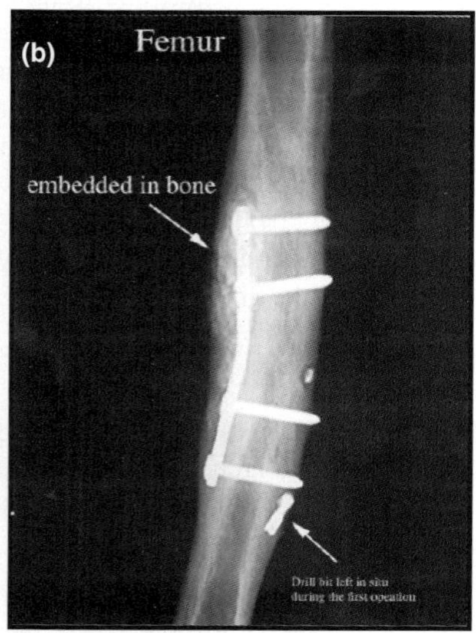

Figure 3–11 (a) Sherman plate and screws removed from a patient after nearly 50 years of service. The 12% Cr plate was badly corroded, while the 304L stainless steel screws were in reasonable condition; (b) X-ray showing that one end of the Sherman plate was covered by bone growth, which protected it from the corrosive environment.

Case Study B

This case study is about fatigue and fatigue corrosion on type 316L straight bone plate [109]. Figure 3–12 shows X-ray images of a plate that was used to treat a pseudarthrosis in the proximal femur. It can be seen that because of an absence of bone in the area between screw hole numbers 5 and 6, no screws were inserted at these locations. In Figure 3–12(a) a wide gap across the fractured bone is visible, which indicates instability. However, since healing did not progress, so the plate was removed and replaced with an angled blade plate so that compression was exerted on the pseudarthrosis site to promote bone healing. Investigation of the removed plate at high magnification revealed fatigue cracks on the top surface of a small section at the fifth screw hole, indicated by a box on Figure 3–12(b). As hole number 5 was located at the transition between the bone and the defect, it was likely to have been exposed to high stress concentrations. However, no damage was seen at the other empty screw hole number 6. It located directly over the bone defect, where elastic deformation could occur more uniformly. Slight fretting corrosion was also found at most of the screw/plate interfaces, being particularly noticeable at hole number 7. This hole was the closest to the fracture and had a relatively short screw, so it was the one likely to undergo the most motion leading to the observed corrosion fatigue.

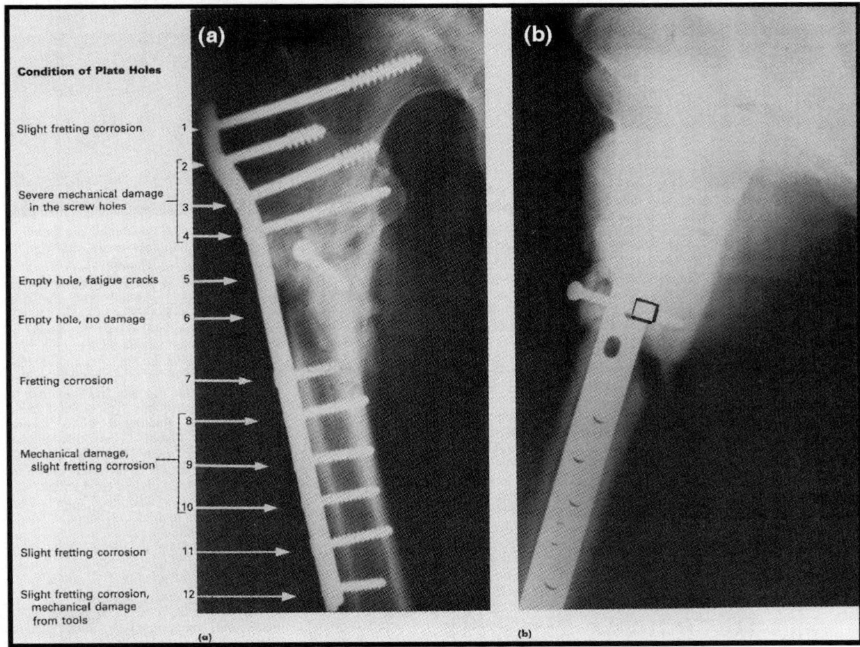

Figure 3–12   Crack initiation on type 316L stainless steel compression plate: (a) anterior-posterior X-ray; (b) lateral view, with a box indicating the location of fatigue crack initiation (Reprinted from reference [109] with permission)

Case Study C

This case study is about fretting and fretting corrosion between screw head and plate, where both components were fabricated from type 316L stainless steel [109]. Figure 3–13(a) shows that only grinding and polishing occurred over most of the contact area. However, at higher magnification in Figure 3–13(b), fine corrosion pits are visible. Evidence of intense mechanical material transfer from fretting in the form of a material tongue can be seen in the upper right corner of Figures 3–13(c) and (d). Figure 3–13(d) also shows a corrosion pit in front of a material tongue surrounded by a burnished surface texture, which may have broken-open at some point. This is consistent with observations from other implants in which material layers are smeared over each other during wear and attacked by pitting corrosion [100]. Subsequently, future wear will cause these pits to be covered by a new burnished material film, which may break-open again. Products of these corrosion and wear processes are then transported to the surrounding tissue.

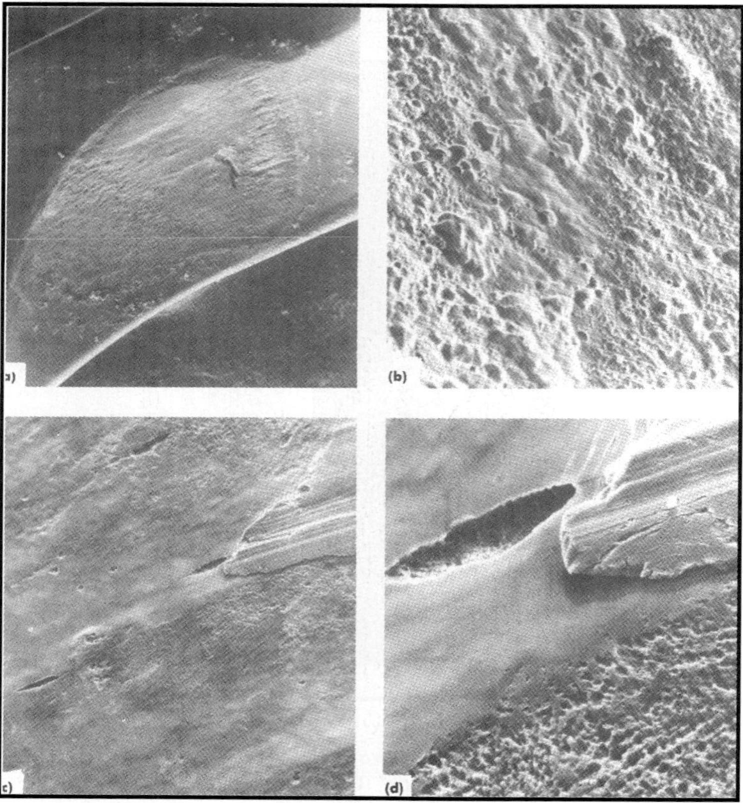

Figure 3–13 Fretting and fretting corrosion between screw head and plate, both components being fabricated from type 316L stainless steel; magnifications: (a) 8x; (b) 190x; (c) 190x; and (d) 345x (Reprinted from reference [109] with permission)

Case Study D

This case is about the broken stem of a femoral head component, which is part of a total hip prosthesis made from Co–Cr–Mo alloy [109]. Five months after implantation into a 65-year-old man, an X-ray showed that radiotranslucency was visible around the collar of the femoral head prosthesis. One month later, failure of the bond cement at the distal end of the stem occurred, and a small notch on the lateral edge of the prosthesis was visible. It was at this point that the stem broke two weeks later. Figure 3–14(a) shows an X-ray of the broken prosthesis. The X-ray reveals the loosening of the implant as a gap between the lateral stem edge and the bone cement. The resultant movement under load bearing led to fatigue and eventually to fracture. Figure 3–14(b) shows the broken prosthesis component. Extensive rubbing against bone cement, due to the loosening, had caused heavy wear at the base of the stem (as marked by the arrow).

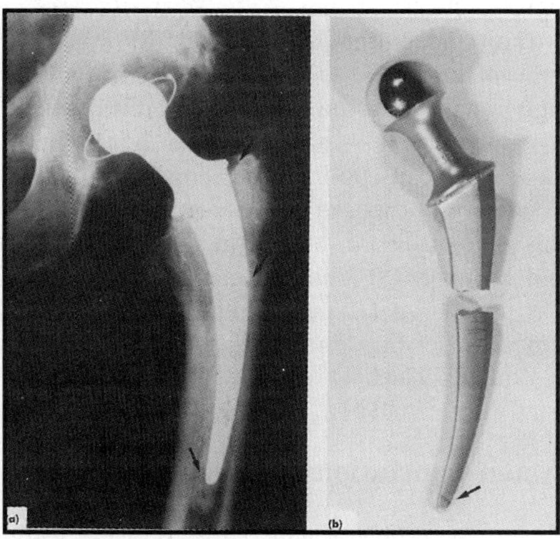

Figure 3–14 Broken Co–Cr–Mo alloy hip prosthesis: (a) X-ray of total hip prosthesis, with arrows showing areas of loosening; (b) fractured stem, with arrow showing area of heavy wear at base of stem (Reprinted from reference [109] with permission)

Case Study E

This case study is about galvanic corrosion in a repaired shoulder [105]. After a patient complained of pain and disability in a repaired shoulder fracture, the screws were removed and analyzed (Figure 3–15). It was found that one screw was made from Co–Cr–Mo alloy, while the others were fabricated from stainless steel. Galvanic corrosion, along with electrical currents generated by the electrochemical cell, was responsible for the patient's pain.

Case Study F

A male patient had previously fractured both his right ulna and radius at the mid-shift region in a road traffic accident. That was around 1960, when both fractures were closed with bone plates and screws. He was 13 years old then. In 1998, he again fractured his right radius and ulna in another road traffic accident. Both fractures were at the distal screws of plate fixation site (Figure

3–16). The old plates were removed, after being *in situ* for about 38 years, and the fracture was closed with two new plate implants. No inflammation or black material in the surrounding soft tissue was noted. The old implants were 4-cm three-hole bone plates, each with three 3-mm diameter screws, and 14 mm in length. Both plates and their respective screws were removed intact with remarkably little corrosion. There were just a few scratches which were incurred during retrieval, and the manufacturer's name "DOWN.A" was still clearly visible (Figure 3–16).

The surgeon who removed the plates and screws was sufficiently impressed to enquire why not all implants were made of such highly corrosion-resistant alloys. Surprisingly, analysis of the plates and screws revealed that both were made from 304L stainless steel — a material that is now considered unsuitable for surgical implants due to its poor track record, particularly in the aspect of pitting corrosion. It was proposed that the low dissolved oxygen levels in human body fluids had made the long-term *in vivo* environment much more benign than would be expected from *in vitro* experiments. Furthermore, the Sherman plate was appropriately small so that the surrounding tissue was not sufficiently perturbed to develop into an environment that would cause pitting corrosion on 304L stainless steel.

3.9 Summary and Conclusions

Corrosion was a serious problem with early implant materials. However, knowledge of corrosion and mechanical properties of biomaterials has enabled the development of a number of extremely successful alloys, e.g., Ti–6Al–4V, 316LVM, and ASTM F1058 Co–Cr–Ni–Mo alloy. It is certain that improved versions of these alloys will continue to be developed in the future. As a result, as long as the chosen material matches the requirements of national and international standards, such as ISO 5832, it is very unlikely that a surgical implant will suffer a corrosion related failure. Most modern failures tend to stem from poor quality control, which can be traced back to either wrong choice of material or use of mismatched materials, which eventually results in galvanic corrosion.

Modern alloys have also reduced the extent to which potentially hazardous metallic ions leach out of biomedical devices. Nevertheless, there remains the concern that extended exposure to even very low levels of corrosion products could result in medical complications. This concern arises in part due to lack of knowledge as to what are the safe levels for transition metal ions to exist in the body. Leveraging on this concern, there is still a continuing need to further reduce passive corrosion rates.

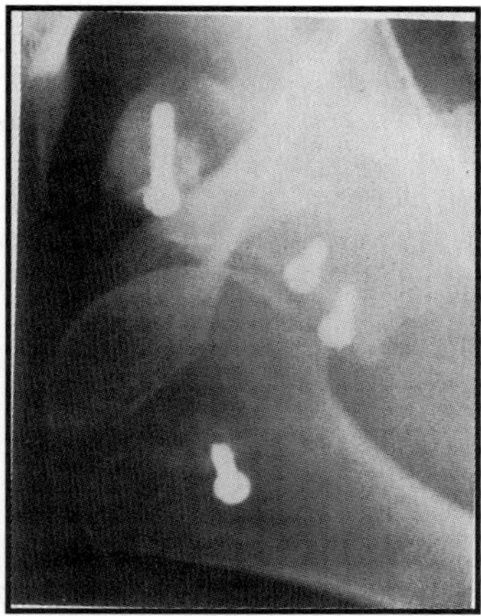

Figure 3–15 X-ray of a repaired shoulder. Examination of the screws revealed one to be made from Co–Cr–Mo alloy and the others from stainless steel; the resulting galvanic corrosion was the cause of the patient's pain. (Reprinted from reference [105] with permission)

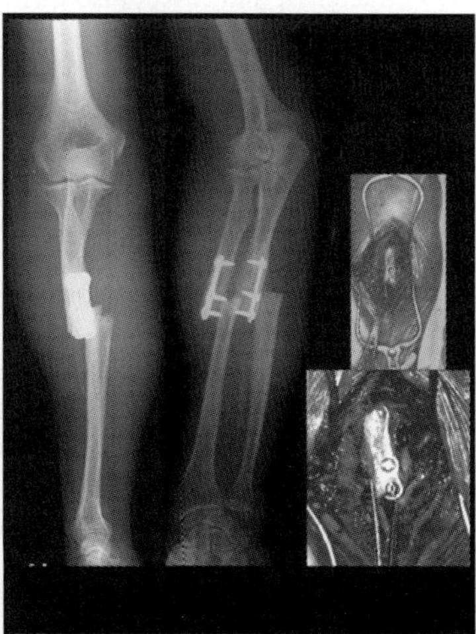
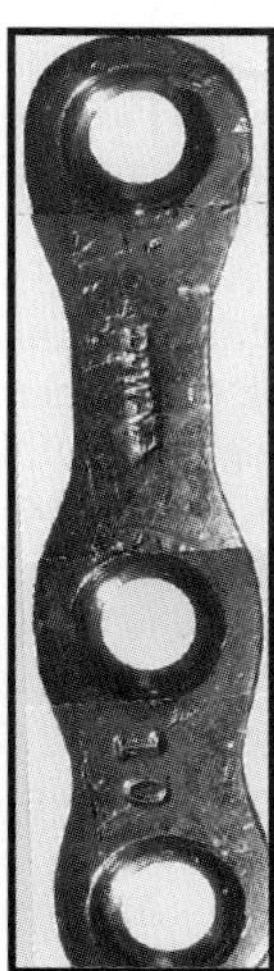

Figure 3–16 (Left) X-ray showing a 304L stainless steel Sherman plate that had to be removed after 38 years as the patient had a second road accident; (right) close-up of the Sherman plate on which the manufacturer's name (DOWN.A) can still be clearly seen

References

1. M. F. LeClerc, Surgical implants, in Corrosion, Vol. 1, 3rd Edition, eds. L. L. Shrier, R. A. Jarman, and G. T. Burstein, (Butterworth Heinemann, Oxford, 1994) Ch. 2.13.

2. P. S. P. Thong, F. Watt, D. Ponraj, S. K. Leong, Y. He, and T. K. Y. Lee, Iron and cell death in Parkinson's disease: a nuclear microscopic study into iron-rich granules in the parkinsonian substantia nigra of primate models, Nucl. Instrum. Methods Phys. Res., Section B, 1999, 158:349–355.

3. I. M. C. Lundstrom, Allergy and corrosion of dental materials in patients with oral lichen planus, Int. J. Oral Surg., 1982, 12:1–9.

4. J. Banoczy, B. Roed-Petersen, J. J. Pindborg, and J. Inovay, Clinical and histologic studies on electrogalvanically induced oral white lesions, Oral Surg., Oral Med., Oral Pathol., 1979, 48:319–323.

5. M. Pourbaix, Atlas of electrochemical equilibria in aqueous solutions, 2nd Edition, (National Association of Corrosion Engineers, Houston, 1974).

6. D. J. Blackwood, R. Peat, and A M Pritchard, *In-situ* imaging of corrosion processes, Mater. Sci. Forum, 1995, 192–193:693–709.

7. L. L. Hench, Bioactive glasses and glass-ceramics, Mater. Sci. Forum, 1999, 293:37–63.

8. Southampton Electrochemistry Group, Instrumental Methods in Electrochemistry, eds. R. Greef, R. Peat, L. M. Peter, D. Pletcher, and J. Robinson, (Ellis Horwood, Chichester, 1985) pp:33–35, pp:233–242.

9. G. T. Burstein, Passivity and localized corrosion, in Corrosion, Vol. 1, 3rd Edition, eds. L. L. Shrier, R. A. Jarman, and G. T. Burstein, (Butterworth Heinemann, Oxford, 1994) Ch. 1.5.

10. L. Young, Anodic Oxide Films, (Academic Press, London, 1961).

11. P. Tengvall and I. Lundstrom, Physico-chemical considerations of titanium as a biomaterial, Clin. Mater., 1992, 9:115–134.

12. N. B. Pilling and R. E. Bedworth, Oxidation of metals at high temperatures, J. Inst. Met., 1923, 29:529–583.

13. D. E. Williams and G. A. Wright, Nucleation and growth of anodic oxide films on bismuth, I. Cyclic voltammetry, Electrochim. Acta, 1976, 21:1009–1019.

14. A. H. Tuthill and R. E. Avery, Specifying stainless steel surface treatments, Adv. Mater. Process, 1992, 12:34–38.

15. G. S. Frankel, Pitting corrosion of metals: A review of the critical factors, J. Electrochem. Soc., 1998, 145:2186–2198.

16. J. A. Disegi, Anodizing treatments for titanium implants, Proc. 16th South. Biomedical Eng. Conf., eds. J. D. Bumgardner and A. D. Pucknett, (Institute of Electrical and Electronics Engineers, New York, 1997) pp:129–132.

17. D. J. Blackwood, L. M. Peter, and D. E. Williams, Stability and open circuit breakdown of passive films on titanium, Electrochim. Acta, 1988, 33:1143–1149.

18. D. A. Jones, Principles and prevention of corrosion, 2nd Edition, (Prentice Hall, New Jersey, 1996) pp:187–188, pp:525–526.

19. M. Traisnel, D. Le Maguer, H. F. Hildebrand, and A. Iost, Corrosion of surgical implants, Clin. Mater., 1990, 5:309–318.

20. K. Endo, Y. Abiko, M. Suzuki, H. Ohno, and T. Kaku, Corrosion resistance and biocompatibility of high-nitrogen stainless steels, Zairyo to Kankyo, 1998, 47:570–576.

21. J. Stewart and D. E. Williams, The initiation of pitting corrosion on austenitic stainless steel: on the role and importance of sulfide inclusions, Corros. Sci., 1992, 33:457–474.

22. M. G. S. Ferreira, T. M. Silva, and A. Catarino, Electrochemical and laser Raman spectroscopy studies of stainless steel in 0.15M sodium chloride solution, J. Electrochem. Soc., 1992, 145:3146–3151.

23. H. Zitter, Case histories on surgical implants and their causes, Werkst. Korros., 1991, 42:455–466.

24. H. J. Mueller and E. H. Greener, Polarization studies on surgical materials in Ringer's solution, J. Biomed. Mater. Res., 1970, 4:29–41.

25. B. C. Syrett and S. S. Wing, Pitting resistance of new and conventional orthopedic implant materials, in Corrosion, 1978, 34:138–145.

26. B. C. Syrett and E. E. Davis, Crevice corrosion of implant alloys: A comparison of the *in-vitro* and *in-vivo* studies, ASTM STP, 1979, 684:229–244.

27. F. R. Morral, Metallurgy of cobalt alloys: 1968 review, JOM., 1968, 20:52–59.

28. J. Cohen and J. Wulff, Clinical failure caused by corrosion of a vitallium plate, J. Bone Jt. Surg., 1972, 54A:617–628.

29. C. O. Clerc, M. R. Jedwab, D. W. Mayer, P. J. Thompson, and J. S. Stinson, Assessment of wrought ASTM F1058 cobalt alloy properties for permanent surgical implants, J. Biomed. Mater. Res., 1997, 38:229–234.

30. L. C. Lucus, R. A. Buchanan, J. E. Lemons, and C. D. Griffin, Susceptibility of surgical cobalt-based alloy to pitting corrosion, J. Biomed. Mater. Res., 1982, 16:799–810.

31. J. Cohen, Corrosion testing of orthopedic implants, J. Bone Jt. Surg., 1962, 44A:307–316.

32. M. Chew, Electrodeposition of calcium phosphate on titanium and its alloys, BSc.(Hons) thesis, (National University of Singapore, 2002) pp:17–18.

33. G. Rondelli, B. Vicentini, and A. Cigada, The corrosion behavior of nickel–titanium shape memory alloys, Corro. Sci., 1990, 30:805–812.

34. D. Mantovani, Shape memory alloys: Properties and biomedical applications, JOM., 2000, 52:36–44.

35. K. H. W. Seah and X. Chen, A comparison between the corrosion characteristics of 316L stainless steel, solid titanium and porous titanium, Corros. Sci., 1993, 34:1841–1851.

36. J. T. Scales, G. D. Winter, and H. T. Shirley, Corrosion of orthopedic implants, J. Bone Jt. Surg., 1959, 41B:810–820.

37. J. A. Disegi and L. D. Zardiackas, Microstructural features of implant quality 316L stainless steel, in Advances in the production and use of steel with improved internal cleanliness, ed. J. K. Mahaney, ASTM STP, 1999, 1361:49–56.

38. J. Galante and W. Rostoker, Corrosion: Related failures in metallic implants and experimental study, Clin. Orthop. Relat. Res., 1972, 86:237–244.

39. K. H. W. Seah, R. Thampuran, and S. H. Teoh, The influence of pore morphology on corrosion, Corros. Sci., 1998, 40:547–556.

40. B. S. Becker and J. D. Bolton, Production of porous sintered Co–Cr–Mo alloys for possible surgical implant applications, Part 2: Corrosion behavior, Powder. Metal., 1995, 38:305–313.

41. R. N. Parkins, Mechanisms of stress corrosion cracking, in Corrosion, Vol. 1, 3rd Edition, eds. L. L. Shrier, R. A. Jarman, and G. T. Burstein, (Butterworth Heinemann, Oxford, 1994) Ch. 8.1.

42. R. H. Jones and B. Craig, Environmentally induced cracking: Stress-corrosion cracking, in Metals Handbook, Vol. 13: Corrosion, 9th Edition, eds. L. J. Korb, D. L. Olson, and J. R. Davis, (ASM, Ohio, 1987) pp:145–163.

43. S. Tsujikawa, Y. Ishihara, and T. Shinohara, Failure analysis of stress corrosion cracking of type 304 steel tubes for hot-water use in Kusatsu town, Gunma Prefecture, Zairyo to Kankyo, 1993, 42:20–26.

44. K. Tamaki, S. Tsujikawa, Y. Hisamatsu, T. Shinohara, and C. Liang, Development of a new test method for chloride stress corrosion cracking of stainless steels in dilute sodium chloride solutions, in NACE 9, Advances in Localized Corrosion: Proc. 2nd Inter. Conf. Localized Corrosion, Orlando, 1987, eds. H. Isaacs, U. Bertocci, J. Kruger, and Z. Szklarska-Smialowska, (National Association of Corrosion Engineers, Houston, 1990) pp:207–214.

45. T. Haruna and T. Shibata, Initiation and growth of stress corrosion cracks in type 316L stainless steel during slow strain rate testing, in Corrosion, 1994, 50:758–791.

46. S. Tsujikawa, T. Shinohara, and Y. Hisamatsu, The role of crevices in comparison to pits in initiating stress corrosion cracks of type 310S steel in different concentrations of magnesium chloride solutions at 80°C, in Corrosion Cracking: Proc. Corros. Cracking Program Relat. Pap. 1985, ed. V. S. Goel, (ASM, Ohio, 1986) pp:35–42.

47. J. R. Cahoon and H.W. Paxton, Metallurgical analysis of failed orthopedic implants, J. Biomed. Mater. Res., 1968, 2:1–22.

48. J. P. Sheehan, C. R. Morris, and K. F. Packer, Study of stress corrosion cracking susceptibility of type 316L stainless steel *in vitro*, in Corrosion and degradation of implant materials, 2nd symposium, eds. A. C. Fraker and C. D. Griffin, ATSM STP, 1985, 859:57–72.

49. B. J. Edwards, M. R. Louthan, and R. D. Sission, Hydrogen embrittlement of Zimaloy: A cobalt–chromium–molybdenum orthopedic implant alloy, in Corrosion and degradation of implant materials, 2nd symposium, eds. A. C. Fraker and C. D. Griffin, ATSM STP, 1985, 859:11–29.

50. K. J. Bundy and V. H. Desai, Studies of stress corrosion cracking susceptibility of type 316L stainless steel *in-vitro*, in Corrosion and degradation of implant materials, 2nd symposium, eds. A. C. Fraker and C. D. Griffin, ATSM STP, 1985, 859:73–90.

51. R. C. Newman and R. P. M. Procter, Stress corrosion ranking: 1965–1990, Br. Corros. J., 1990, 25:259–269.

52. M. F. Leclerc, A review of the factors influencing the mechanical failure of the femoral component used in total hip replacement, Proc. Eng, Ortho. Surg. Rehab., (Bioengineering Unit, Princess Margaret Rose Hospital, Edinburgh, 1982) pp:36–48.

53. M. Morita, T. Sasada, H. Hayashi, and Y. Tsukamoto, The corrosion fatigue properties of surgical implants in a living body, J. Biomed. Mater. Res., 1988, 22:529–540.

54. C. O. Bechtol, Failure of femoral implant components in total hip replacement operations, Orthop. Rev., 1975, 4:23–29.

55. M. von Knoch, A. Bluhm, M. Morlock, and G. von Förster, Surface roughness changes of non-polished femoral components of artificial hip joints during two to 15 years in service, J. Arthroplasty, 2003, 18:471–477.

56. A. N. Hughes, B. A. Jordan, and S. Orman, The corrosion fatigue properties of surgical implant materials: Third progress report — May 1973, Eng. Med., 1978, 7:135–141.

57. J. Yu, Z. J. Zhao, and L. X. Li, Corrosion fatigue resistances of surgical implant stainless steels and titanium alloy, Corros. Sci., 1993, 35:587–597.

58. H. R. Piehler, M. A. Portnoff, L. E. Sloter, E. J. Vegdahl, J. L. Gilbert, and M. J. Weber, Corrosion-fatigue performance of hip nails: The influence of materials selection and design, in Corrosion and degradation of implant materials, 2nd symposium, eds. A. C. Fraker and C. D. Griffin, ATSM STP, 1985, 859:93–104.

59. B. C. Syrett and S. S. Wing, An electrochemical investigation of fretting corrosion of surgical implant materials, in Corrosion, 1978, 34:379–386.

60. M. G. Fontana, Corrosion Engineering, 3rd Edition, (McGraw–Hill, Singapore, 1987) pp:109.

61. J. Rieu, L. M. Rabbe, and P. Combrade, Fretting wear corrosion of surgical implant alloys: Effects of ion implantation and ion nitriding on the fretting behavior of metals/PMMA contacts, in Proc. 8th Inter. Conf. Surf. Modification Tech., Nice, 1994, eds. T. S. Sudarshan and M. Jeandin, (Institute of Materials, London, 1995) pp:43–52.

62. R. A. Buchanan, E. D. Rigney, and J. M. Williams, Ion implantation of surgical Ti–6Al–4V for improved resistance to wear-accelerated corrosion, J. Biomed. Mater. Res., 1987, 21:355–366.

63. A. Shenhar, I. Gotman, S. Radin, P. Ducheyne, and E. Y. Gutmanas, Titanium nitride coatings on surgical titanium alloys produced by powder immersion reaction assisted coating method: Residual stresses and fretting behaviour, Surf. Coat. Technol., 2000, 126:210–218.

64. D. Starosvetsky, A. Shenhar, and I. Gotman, Corrosion behavior of PIRAC nitrided Ti–6Al–4V surgical alloy, J. Mater. Sci.: Mater. Med., 2001, 12:145–150.

65. J. A. von Fraunhofer, Corrosion in the oral cavity, in Corrosion, Vol. 1, 3rd Edition, eds. L. L. Shrier, R. A. Jarman, and G. T. Burstein, (Butterworth Heinemann, Oxford, 1994) Ch. 2.14.

66. H. P. Hack and D. Taylor, Evaluation of galvanic corrosion, in Metals Handbook, Vol. 13: Corrosion, 9th Edition, eds. L. J. Korb, D. L. Olson, and J. R. Davis, (ASM, Ohio, 1987) pp:234–241.

67. M. J. Pryor and D. J. Astley, Bimetallic corrosion, in Corrosion, Vol. 1, 3rd Edition, eds. L. L. Shrier, R. A. Jarman, and G. T. Burstein, (Butterworth Heinemann, Oxford, 1994) Ch. 1.7.

68. W. Rostoker, C. W. Pretzel, and J. O. Galante, Couple corrosion among alloys for skeletal prostheses, J. Biomed. Mater. Res., 1974, 8:407–419.

69.   D. C. Mears, The use of dissimilar metals in surgery, J. Biomed. Mater. Res. (Symp.), 1975, 6:133–148.

70.   H. Jackson-Burrows, J. N. Wilson, and J. T. Scales, Excision of tumors of humerus and femur with restoration of internal prostheses, J. Bone Jt. Surg., 1975, 57B:148–159.

71.   J. A. von Fraunhofer and P. J. Staheli, Corrosion of dental amalgam, in Nature, 1972, 240:304–306.

72.   N. K. Sarkar and C. S. Eyer, The microstructural basis of creep-in dental amalgam, J. Oral Rehab., 1987, 14:27–33.

73.   B. M. Eley, The future of dental amalgam: a review of the literature, Part 1: Dental amalgam structure and corrosion, Brit. Dent. J., 1997, 182:247–249.

74.   T. Newton, Dental fillings, Chem. Br., 2002, 38(10):24–27.

75.   P. Mueller and C. Rodig, Dispersion hardening behavior of cold-formed X2CrNiMoN18.12 steel for surgical implants, Neue Huette, 1989, 34:378–381.

76.   R. J. Solar, Corrosion resistance of titanium surgical implant alloys: A review, in Corrosion degradation implant materials, eds. B. C. Syrett and A. Acharya, ASTM STP, 1979, 684:259–273.

77.   B. Jacobson and J. B. Webster, Surgery, in Medicine and clinical engineering, eds. B. Jacobson and J. B. Webster, (Prentice–Hall, New Jersey, 1977) Ch. 10.

78.   P. G. Liang, Compatibility of biomaterials, Orthop. Clinc. Nor. Am., 1973, 4:249–273.

79.   P. Thomsen and L. E. Ericson, in The bone-biomaterial interface, ed. J. E. Davis, (University of Toronto Press, Toronto, 1991) pp:153–164.

80.   N. D. Greene, Corrosion of surgical alloys: A few basic ideas, in Corrosion and degradation of implant materials, 2nd symposium, eds. A. C. Fraker and C. D. Griffin, ATSM STP, 1985, 859:5–10.

81.   S. Ciolac, E. Vasilescu, P. Drob, M. V. Popa, and M. Anghel, Long-term *in vitro* study of titanium and some titanium alloys used in surgical implants, Rev. Chim. (Bucharest), 2000, 51:36–41.

82.   R. Schenk, Titanium in medicine: material science, surface science, engineering, biological responses, and medical applications, eds. D. M. Brunette, P. Tengvall, M. Textor, and P. Thomsen, (Springer, Berlin, 2001) pp:145–170.

83.   T. Fusayama, T. Katayori, and S. Nomoto, Corrosion of gold and amalgam placed in contact with each other, J. Dent. Res., 1963, 42:1183–1197.

84.   A. U. J. Yap, B. L. Ng, and D. J. Blackwood, Corrosion behavior of high-copper dental amalgams, J. Oral Rehab., 2003, (in press).

85.   S. Joyston-Bechal and E. A. M. Kidd, Update on the appropriate uses of fluoride, Dental Update, 1994, 21:366–371.

86.   A. C. Fraker, Corrosion of metallic implants and prosthetic devices, in Metals Handbook, Vol. 13: Corrosion, 9th Edition, eds. L. J. Korb, D. L. Olson, and J. R. Davis, (ASM, Ohio, 1987) pp:1325-1335.

87.   G. H. Hille, Titanium for surgical implants, J. Materials, 1966, 1:373–383.

88.   M. Spector, M. J. Michno, W. H. Smarook, and G. T. Kwiatkowski, A high-modulus polymer for porous orthopedic implants: biomechanical compatibility of porous implants, J. Biomed. Mater. Res., 1978, 12:665–677.

89. K. H. W. Seah, R. Thampuran, X. Chen, and S. H. Teoh, A comparison between the corrosion behavior of sintered and unsintered porous titanium, Corros. Sci., 1995, 37:1333–1340.

90. D. J. Blackwood, A. W. C. Chua, K. W. H. Seah, R. Thampuran, and S. H. Teoh, Corrosion behavior of porous titanium–graphite composites designed for surgical implants, Corros. Sci., 2000, 42:481–503.

91. D. J. Blackwood and S. K. M. Chooi, Stability of protective oxide films formed on porous titanium, Corros. Sci., 2002, 44:395–405.

92. F. X. Gil, J. M. Manero, and J. A. Planell, Relevant aspects in the clinical applications of Ni–Ti shape memory alloys, J. Mater. Sci.: Mater. Med., 1996, 7:403–406.

93. J. Ryhänen, E. Niemi, W. Serlo, E. Niemelä, P. Sandvik, H. Pernu, and T. Salo, Biocompatibility of nickel–titanium shape memory metal and its corrosion behavior in human cell cultures, J. Biomed. Mater. Res., 1997, 35:451–457.

94. R. D. Barrett, S. E. Bishara, and J. K. Quinn, Biodegradation of orthodontic appliances, Part 1: Biodegradation of nickel and chromium *in vitro*, Am. J. Orthod. Dentofacial. Orthop., 1993, 103:8–14.

95. G. Rondelli, Corrosion resistance tests on Ni–Ti shape memory alloy, Biomaterials, 1996, 17:2003–2008.

96. L. Reclaru and J. M. Meyer, Effects of fluorides on titanium and other dental alloys in dentistry, Biomaterials, 1998, 19:85–92.

97. E. Lenz, Der einfluss von fluoriden auf das korrosionsverhalten von titan, Dtsch. Zahnärztl. Z., 1997, 52:351–354.

98. R. G. Kelly, J. R. Scully, D. W. Shoesmith, and R. G. Buchheit, Electrochemical techniques in corrosion science and engineering, (Marcel Dekker, New York, 2002).

99. K. R. Trethewey and J. Chamberlain, Corrosion for science and engineering, 2nd Edition, (Longman Harlow, Essex, 1995).

100. U. Kamachi Mudali, T. M. Sridhar, N. Eliaz, and B. Raj, Failure of stainless steel implants: Causes and remedies, Corrosion Reviews, 2003, 21:231–267.

101. D. Sharan, The problem of corrosion in orthopedic implant materials, Orthop. Update (India), 1999, 9:1–5.

102. D. Starosvetsky and I. Gotman, Corrosion behavior of titanium nitride coated Ni–Ti shape memory surgical alloy, Biomaterials, 2001, 22:1853–1859.

103. R. Hubler, Hardness and corrosion protection enhancement behavior of surgical implant surfaces treated with ceramic thin films, Surf. Coat. Technol., 1999, 116–119:1111–1115.

104. C. D. Griffin, R. A. Buchanan, and J. E. Lemons, *In vivo* electrochemical corrosion study of coupled surgical implant materials, J. Biomed. Mater. Res., 1983, 17:489–500.

105. J. B. Park and R. S. Lakes, Metallic implant materials, in Biomaterials: An introduction, (Plenum Press, New York, 1992) pp:75–115.

106. B. Normand, F. Renaud, C. Coddet, and F. Tourenne, The effect of spraying conditions on the corrosion resistance of titanium coatings for surgical implants, Proc. 9th National Thermal Spraying Conference, ed. C. S. Berndt, (ASM, Materials Park, Ohio, 1996) pp:73–78.

107. J. E. Lemons, Surface modifications of surgical implants, Surf. Coat. Technol., 1998, 103–104:135–137.
108. K. Hayashi, T. Mashima, and K., Uenoyama, The effect of hydroxyapatite coating by bony ingrowth into grooved titanium implants, Biomaterials, 1999, 20:111–119.
109. E. M. Ortrun, Failures of metallic orthopedic implants, in Metals Handbook, Vol. 11: Failure analysis and prevention, 9th Edition, eds. R. J Shipley and W. T. Becker, (ASM, Ohio, 1986) pp:670–694.

CHAPTER 4

SURFACE MODIFICATION OF METALLIC BIOMATERIALS

Takao Hanawa

Institute of Biomaterials and Bioengineering
Tokyo Medical and Dental University
2–3–10 Kanda-Surugadai, Chiyoda-ku, Tokyo 101–0062
E-mail: hanawa.met@tmd.ac.jp

When a metallic material is implanted into a human body, immediate reaction occurs between its surface and the living tissues. In other words, immediate reaction at this initial stage straightaway determines and defines a metallic material's tissue compatibility. Since conventional metallic biomaterials are usually covered with metal oxides, surface oxide films on metallic materials play an important role not only against corrosion but also in tissue compatibility. Surface properties of a metallic material may be controlled with surface modification techniques. To develop and apply the appropriate surface modification technique, knowledge of the material's surface composition is absolutely necessary. This is because surface modification is a process that improves surface property by changing the composition and structure, while leaving the mechanical properties of the material intact. Since surface properties are critically important in biomaterials, issues closely related to this aspect of metallic biomaterials are discussed here: Surface compositions of metallic biomaterials; How surface compositions change due to interaction with human tissues; and How to control surface compositions and morphologies using surface modification techniques.

4.1 Surface of Metals

The definition of "surface" varies in situations. In this section, only the general concept will be explained.

Atoms in metallic materials located at the surface are considered partly reactive to the environment because atomic configuration terminates at the surface. The surface represents a property different from that inside the material. Due to high surface energy, a single molecular layer forms easily on solid surface where gas molecules are adsorbed at 1 Pa in 10^{-4} seconds. For example, in the presence of oxygen atoms, oxygen atoms and metal atoms chemically bond together to form an oxide layer. This phenomenon occurs even at the surface of gold — which is the most noble metal. Unlike ceramics and polymers, enrichment of component elements occurs easily at metal surfaces. This means that the surface composition of a metal is different from its inside composition in the order of nanometers. Therefore the variant surface composition of a metallic material contributes significantly to defining the overall properties of the material.

A metal surface is usually covered with a surface oxide film. The surface oxide layer, on the other hand, is always covered with surface hydroxyl groups that are adsorbed by water (Figure 4–1). Of particular interest in this chapter is the surface oxide film.

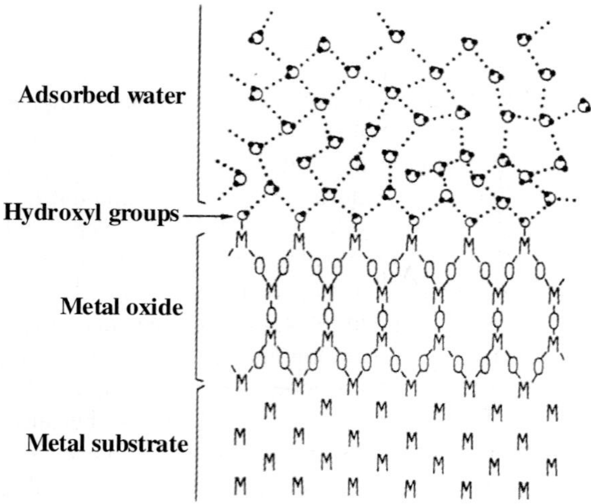

Figure 4–1   Schematic model of the structure of surface layer consisting of oxide layer hydroxyl group layer and adsorbed water layer on metals and alloys

4.2   Surface Oxide Film

Except in reduction environments, the corrosion process always causes a reaction film to form on metallic materials. Passive film is one such reaction film and is particularly significant for corrosion protection. When solubility is extremely low and pores are absent, adhesion of film — which is formed in an aqueous solution —to the substrate will be strong. The film then becomes a corrosion-resistant or passive film. Passive film is about 1–5 nm thick and transparent. Due to the tremendously fast rate at which it is formed, passive film readily becomes amorphous. For example, film on a titanium metal substrate was generated in 30 seconds. This was estimated from the time transient of current of titanium at 1 V vs. SCE after exposing the metal surface as shown in

Figure 4–2.   Since amorphous films hardly contain grain boundary and structural defects, they are corrosion-resistant.   However, corrosion resistance decreases with crystallization.   Fortunately, passive films contain water molecules that promote and maintain amorphousness.

Metallic materials — such as stainless steels, cobalt–chromium alloys, commercially pure titanium, and titanium alloys — used for biomedical devices are covered by their characteristic passive films.   These films self-repair when they are disrupted by some causes (as given in Figure 4–2).   Noble metals and alloys such as dental alloys are also covered with an oxide layer.   While the oxide layer protects against corrosion, it is not chemically strong like the passive film.

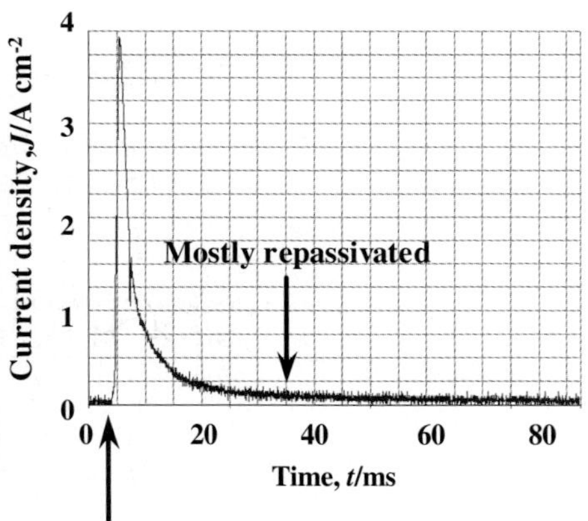

Figure 4–2 Time transient of anodic current of titanium in Hanks' solution under 1 V charge versus a saturated calomel electrode (SCE); anodic current is generated with the dissolution and repassivation of titanium

4.2.1 Titanium

When titanium was polished in de-ionized water and analyzed using X-ray photoelectron spectroscopy (XPS), the Ti 2p spectrum obtained from the titanium gave four doublets according to valence: Ti^0, Ti^{2+}, Ti^{3+}, and Ti^{4+}. Published data [1] were used to determine the binding energy of each valence. Figure 4–3 shows an example of the decomposition of Ti 2p spectrum.

A distinct Ti^0 peak at metallic state was observed, which accounted for a very thin surface oxide film at less than a few nanometers only. Besides, Ti^{4+} (TiO_2), Ti^{3+} (Ti_2O_3), and Ti^{2+} (TiO) were detected. Though Ti^{2+} oxide existed in the surface oxide film, Ti^{2+} formation is always thermodynamically less favorable than Ti^{3+} formation at the surface. The surface film on titanium consisted mainly of amorphous or low-crystalline and non-stoichiometric TiO_2, and the film stood firm against chloride ions.

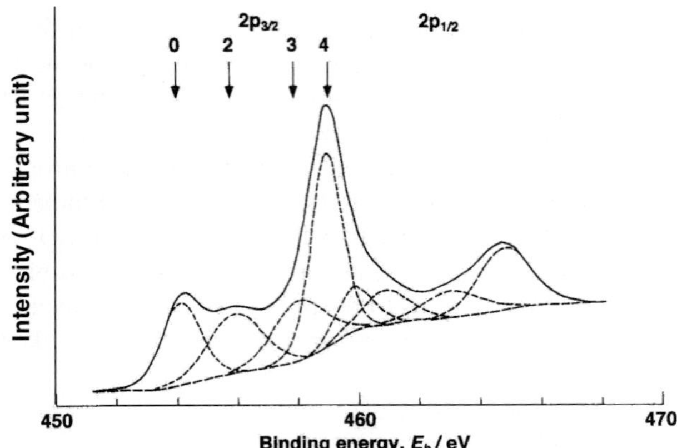

Figure 4–3 Decomposition of Ti 2p XPS spectrum obtained from titanium abraded and immersed for 300 seconds in water into eight peaks ($2p_{3/2}$ and $2p_{1/2}$ electron peaks in four valences); numbers with arrows are valence numbers

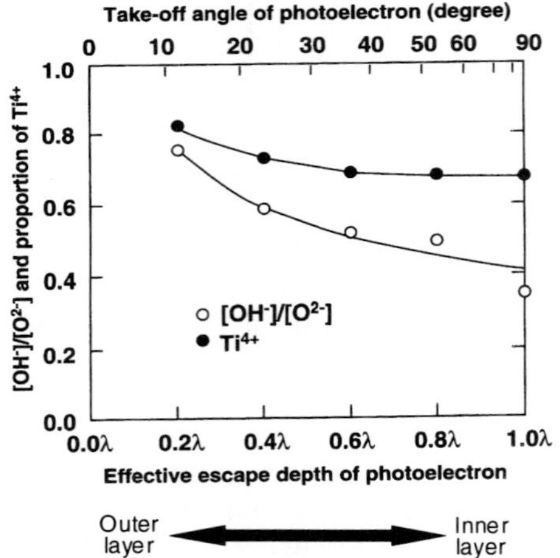

Figure 4–4 The proportional ratio of OH^- concentration to that of O^{2-} (*i.e.*, $[OH^-]/[O^{2-}]$), and the proportion of cationic fraction of Ti^{4+} among titanium species in surface oxide film of titanium polished in water plotted against the average effective escape depth of photoelectrons for angle-resolved XPS measurements [2]. Lambda (λ) is the average escape depth of O 1s and Ti $2p_{3/2}$ photoelectrons, and the effective escape depth is obtained by (escape depth x sine[take-off-angle]). The values at small take-off angles of photoelectron (or effective escape depths of photoelectron) represent outer region information and those larger ones represent inner region information.

Since a considerable portion of oxidized titanium stayed as Ti^{2+} and Ti^{3+} in the surface film, the oxidation process might proceed to the end just at the uppermost part of the surface film. As shown in Figure 4–4, the proportion of Ti^{4+} among titanium cations (Ti^{2+}, Ti^{3+} and Ti^{4+}) in the film decreased with increase of photoelectron take-off angle [2], indicating that more Ti^{4+} existed near the outer layer in the film. Deducing from the take-off angle dependence of $[OH^-]/[O^{2-}]$ in Figure 4–4, oxygen atoms in the hydroxyl group were mainly located in the outer part of the surface film. This means that dehydration proceeded inside the surface film, and only partly for Ti^{4+} oxide.

Thickness of the film was about 2 nm just after polishing, and about 5 nm at one week after polishing (as shown in Figure 4–5). Note too that thickness of the surface oxide film increased according to the logarithmic rule which is common in the initial growth of oxide films of metallic materials.

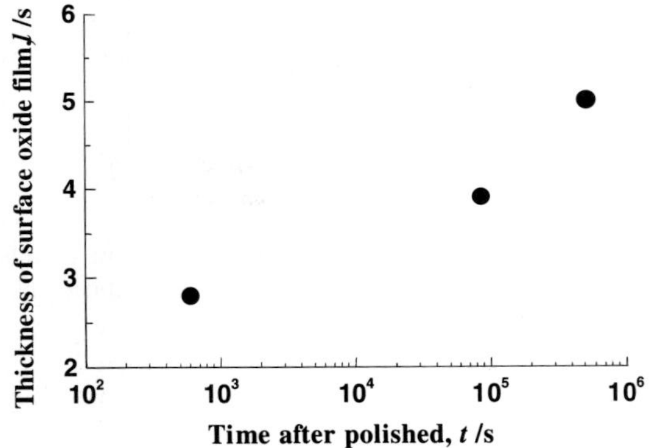

Figure 4–5 Thickness of the surface oxide film on titanium as a function of time after polishing

4.2.2 Titanium Alloys

The film on Ti–6Al–4V alloy was almost the same as that on titanium, containing a small amount of aluminum oxide [3,4]. In other words, the surface oxide film on Ti–6Al–4V was a TiO_2 containing small amounts of Al_2O_3, hydroxyl groups, and bound water. Vanadium contained in the alloy was not detected in the oxide film after the alloy was polished.

The Ti–56Ni shape memory alloy was covered by TiO_2-based oxide, with minimal amounts of nickel in both the oxide and metallic states [3,4]. The film on Ti–56Ni was a TiO_2 containing small amounts of metallic nickel, NiO, hydroxyl groups, and bound water.

In Ti–Zr alloy, the surface oxide film consisted of titanium and zirconium oxides [5]. The relative concentration ratio of titanium to zirconium in the film was almost the same as that in the alloy (Figure 4–6). In the surface oxide film, titanium and zirconium were uniformly distributed along the depth. The thickness of the film increased with increase of zirconium content. The chemical state of zirconium was more stable than that of titanium in the film.

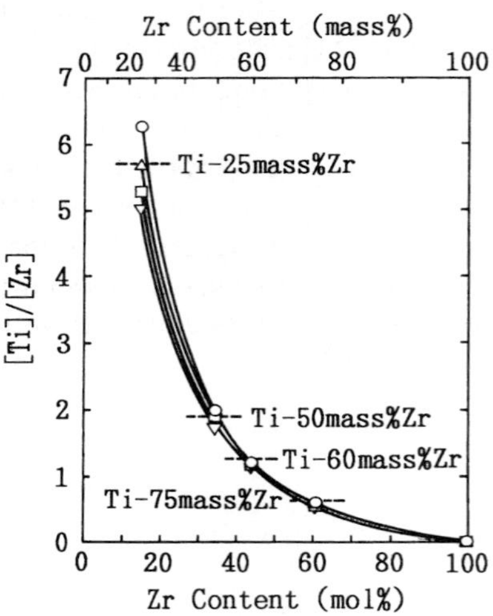

Figure 4–6 Change in ratio of the concentration of titanium to that of zirconium, [Ti]/[Zr], as the zirconium content increases [5]; dashed lines indicate the [Ti]/[Zr] values from nominal compositions of specimens

4.2.3 Stainless Steel

Compositions of surface oxide films on stainless steels are well understood in the field of engineering. In an austenitic stainless steel, the surface oxide film consists of iron, chromium, and a small amount of molybdenum. But it does not contain nickel while in the air and in chloride solutions [6,7].

On the other hand, surface oxide film on 316L steel polished mechanically in de-ionized water consists of oxide species of iron, chromium, nickel, molybdenum and manganese, and its thickness is about 3.6 nm [8]. The surface film contains a large amount of OH^- — the oxide which is hydrated or oxyhydroxidized (Figure 4–7). The surface oxide film is also enriched with iron, while the alloy substrate just under the film is enriched with nickel, molybdenum, and manganese.

4.2.4 Co–Cr–Mo Alloy

Surface oxide film of a Co–Cr–Mo alloy is characterized as containing oxides of cobalt and chromium without molybdenum [9].

On the other hand, the surface oxide film on another Co–Cr–Mo alloy polished mechanically in de-ionized water consists of oxide species of cobalt, chromium and molybdenum, and its thickness is about 2.5 nm [10]. This surface film contains a large amount of OH⁻ — the oxide which is hydrated or oxyhydroxidized. There are also more traces of chromium and molybdenum distributed at the inner layer of the film.

4.2.5 Noble Metal Alloys

Au–Cu–Ag alloys and Ag–Pd–Cu–Au alloys for dental restoration are covered by copper oxide and/or silver oxide [11]. An Ag–In alloy is covered by zinc oxide and indium oxide, and an Ag–Sn–Zn alloy is covered by tin oxide and zinc oxide. Dental amalgams (Ag–Sn–Cu–Hg alloys) are covered by tin oxide [12]. While these oxides serve as a protective film against corrosion, they are not as chemically strong as the passive film.

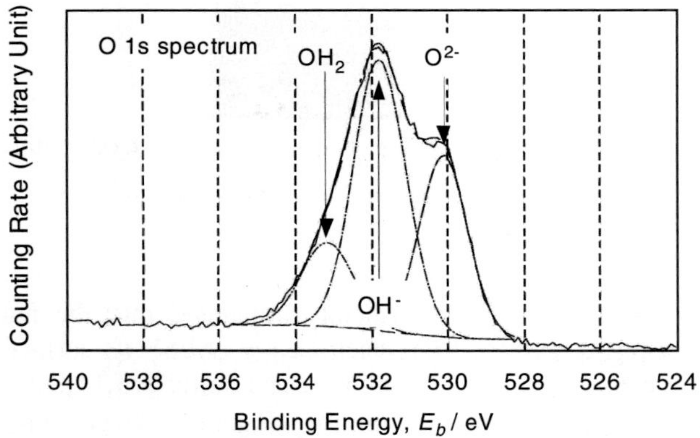

Figure 4–7 Typical O 1s spectrum obtained from 316L austenitic stainless steel and its de-convolution into O^{2-}, OH^- and H_2O components

4.3   Reconstruction of Surface Oxide Film

Composition of surface oxide film varies according to environmental changes, though the film is macroscopically stable. Passive surfaces co-exist in close contact with electrolytes, undergoing a continuous process of partial dissolution and re-precipitation from the microscopic viewpoint. In this sense, surface composition is always changing according to the environment (Figure 4–8).

Due to abrasion with bone and other materials, surface oxide film may be scratched and destroyed during insertion and implantation into living tissues. Fretting corrosion also leads to film destruction. Fortunately, surface oxide is immediately regenerated in a biological environment where biofluid surrounds the metallic material. However, the composition and properties of the oxide film regenerated in a biological environment may be different from those in water.

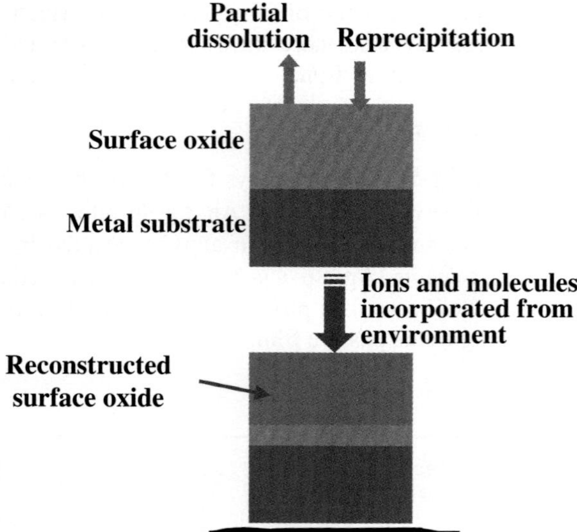

Figure 4–8   Schematic reconstruction model of surface oxide film on metallic biomaterials

4.3.1 Titanium

When titanium which has been surgically implanted into the human jaw is characterized using Auger electron spectroscopy (AES), its surface oxide film reveals constituents of calcium, phosphorus, and sulfur [13,14]. By immersing titanium and its alloys in Hanks' solution (Figure 4–9) and other solutions [3–5,15], preferential adsorption of phosphate ions occurs — leading to formation of calcium phosphate on their surfaces [16].

Hanks' solution, whose pH is 7.4, is an artificial biofluid. Its inorganic composition is similar to extracellular fluid. Hydrated phosphate ions are adsorbed by a hydrated titanium oxide surface during the release of protons [15]. Calcium ions are then adsorbed by phosphate ions — which are adsorbed on the titanium surface, thus leading to calcium phosphate being formed eventually. On the same note, when titanium is immersed in Hanks' solution containing albumin, a non-uniform and porous albumin-containing apatite[*] is formed [17]. The above phenomena are characteristic of titanium and its alloys [4].

---

*Apatite is a general term referring to similar crystals, and the predominant apatite is hydroxyapatite. Here, apatite refers to hydroxyapatite.

The surface oxide film regenerated in Hanks' solution contains phosphate ions in the outermost layer. Phosphate ions are preferentially taken up during regeneration of surface oxide film on titanium. The resultant film comprises titanium oxide and titanium oxyhydroxide — and the latter contains titanium phosphate. Following regeneration, calcium and phosphate ions are adsorbed to the film, thus forming calcium phosphate or calcium titanium phosphate on the outermost surface as shown in Figure 4–10 [2].

Calcium phosphate precipitates faster on a surface film regenerated in a biological system than that in water because seeds of calcium phosphate already exist on the regenerated film. Extrapolating from here, it can be assumed that bone formation is faster on titanium implanted in hard tissue simply because the surface oxide film is titanium oxide. On this basis, surface modification was attempted on titanium using this repassivation reaction [18].

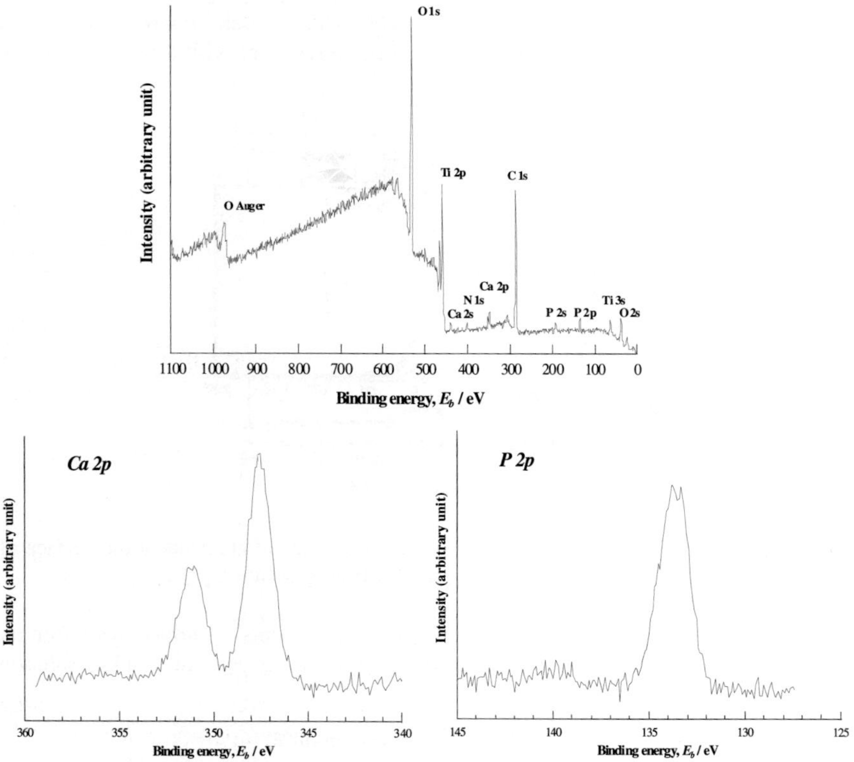

Figure 4–9 XPS spectra of survey: Ca 2p and P 2p regions obtained from titanium immersed in Hanks' solution for one day. Peak binding energies of Ca 2p and P 2p regions reveal that calcium and phosphorus exist as calcium phosphate.

                                    T. Hanawa

4.3.2 Titanium Alloys

Calcium phosphate is also formed on Ti–6Al–4V and Ti–56Ni alloys after immersion in Hanks' solution, but the [Ca]/[P] ratios are smaller than that in titanium [3,4]. On the other hand, only phosphate without calcium is formed on Ti–Zr alloys that contain over 50mass%Zr [5].

Ti–6Al–4V, Ti–56Ni, and Ti–xZr (x=0, 25, 50, 60, 75, 100 in mass%) alloys were abraded and kept for 300 seconds in water and Hanks' solution [19]. The regenerated surface oxide film in Hanks' solution was characterized using XPS. As summarized in Tables 4–1 to 4–3, phosphate ions are preferentially taken up in the surface oxide film during regeneration. Besides calcium and phosphate, other ionic constituents of Hanks' solution were absent from the surface oxide film. In the case of titanium and Ti–6Al–4V, calcium phosphate was found in the surface oxide film regenerated in Hanks' solution. However, for Ti–56Ni, Ti–Zr and zirconium, phosphate without calcium was formed on the surfaces instead. These results are in good agreement with those of titanium alloys immersed in Hanks' solution.

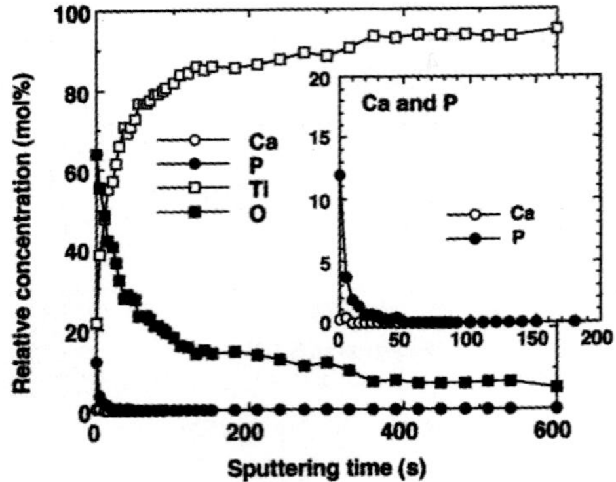

Figure 4–10 AES depth profiles of relative concentrations of elements at the surface of titanium abraded and immersed for 300 seconds in Hanks' solution [2]

Table 4–1 XPS results for relative concentrations of elements in surface oxide film on Ti–6Al–4V (Ti–10.2at%Al–3.6at%V) regenerated in water and in Hanks' solution during 300-s immersion [33]

Abraded in	Relative concentration (at%)					
	Ti	Al	V	O	Ca	P
Water	24.5 (0.9)*	3.8 (1.1)	0.0 (0.0)	71.8 (0.1)	0.0 (0.0)	0.0 (0.0)
Hanks	21.4 (0.1)	3.2 (0.2)	0.0 (0.0)	73.2 (0.3)	0.1 (0.0)	2.2 (0.0)

* Standard deviations

Table 4–2 XPS results for relative concentrations of elements in surface oxide film on Ti–56Ni (Ti–50at%Ni) regenerated in water and in Hanks' solution during 300-s immersion [33]

Abraded in	Relative concentration (at%)				
	Ti	Ni	O	Ca	P
Water	23.4 (0.1)*	7.2 (0.7)	69.4 (0.6)	0.0 (0.0)	0.0 (0.0)
Hanks	24.0 (0.4)	5.6 (0.7)	69.0 (0.6)	0.0 (0.0)**	1.4 (0.2)

*   Standard deviations
** Trace amount

Table 4–3 XPS results for relative concentrations of elements in surface oxide film on titanium, zirconium, and Ti–Zr alloys regenerated in water (top values) and in Hanks' solution (bottom values) during 300-s immersion [33]

	Relative concentration (at%)				
	Ti	Zr	O	Ca	P
Ti	29.6	0.0	70.4	0.0	0.0
	28.6	0.0	70.6	0.2	0.7
Ti–mass25Zr	29.4	4.7	65.9	0.0	0.0
(18.7at%Zr)	24.1	4.0	70.2	0.0	1.7
Ti–mass50Zr	23.7	12.0	64.3	0.0	0.0
(40.8at%Zr)	18.2	9.1	70.7	0.0	1.9
Ti–mass60Zr	18.6	15.5	65.9	0.0	0.0
(50at%Zr)	16.1	11.8	70.5	0.0	1.7
Ti–mass75Zr	12.7	20.9	66.4	0.0	0.0
(67.4at%Zr)	10.0	15.5	72.4	0.0	2.1
Zr	0.0	32.1	67.9	0.0	0.0
	0.0	20.6	77.5	0.0	1.9

4.3.3 Stainless Steel

In pins and wires made from 316L austenitic stainless steel, calcium and phosphorus are present in the surface oxide [20]. The corrosion product of 316L steel implanted in the femur — as part of an artificial hip joint — consists of chromium combined with sulfur, and/or iron combined with phosphorus (where the latter contains calcium and chlorine) [21].

Five surface oxide specimens of stainless steel were prepared according to the following methods [8]:

- Polishing in de-ionized water;
- Autoclaving;
- Immersion in Hanks' solution;

- Immersion in cell culture medium; and
- Incubation with cultured cells.

Next, XPS was performed to find out the following:
- Composition of surface oxide film;
- Composition of substrate; and
- Thickness of surface oxide film.

For 316L steel polished in de-ionized water, the surface oxide film consisted of iron and chromium oxides which contained small amount of nickel, molybdenum and manganese oxides. The surface oxide also contained a large amount of OH^-.

For specimens immersed in Hanks' solution and in cell culture medium, as well as incubated with culture cells, calcium phosphate was formed. Sulfate was adsorbed by the surface oxide film and reduced to sulfite in cell culture medium and with the cultured cells. The results in this study suggest that nickel and manganese are depleted in the oxide film. The surface oxide changes into iron and chromium oxides, where a small amount of molybdenum oxide will be present in the human body.

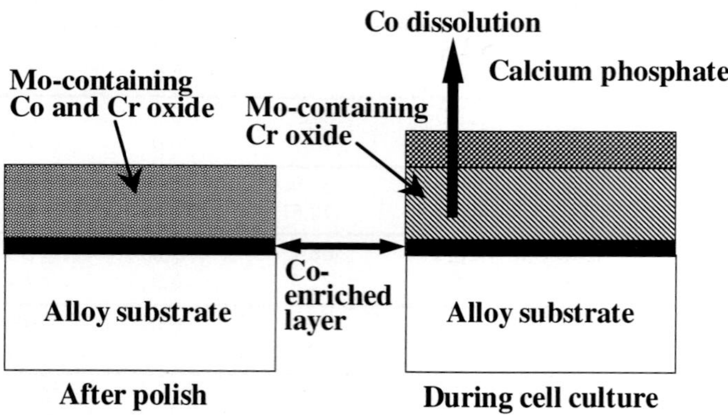

Figure 4–11   Schematic illustration of reconstruction of surface oxide film on a Co–Cr–Mo alloy after polishing and during cell culture [10]

4.3.4 Co–Cr–Mo Alloy

In Co–Cr–Mo alloy, cobalt was dissolved during immersion in the Hanks' solution and in cell culture medium, as well as during incubation in a cell culture [10]. After dissolution, the surface oxide consisted of chromium oxide (Cr^{3+}) which contained molybdenum oxide (Mo^{4+}, Mo^{5+}, and Mo^{6+}). Results from angle-resolved XPS revealed that chromium and molybdenum were more widely distributed in the inner layer than in the outer layer of the oxide film.

In body fluids, cobalt is completely dissolved. The surface oxide changes into chromium oxide containing a small amount of molybdenum oxide. Calcium phosphate is also formed on the top surface. The above process is shown using a schematic illustration in Figure 4–11.

4.4   Adsorption of Proteins

When a metallic material is implanted into a human body and in contact with its living tissues, proteins are immediately adsorbed by the material (as shown in Figure 4–12).

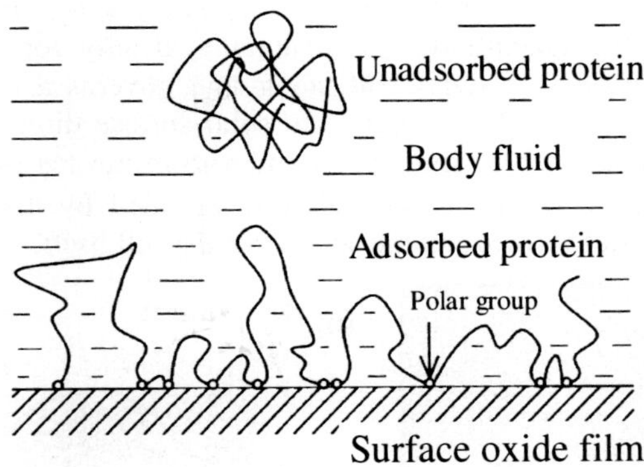

Figure 4–12 Possible model of protein adsorption by metals

Proteins adsorption influences material corrosion, and subsequently cells adhesion. Likewise, proteins denaturalization and fragmentation (which occur due to adsorption) may affect the function of the host body. To characterize proteins adsorbed to metals and metal oxides, various techniques can be used [22], especially that of ellipsometry [23]. To predict proteins adsorption, the wettability test is used where a liquid droplet is applied to the material [24].

Adsorption behavior of albumin to a metal surface varies according to the metallic element as follows [25]:

- Titanium, aluminum, molybdenum, cobalt, nickel, and tantalum — adsorption amount of albumin is small both at the initial and later stages.
- Vanadium — small adsorption amount at the initial stage, but amount increases at the later stage.
- Silver, gold, and copper — large adsorption amount at the initial stage, and amount increases further at the later stage.

These results reveal that proteins adsorption is governed not only by surface energy, but also by a metal's electrostatic force. The adsorption of fibronectin, α-lacto albumin, α-amilaze and albumin, bovine serum albumin, and glycosaminogrycan by titanium or titanium dioxide were investigated. Serum proteins were adsorbed by titanium surface through cations such as calcium ions in a CaCl$_2$ solution. Adsorption amount of albumin by titanium dioxide, on the other hand, was controlled by Ca^{2+} and HPO_4^{2-}.

4.5   Adhesion of Cells

Affinity for cells is one important property for biomaterials, because they are always used adjacent to living tissues. Qualitatively, cells adhesion is evaluated by observing the cells adhering to the surface under a microscope. However, to develop new biomaterials with superior biocompatibility, it is absolutely necessary to evaluate quantitatively a material's affinity for cells. This is because cells adhesion is a significant factor that governs a material's tissue compatibility. Since cells do not adhere to solid surface directly, but through cell adhesion proteins such as fibronectin and vitronectin (as shown in Figure 4–13), the adhesion force to a material is determined by the adsorption of proteins to the material surface and the activity of the cell itself.

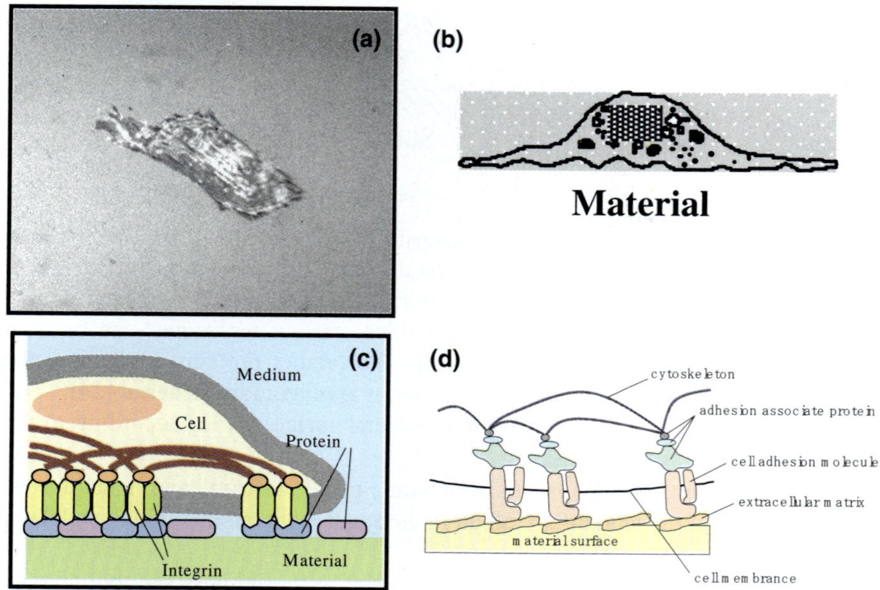

Figure 4–13 (a) Interference reflection microscopic image of human fibroblast cells IMR–90 adhered to a glass surface; (b) schematic image of cell adhesion to a material; (c) & (d) schematic models of cell adhesion mechanism to a material

Adhesion of osteoblasts and fibroblasts to titanium, titanium alloys and a Co–Cr alloy were investigated from the viewpoint of hard tissue compatibility [26]. Adhesion of epitherial cells to titanium was investigated from the viewpoint of dental implant [27]. In these studies, effects of surface roughness, pores, grooves, and surface treatment on cells adhesion were investigated — a stretch of cells, for example, resided in the grooves [26]. In the case of osteoblasts and osteoblastic cells, osteiod tissue formation was also investigated [28].

One method to quantitatively evaluate a material's affinity for cells is to measure the detachment force of an adherent cell on the material. A new system was developed to measure directly the shear force required to detach a cell from a material [29]. Using a micro-cantilever, the detachment force was measured in the cell culture medium by applying a lateral load to the cell which adhered to the material. The schematic illustration of the system is shown in Figure 4–14. Adhesive properties of L929 to sputter-deposited metal films depend on the types of metal to which they adhere (as shown in Figure 4–14). Among titanium, chromium, aluminum, gold, silver, and palladium, cells on chromium and titanium had the highest cell adhesive shear strength and cell detachment surface energy — almost close to those of glass materials [30].

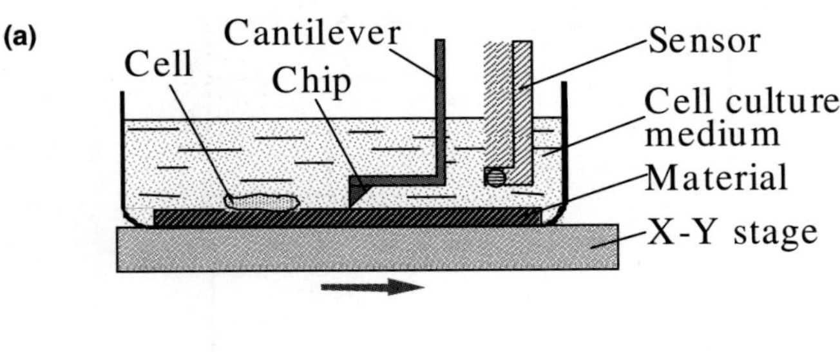

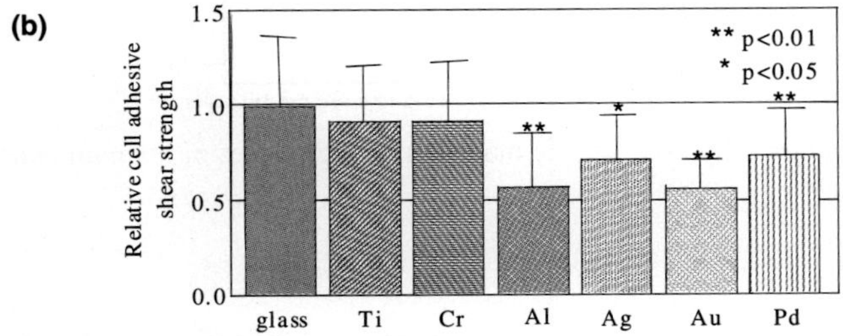

Figure 4–14 (a) Principle of shear force measurement for cell detachment from a material using a newly developed instrument, and force displacement curves obtained with the instrument [29]; (b) relative cell adhesive shear strength of L929 to thin metal films normalized by cell adhesive shear strength of L929 to glass [30]

4.6   Surface Modification

Surface modification is a process that changes a material's surface composition, structure and morphology, leaving the bulk mechanical properties intact. With surface modification, chemical and mechanical durability, as well as tissue compatibility of surface layer could be improved. Surface property is particularly significant for biomaterials, and thus surface modification techniques are particularly useful to biomaterials. Dry-process (using ion beam) and hydro-process (which is performed in aqueous solutions) are predominant surface modification techniques. Apatite coating on titanium with plasma spray, titanium nitride coating with sputter deposition, and titanium oxide growth with morphological control by electrolysis are already available for commercial use (as shown in Figure 4–15).

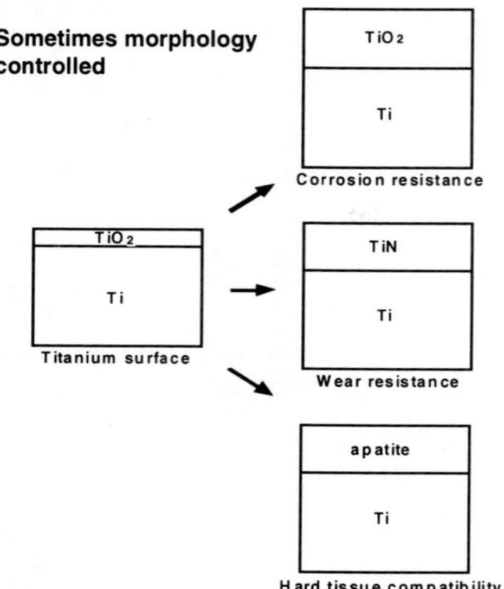

Figure 4–15 Commercially used surface modification techniques of titanium (when it is used as biomaterial)

4.6.1 Purpose

In biomaterials, the chief purpose of surface modification is to improve corrosion resistance, wear resistance, antibacterial property, and tissue compatibility. Shown in Figure 4–16 are schematic illustrations of artificial hip joint, bone plate, and screws.

When the sliding interface between head and socket is worn, wear debris will be generated. Fretting fatigue and crevice corrosion may occur at fixation site of plate with screws. Metallic elements are released as ions and wear debris due to corrosion and wear, causing metallosis of the surrounding tissue and loosening at the fixation site. Although commercial metallic biomaterials are corrosion-resistant, trace metal ions may be released because of characteristic corrosion mechanism in the human body. In bone implant materials, rapid bone conductivity is required. In cardiovascular devices, blood compatibility or antithrombogenecity is required. In dental implants, soft tissue compatibility is required to prevent bacteria invasion from the crevice — which is between the dental implant and gingival epithelium (Figure 4–17).

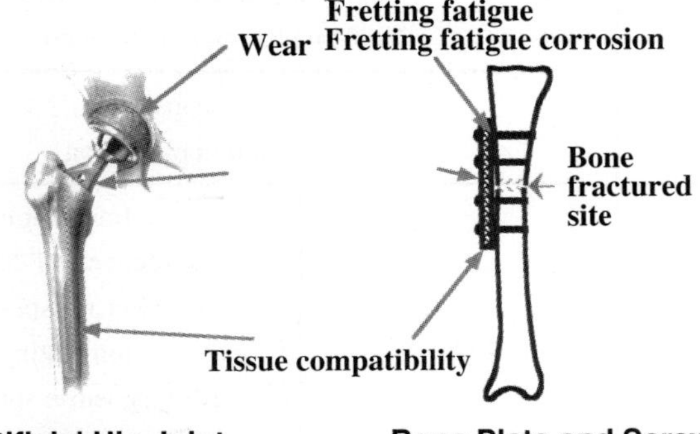

Figure 4–16 Schematic illustrations of artificial hip joint, bone plate and screws, and problems sometimes occurring in clinical use

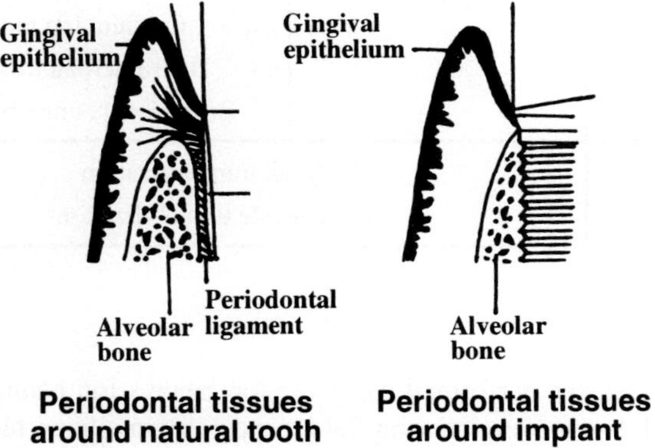

Figure 4–17 Schematic illustrations of periodontal tissues around natural tooth and dental implant material — bacteria may invade from the pocket between gingival epithelium and dental implant. Dental implant must fix with alveolar bone.

Surface modification processes are categorized into dry processes and hydro-processes.　Surface modification techniques being investigated are summarized in Table 4–4 according to their objectives.

Table 4–4 Surface modification techniques for metallic biomaterials

Purpose	Techniques	
Improve corrosion resistance	Immersion Anodic polarization or electrolysis Noble metal ion implantation	
Improve wear resistance	TiN layer deposition Nitrogen ion implantation	
Improve hard tissue compatibility	Apatite layer formation	Immersion Electrochemical deposition Plasma spray Ion plating RF magnetron sputtering Pulse laser deposition
	Non-apatite layer formation	Immersion in alkaline solution and heating Immersion in H_2O_2 Calcium ion implantation Calcium ion mixing Hydrothermal treatment Biomolecule unmobilization
Improve blood compatibility	Polymer unmobilization Biomolecule unmobilization	

4.6.2 Dry Process

Most dry processes are performed using the ion beam.　Ion beam technology is particularly useful in the engineering field, especially in silicon technology.　Ion beam technology permits the formation of thin films at atomic and molecular levels, as well as low temperature syntheses utilizing ionic effects.　The process is thermal-unequilibrium, thus making it possible to synthesize unnatural substances.

Ion beam technology has contributed significantly to the modification of biomaterial surfaces.　It can be classified according to the effects on solid surface: film formation, sputtering, and ion implantation. When ion impacts a material surface, attaching, sputtering and implantation effects occur according to the ion's energy (Figure 4–18).

By utilizing these effects, thin film formation, graded-composition layer, and unequilibrium layer are obtained. Figure 4–18 also presents surface modification techniques as a function of ion energy and thickness of the resultant surface-modified layer. This figure serves only as a guide and need not be true for advanced techniques. Figure 4–19 shows the key principles of predominant dry processes, plasma spray, and ion implantation.

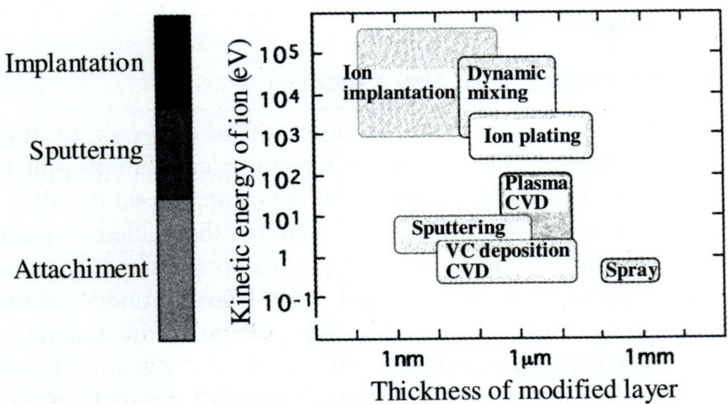

Figure 4–18 Effects of ion irradiation on solid surface due to ion energy (hence the ion beam technique as a function of kinetic ion energy), and the resultant thickness of modified layer

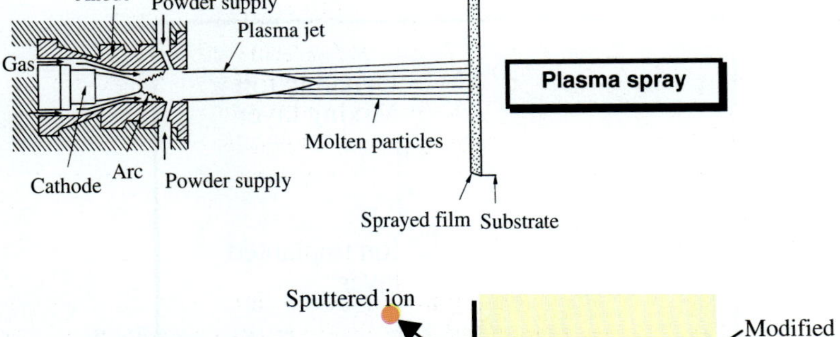

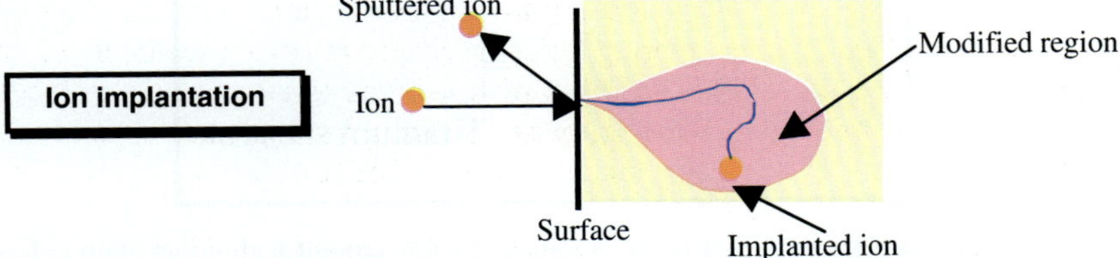

Figure 4–19 Principles of plasma spray and ion implantation

4.6.3 Hydro-Process

Hydro-process is performed in aqueous solutions. This process does not require large facilities and cost as immersion or electrolysis in aqueous solutions is a basic process. The resultant modified layer changes according to changes in the following parameters:

- Composition and pH of aqueous solution;
- Potential gain due to electrolysis; and
- Current density of electrolysis.

4.7　Apatite Film Formation

4.7.1 Apatite Formation with Dry Process

The chief purpose for surface modification of titanium is to improve its hard-tissue compatibility. This is done by forming a calcium phosphate film on the titanium surface. Currently, plasma spraying of apatite on metallic materials is widely used to form the apatite layer — which is the nucleus for active bone formation and conductivity. In the case of plasma-sprayed apatite, however, the apatite-titanium interface or apatite itself may fracture under relatively low stress because of low interface bonding strength and low toughness of the sprayed layer itself [31]. To overcome this weakness, dynamic ion mixing is applied to form an apatite with high interface bonding strength. Calcium ions are implanted during the mixing process to induce strong bonding between the apatite film and the titanium substrate, with implanted calcium ions serving as a binder (as shown in Figure 4–20). Sputter deposition of apatite is now done by using RF magnetron sputtering and laser-pulse deposition.

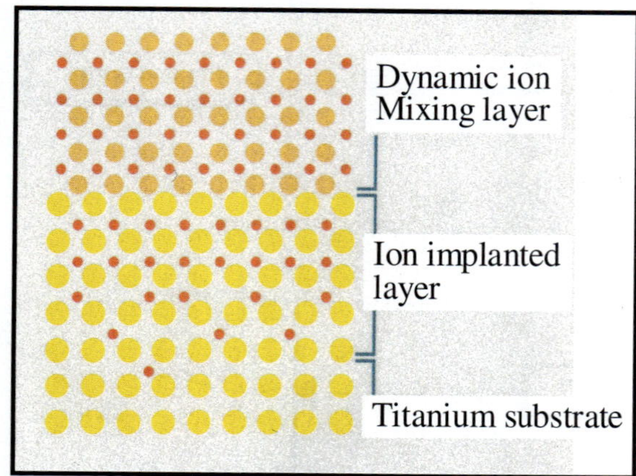

Figure 4–20　Surface-modified layer produced by ion mixing techniques with calcium ion implantation and sputter deposition of hydroxyapatite

Solubility of ceramics increases as its crystallinity decreases. The crystallinity of a thin film formed with ion beam is low and the solubility is high. The crystallinity of coated apatite is an important factor because crystallinity governs solubility in the human body. Low-crystalline film on titanium dissolves rapidly when the titanium is implanted into a human body. This is because the pH of body fluid can reach as low as 5. Thus heat treatment of apatite film is necessary to increase its crystallinity and reduce its solubility [31]. Therefore based on the discussion thus far in this section, the following issues must be carefully considered when ion beam technique is to be used to form the apatite layer:

- Composition of apatite layer;
- Coating efficiency;
- Bonding strength of apatite to substrate; and
- Crystallinity of apatite.

4.7.2 Apatite Formation with Hydro-Process

Titanium has a unique property that enables calcium phosphate to form on its surface in simulated biofluids [3–5,15]. When both the composition and pH of a solution are selected properly, apatite can be formed on titanium in the solution. The apatite formed by this technique contains a large amount of carbonate. Control of morphology, volume, and composition in the precipitate is difficult. Moreover, the apatite film is mechanically weak.

Electrochemical treatment [32,33] is used commonly to form an apatite layer on titanium. Through an electrochemical process, carbonate-containing apatite with desirable morphology such as plate, needle, and particle could be precipitated on titanium substrate. Figure 4–21 shows an example of morphology control using electrolysis techniques [32]. This process could also be used to coat substrates of complex design. When titanium with apatite fabricated by this process is implanted into rat femur, apatite-formed titanium shows larger bonding strength than untreated titanium.

4.8   Surface-Modified Layer for Bone Formation

Hard-tissue compatibility can be improved by modifying the titanium surface instead of the apatite film. In this section, various techniques to modify the titanium surface are given as follows:

- Immersion in alkaline solution and heating;
- Immersion in hydrogen peroxide solution;
- Immersion and hydrothermal treatment in calcium-containing solution; and
- Calcium ion implantation.

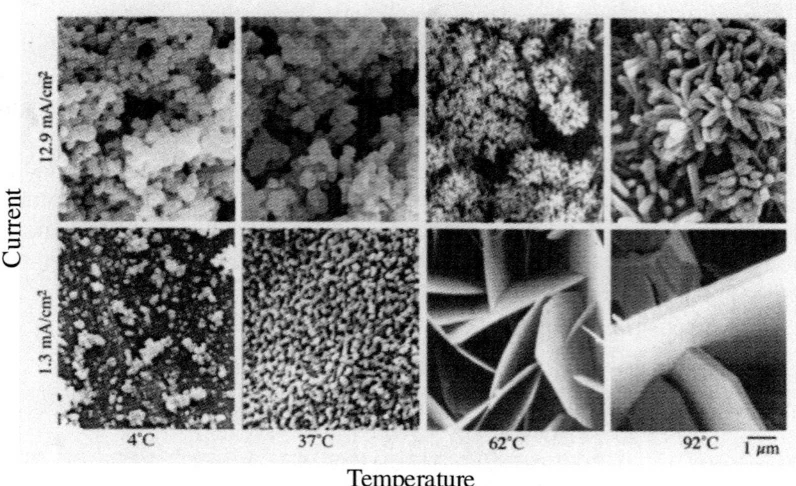

Figure 4–21   Hydroxyapatite precipitates with various morphologies according to different current and temperature readings in electrolysis [32]

4.8.1 Immersion in Alkaline Solution and Heating

When titanium is immersed in NaOH or KOH alkaline solution, a hydrated titanium oxide gel containing alkaline ions (gel-like titanium oxide containing hydroxyl groups) with 1 µm thickness is formed on the titanium substrate, as shown in Figure 4–22 [34]. Upon heating, the gel layer condenses and the gel bonds to the substrate strongly.

When titanium with the gel is immersed in a simulated biofluid, alkaline ions are released from the layer to the solution. Simultaneously hydronium ions are soaked up by the layer, eventually forming titania-hydrogel. This increases the magnitude of supersaturation of hydroxyapatite in the solution near the surface. The gel induces apatite nucleation, and the apatite layer is rapidly formed. This process is expected to accelerate bone formation on titanium in hard tissue.

4.8.2 Immersion in Hydrogen Peroxide Solution

When a material is implanted into a human body, macrophages will attach themselves to the material. The macrophages generate active oxygen species, which then react with the material. When titanium was incubated with macrophages, titanium dissolution was significantly accelerated in the presence of macrophages [35]. Hydrogen peroxide is an active oxygen species, and reaction between titanium and hydrogen peroxide was investigated [36]. As shown in Figure 4–23, this reaction was applied to induce the formation of a titanium oxide gel on titanium [37].

Immersion of titanium in $TaCl_2$-containing H_2O_2 accelerates apatite formation in a simulated body fluid. Pull-out test of specimens from rat tibia reveals increased bonding strength of titanium to the bone.

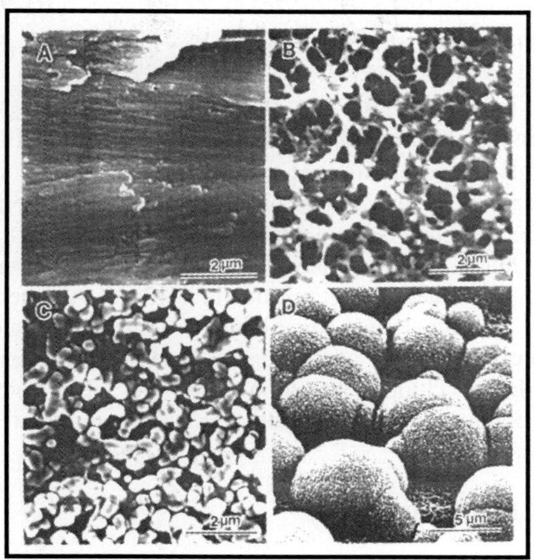

Figure 4–22　(a) Titanium surface before treatment; (b) after alkaline treatment; (c) after heat treatment; and (d) after immersion in a simulated body fluid in alkaline and heat treatments [34]

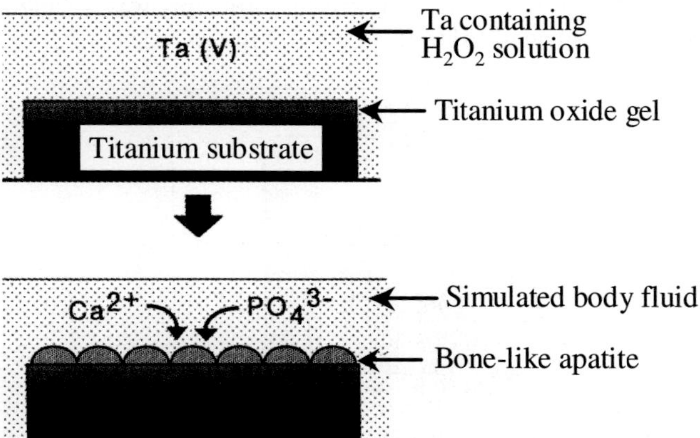

Figure 4–23　Schematic illustration of treating titanium with tantalum-containing hydrogen peroxide [37]

4.8.3 Immersion and Hydrothermal Treatment in Calcium-Containing Solution

A titanium oxide layer, which contains calcium hydroxide, is formed whenever titanium is immersed in any of the following calcium-containing solutions [38]:

- Calcium nitrate (pH 3.9);
- Calcium chloride (pH 7.4); and
- Calcium hydroxide (pH 12.6).

The oxide layer catalyzes the precipitation of calcium phosphate on titanium when immersed in Hanks' solution. As shown in Figures 4–24 and 4–25, the catalytic function was confirmed by mass changes, X-ray diffractometry, and XPS. It was also observed that the most effective means to precipitate apatite was immersion in alkaline solutions.

While in identical calcium-containing solutions, hydrothermal modification of titanium was performed using an autoclave [39]. Apatite precipitation in Hanks' solution was the largest on titanium modified in calcium hydroxide solution. On the other hand, apatite precipitation was prevented on titanium modified in calcium chloride solution. It was also noted that surface modification of titanium in calcium hydroxide was more effective with increase in temperature or pressure.

4.8.4 Calcium Ion Implantation

Calcium ion implantation is another surface modification technique used to improve the hard-tissue compatibility of titanium. When calcium ions are implanted into titanium, calcium phosphate precipitation in an electrolyte was speeded up [40] (as shown in Figure 4–26). MC3T3–E1 cells on titanium were activated to form osteoid tissue, and tissue formation was accelerated when calcium ions were implanted [41].

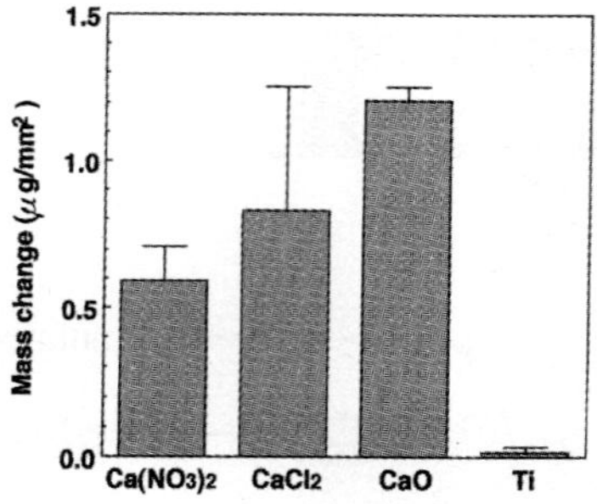

Figure 4–24 Mass changes of titanium specimens with and without modification in calcium nitrate, calcium chloride, and calcium oxide solutions before and after immersion in Hanks' solution [38]

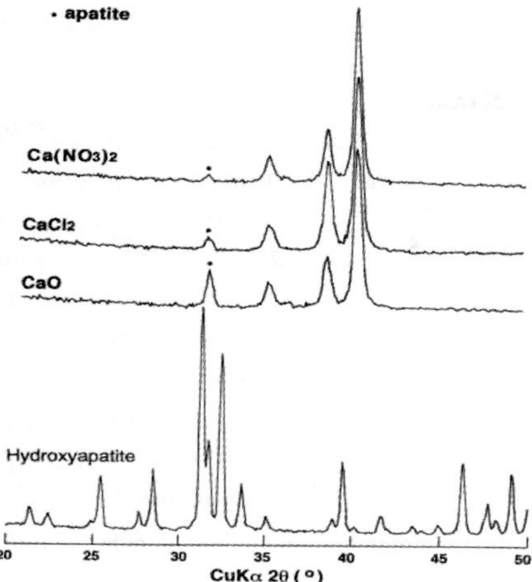

Figure 4–25 X-ray diffraction patterns of surface-modified titanium immersed in Hanks' solution at 37°C for 30 days and heated at 600°C for 30 minutes under a reduced pressure of 100 Pa [38]

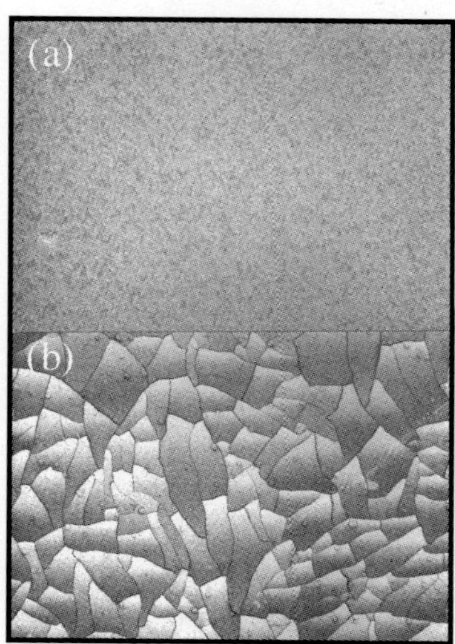

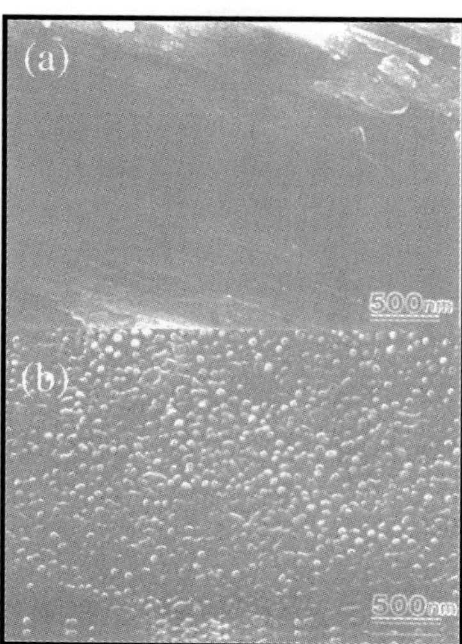

Figure 4–26 Scanning electron micrographs of (a) titanium; and (b) calcium-ion-implanted titanium [40]

Figure 4–27 Surfaces of (a) titanium; and (b) calcium-ion-implanted titanium after scraping off osteogenic cells with which these specimens are incubated for 14 days [41]

In Figure 4–27, both un-implanted titanium and calcium-ion-implanted titanium were incubated with MC3T3–E1 cells. Calcium phosphate formed only on calcium-ion-implanted titanium, but not on un-implanted titanium. Moreover, new osteoid tissue was formed earlier on calcium-ion-implanted titanium than on un-implanted titanium — as early as two days after implantation into rat tibia [42]. This superiority of calcium-ion-implanted titanium is due to the modified surface by calcium ion implantation.

In Figure 4–28, the depth distribution of substances on calcium-ion-implanted titanium is illustrated schematically. The modified surface of calcium-ion-implanted titanium comprised titanium oxide, which contained calcium in the chemical state of calcium titanate [43]. Compared to the un-implanted titanium surface, the calcium-ion-implanted titanium surface was more positively charged due to the dissociation of hydroxyl radicals [44], as schematically illustrated in Figure 4–29. As a result, the number of charging sites was bigger.

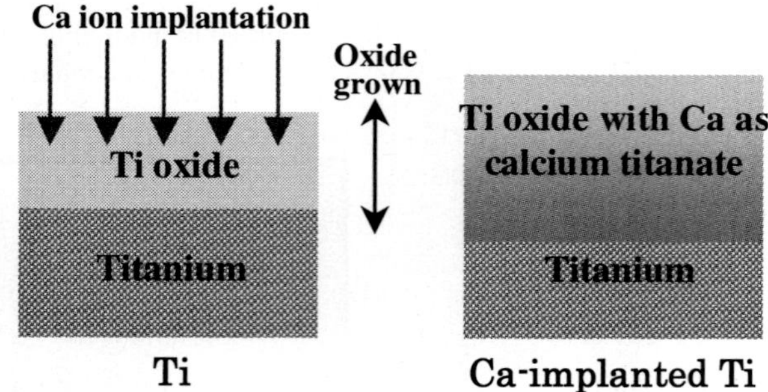

Figure 4–28 Change in surface layer of titanium with calcium ion implantation

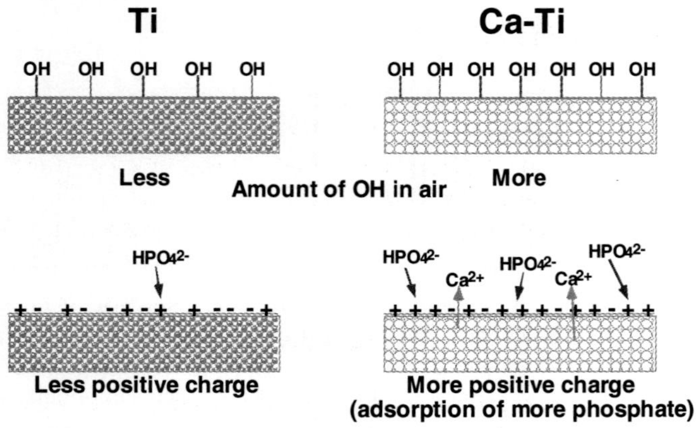

Figure 4–29 Acceleration mechanism of calcium phosphate precipitation on titanium with calcium ion implantation

More phosphate ions in the body fluid adsorb onto the calcium-ion-implanted titanium surface because of electric charge attraction. The more phosphate ions adsorbed, the more calcium ions attracted, and the more calcium phosphate is precipitated. Simultaneously, calcium ions are released from the surface of calcium-ion-implanted titanium [45,46], leading to supersaturation of calcium ions in body fluid near the surface and resulting in accelerated calcium phosphate precipitation.

To obtain a surface composition which is the same as a modified layer (where the latter is modified by calcium ion implantation), advanced techniques such as $CaTiO_3$ sputter deposition with argon ion or titanium ion mixing can be used.

4.9　Titanium Oxide Layer Formation

The easiest way to increase the corrosion resistance of titanium is either by anodic oxidation in an acidic solution or by high-temperature oxidation in the air (see Figure 4–15). Sputter deposition of a thin TiO_2 film is also effective in improving corrosion resistance. By iridium ion implantation into Ti–6Al–4V, electrochemical properties of the alloy approached those of iridium, eventually improving corrosion resistance. Improving corrosion resistance, however, does not always ensure bone conductivity.

Electrolysis in aqueous solution is effective for forming porous or irregular-shaped titanium oxide layer on titanium substrate (as shown in Figure 4–30). This technique is already applied to control the surface morphology of dental implants. Recently, titanium oxide film is used as coloring to categorize devices.

4.10　Titanium Nitride Layer Formation

Nitrogen ions are implanted onto titanium to improve wear resistance and hard-tissue compatibility, and into Ti–6Al–4V to improve corrosion resistance. A thin nitride film formed on titanium with high wear resistance is already used commercially in bone plates, dental implants, and artificial hip joints (see Figure 4–15). Thin films of TiN show gold color — the film is used to categorize devices.

4.11　Modification with Biomolecules and Polymers

In the design of bone-substituting and blood-contacting materials for both medical implants and bioaffinity sensors, it is a major challenge to generate surfaces and interfaces that are able to withstand proteins adsorption.

To accelerate bone formation surrounding implant materials, the materials are modified with biomolecules. Several phospholic acids were synthesized and grafted onto titanium. Proliferation, differentiation, and protein production of rats' osteoblastic cells on the titanium were then investigated [47]. Type I collagen production increased with modification by ethane–1,1,2–triphospholic acid and methylenediphosphonic acid. To improve hard tissue response, bone morphogenetic protein–4 (BMP–4) was immobilized on Ti–6Al–4V alloy through lysozyme [48]. To improve tissue compatibility, attempts were made for silane chemistry to couple proteins to the oxidized metal surfaces of Co–Cr–Mo, Ti–6Al–4V, Ti, and Ni–Ti [49].

Platelets adhesion, adsorption of proteins, peptides and antibodies, and DNA can likewise be controlled by modifications. A class of copolymers based on poly(L–lysine)–g–poly(ethylene glycol), PLL–g–PEG, was found to spontaneously adsorb from aqueous solutions onto TiO_2, $Si_{0.4}Ti_{0.6}O_2$, and Nb_2O_5 to develop blood-contacting materials and biosensors [50]. Poly(ethylene glycol)–poly(DL–lactic acid) (PEG–PLA) copolymeric micelles were attached on functionalized TiO_2 and Au. The micelle layer enhanced the protein resistance of the surfaces by up to 70 percent.

Silicon and titanium oxide surfaces (SiO_2/Si and TiO_2/Ti) were covalently modified with bioactive molecules (e.g., peptides) in a simple three-step procedure to control cellular and biomolecular functions on the surfaces. Bioactive surfaces were synthesized by first immobilizing N–(2–aminoethyl)–3–aminopropyl–trimethoxysilane (EDS) to polished quartz disks, polished silicon wafers, or sputter-deposited titanium films. Subsequently, a maleimide-activated surface — amenable to tethering molecules — with a free thiol (e.g., cysteine) was created by coupling sulfosuccinimidyl 4–(N–maleimidomethyl) cyclohexane–1–carboxylate (sulfro–SMCC) to the terminal amine on EDS. Peptides with terminal cysteine residues were immobilized on maleimide-activated oxides [51].

The surface of stainless steel was first modified by the silane coupling agent (SCA), (3–mercaptopropyl)trimethoxysilane. The silanized stainless steel surface (SCA–SS surface) was subsequently activated by argon plasma and then subjected to UV-induced graft polymerization of poly(ethylene glycol)methacrylate (PEGMA). The PEGMA graft-polymerized stainless steel couple (PEGMA–g–SCA–SS) with a high graft concentration, and thus a high PEG content, was found to be very effective in preventing bovine serum albumin and γ-globulin adsorption [52].

Metal oxide surfaces (Ta_2O_5, Al_2O_3, Nb_2O_5, ZrO_2, SiO_2) were coated by self-assembled monolayers (SAMs) of dodecyl phosphate ($DDPO_4$) and 12–hydroxy dodecyl phosphate ($OH–DDPO_4$). The coating was done by a novel surface modification protocol based on the adsorption of alkyl phosphate ammonium salts from aqueous solution for application to biochemical analyses and biosensors [53]. To apply a surface plasmon resonance (SPR) to biosensors, a sandwich immunoassay was performed on a thin gold film set in SPR cell. The molecular motion of self-assembled monolayers on gold was examined using SPR under an electric field. Two examples of polymer modification of TiO_2 are shown in Figure 4–31.

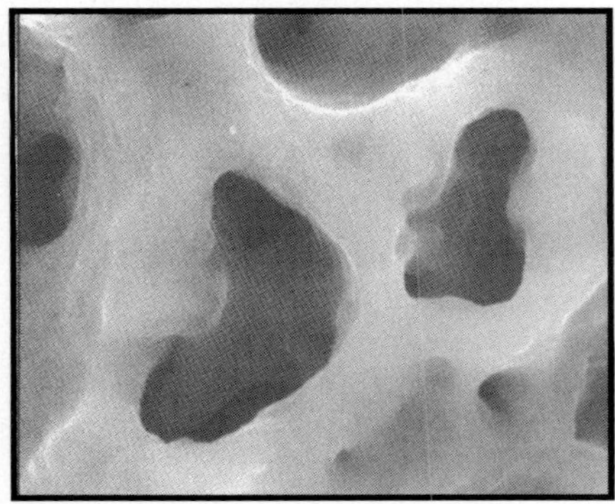

Figure 4–30 Porous titanium oxide surface [from Brånemark System® TiUnite™ Catalogue, Nobel Biocare]

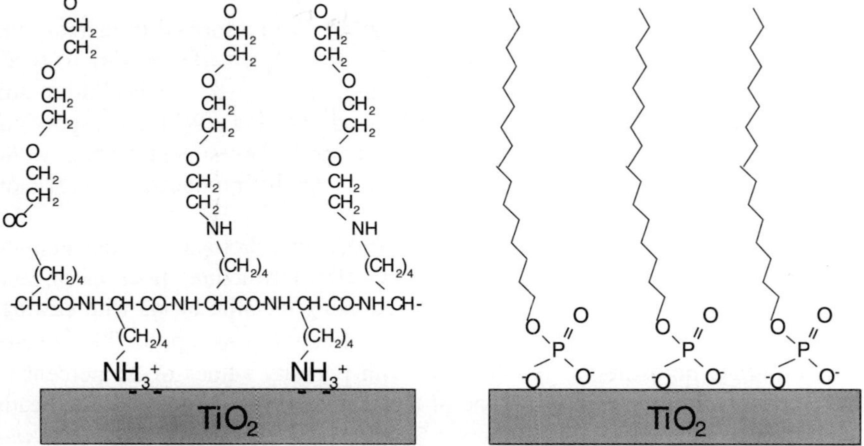

Figure 4–31 Examples of polymer immobilization model on titanium [53]

4.12 Morphological Modification

Morphology of an implant surface influences the bonding strength of bone-implant interface. In other words, the surface structure of an implant has a significant influence on both its anchorage and strength of adhesion to the tissue. A smooth implant surface with a small contact area with the tissue will show lower adhesion strength than a rough surface. Ingrowth of bone into surface cavities has a favorable influence on adhesion strength. Cell growth is unaffected by grooves or pores on the implant surface. Figure 4–32 shows how cell growth was expanded alongside the grooves on titanium — which was vaporized on silicon substrate.

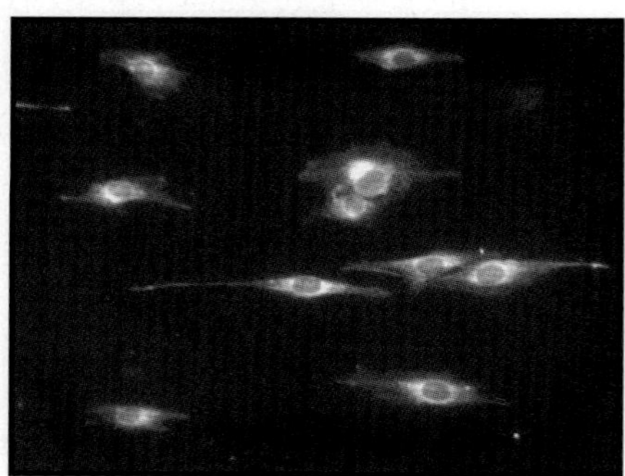

Figure 4–32 Fluorescent microscopic image of human endotherial cell type HGTFN expanding along to fill grooves present in gold, which is deposited on silicon substrate. Grooves are not apparent in this picture, but transverse directional grooves exist on gold.

Surface structuring or morphological control was performed to increase the anchoring or bonding of bone to implants. For structured surfaces, various types were formed by casting, surface roughening, or through lacunae holes and porous coating produced by sintering or plasma spraying. With corresponding wax models, a roughened surface can be produced by investment casting, while a special open-cell, porous, sponge structure can be produced by precision casting.

In terms of morphological control, various morphologies of the implant surface were designed: beads, grooves, cancellous structure, fiber mesh, and porous coating. Rough pores were prepared using metallic beads with casting. The pore size was 0.4–1.5 mm, and pore fraction was up to 70 percent. Micro-porous porosities of 0.1–0.4 mm with porosity values of 35 percent to 50 percent were produced using one of these methods: sintering of metal beads or diffusion welding of metal fibers. Smaller pore size of 0.02–0.2 mm was obtained through plasma spraying of titanium powder. To evaluate the effect of porous surface structures on fatigue strength, a surface layer consisting of beads or wires and which corresponded to a porous coating was used. All pores were interconnected and superficially linked to the outer demarcation of the coating. Typical surface patterns are shown in Figure 4–33.

Many studies were conducted to examine the effect of pores (see Figure 4–30) on the ingrowth of tissues or cells to titanium. The host bone came into contact with a surface relief of the plasma-sprayed coating, which was then characterized using an open microstructure with variable height at any part of a surface. Animal tests confirmed the advantage of a rough surface. Several studies have been made on bone ingrowth into porous systems with different pore sizes. The diameter of interconnecting pores seems to dictate the quality of tissue growing into porosity space. When pore sizes were down to 50 μm, there was effective bone ingrowth into porous coatings. However, for regeneration of mineralized bone, the interconnections of porosity must be larger than 100 μm. When the pore size was larger than 1 mm, fibrous tissues were sometimes formed. Based on these readings, the optimal pore size for mineralized bone ingrowth was concluded at 100–400 μm [54].

Titanium fiber mesh (see Figure 4–30) was used as a scaffold for tissue engineering with cultured osteogenic cells [47,55]. After titanium fiber mesh was seeded with osteogenic cells, bone formation was generated more effectively in a shorter culture time.

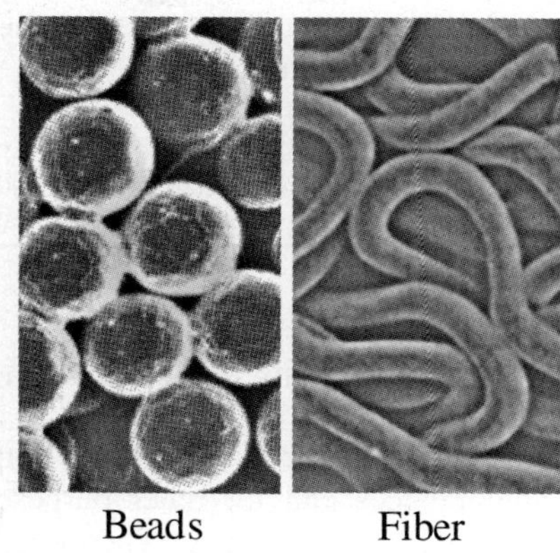

Figure 4–33 Beads and fibers of titanium

4.13 Surface Analysis

Surface analysis and surface modification are inseparably related to each other. Following surface modification, surface analysis techniques will be used to characterize composition, crystallinity, and other critical surface properties of modified surfaces.

A surface analysis technique consists of two components. The first component is the probe that irradiates a material surface. The second component refers to the signal used for analysis. Summarized in Table 4–5 are the probe-signal permutations of various surface analytical instruments.

XPS, AES, SIMS, and RBS are surface-sensitive techniques used to characterize thin films and layers at nanometer level. On the other hand, SEM, EDS, and EPMA are conventional tools that analyze specimens' morphologies and compositions.

Table 4–5 Examples of surface analysis instrument: original probe and detected signal

Signal	Probe		
	(a) X-ray or Light	(b) Electron	(c) Ion
1. Photoelectron	X-ray Photoelectron Spectroscopy (XPS)		
2. Auger electron		Auger Electron Spectroscopy (AES)	
3. Secondary electron		Scanning Electron Spectroscopy (SEM)	
4. Ion	Laser Microprobe Mass Spectrometry (LAMMA)		Secondary Ion Mass Spectroscopy (SIMS)
5. X-ray or Light	X-ray Diffractometry (XRD)	Energy Dispersive Spectroscopy (EDS) Electron Probe Microanalysis (EPMA)	Particle Induced X-ray Emission (PIXE)
6. Back scattering ion		Scanning Electron Spectroscopy (SEM)	Rutherford Back Scattering (RBS)

4.14 Future of Surface Engineering of Metallic Biomaterials

Metallic materials are widely used in medicine not only for orthopedic implants, but also as cardiovascular devices and for other purposes. Biomaterials are always used in close contact with living tissues. Therefore, interactions between material surfaces and living tissues must be well understood. This knowledge is essential to developing new novel materials.

In particular, metal surface-biomolecule reactions and/or metal surface-cell reactions are important. A good knowledge of these reactions can help to add biofunctions to metallic materials that already have excellent mechanical properties. Finally, through surface modification techniques such as multi-layer coating and patterning of multi-functional layers, it is possible to arrive at an optimal range of biofunctions in a biomaterial.

References

1. K. Asami, S. C. Chen, H. Habazaki, and K. Hashimoto, The surface characterization of titanium and titanium–nickel alloys in sulfuric acid, Corros. Sci., 1993, 35:43–49.
2. T. Hanawa, K. Asami, and K. Asaoka, Repassivation of titanium and surface oxide film regenerated in simulated bioliquid, J. Biomed. Mater. Res., 1998, 40:530–538.
3. T. Hanawa and M. Ota, Calcium phosphate naturally formed on titanium in electrolyte solution, Biomaterials, 1991, 12:767–774.
4. T. Hanawa, Titanium and its oxide film: a substrate for formation of apatite, in The bone-biomaterial interface, ed. J. E. Davies, (University of Toronto Press, Toronto, 1991) pp:49–61.
5. T. Hanawa, O. Okuno, and H. Hamanaka, Compositional change in surface of Ti–Zr alloys in artificial bioliquid, J. Jpn. Inst. Met., 1992, 56:1168–1173.
6. P. Bruesch, K. Muller, A. Atrens, and H. Neff, Corrosion of stainless steels in chloride solution — an XPS investigation of passive films, Appl. Phys., 1985, 38:1–18.
7. S. Jin and A. Atrens, ESCA-studies of the structure and composition of the passive film formed on stainless steels by various immersion times in 0.1 M NaCl solution, Appl. Phys., 1987, A42:149–165.
8. T. Hanawa, S. Hiromoto, A. Yamamoto, D. Kuroda, and K. Asami, XPS characterization of the surface oxide film of 316L stainless samples that were located in quasi-biological environments, Mater. Trans., 2002, 43:3088–3092.
9. D. C. Smith, R. M. Pilliar, J. B. Metson, and N. S. McIntyre, Preparative procedures and surface spectroscopic studies, J. Biomed. Mater. Res., 1991, 25:1069–1084.
10. T. Hanawa, S. Hiromoto, and K. Asami, Characterization of the surface oxide film of a Co–Cr–Mo alloy after being located in quasi-biological environments using XPS, Appl. Surf. Sci., 2001, 183:68–75.
11. K. Endo, Y. Araki, and H. Ohno, *In vitro* and *in vivo* corrosion of dental Ag–Pd–Cu alloys, Transaction of International Congress on Dental Materials, 1989, 226–227.
12. T. Hanawa, H. Takahashi, M. Ota, R. F. Pinizzotto, J. L. Ferracane, and T. Okabe, Surface characterization of amalgams using X-ray photoelectron spectroscopy, J. Dent. Res., 1987, 66:1470–1478.
13. J. E. Sundgren, P. Bodo, and I. Lundstrom, Auger electron spectroscopic studies of the interface between human tissue and implants of titanium and stainless steel, J. Colloid Interface Sci., 1986, 110:9–20.
14. M. Espostito, J. Lausmaa, J. M. Hirsch, and P. Thomsen, Surface analysis of failed oral titanium implants, J. Biomed. Mater. Res. Appl. Biomater., 1999, 48:559–568.
15. T. Hanawa and M. Ota, Characterization of surface film formed on titanium in electrolyte, Appl. Surf. Sci., 1992, 55:269–276.
16. K. E. Healy and P. Ducheyne, The mechanisms of passive dissolution of titanium in a model physiological environment, J. Biomed. Mater. Res., 1992, 26:319–338.
17. A. P. Serro, A. C. Fernandes, B. Saramago, J. Lima, and M. A. Barbosa, Apatite desorption on titanium surfaces — the role of albumin adsorption, Biomaterials, 1997, 18:963–968.

18. T. Hanawa, S. Hiromoto, K. Asami, H. Ukai, and K. Murakami, Surface modification of titanium utilizing a repassivation reaction in aqueous solutions, Mater. Trans., 2002, 43:3005–3009.

19. T. Hanawa, S. Hiromoto, K. Asami, O. Okuno, and K. Asaoka, Surface oxide films on titanium alloys regenerated in Hanks' solution, Mater. Trans., 2002, 43:3000–3004.

20. J. E. Sundgren, P. Bodo, I. Lundstrom, A. Berggren, and S. Hellem, Auger electron spectroscopic studies of stainless steel implants, J. Biomed. Mater. Res., 1985, 19:663–671.

21. J. Walczak, F. Shahgaldi, and F. Heatley, *In vivo* corrosion of 316L stainless steel hip implants: morphology and elemental compositions of corrosion products, Biomaterials, 1998, 19:229–237.

22. B. Ivarsson and I. Lundström, Physical characterization of protein adsorption on metal and metal oxide surfaces, CRC Critic. Rev. Biocompatibility, 1986, 2:1–96.

23. H. Elwing, Protein adsorption and ellipsometry in biomaterial research, Biomaterials, 1998, 19:397–406.

24. R. D. Bagnall and P. A. Arundel, A method for the prediction of protein adsorption on implant surfaces, J. Biomed. Mater. Res., 1983, 17:459–466.

25. R. L. Williams and D. F. Williams, Albumin adsorption on metal surfaces, Biomaterials, 1988, 9:206–212.

26. M. Ahmad, D. Grawronski, J. Blum, J. Goldberg, and G. Gronowicz, Differential response of human osteoblast-like cells to commercially pure (CP) titanium grades 1 and 4, J. Biomed. Mater. Res., 1999, 46:121–131.

27. L. Raisanen, M. Kononen, J. Juhanoja, P. Varpavaara, J. Hautaniemi, J. Kivilahti, and M. Hormia, Expression of cell adhesion complexes in epithelial cells seeded on biomaterial surfaces, J. Biomed. Mater. Res., 2000, 49:79–87.

28. J. E. Davies, B. Lowenberg, and A. Shiga, The bone-titanium interface *in vitro*, J. Biomed. Mater. Res., 1990, 24:1289–1306.

29. A. Yamamoto, S. Mishima, N. Maruyama, and M. Sumita, A new technique for direct measurement of the shear force necessary to detach a cell from a material, Biomaterials, 1998, 19:871–879.

30. A. Yamamoto, S. Mishima, M. Sumita, and T. Hanawa, Measurement of cell adhesive shear strength and cell detachment surface energy of a single murine fibroblast adhering to thin metal films, J. Jpn. Soc. Biomater., 2000, 18:87–94.

31. J. L. Ong and L. C. Lucas, Post-deposition heat treatment for ion beam sputter deposited calcium phosphate coatings, Biomaterials, 1994, 15:337–341.

32. S. Ban and S. Maruno, Morphology and microstructure of electrochemically deposited calcium phosphates in a modified simulated body fluid, Biomaterials, 1998, 19:1245–1253.

33. H. Ishizawa and M. Ogino, Formation and characterization of anodic titanium oxide films containing Ca and P, J. Biomed. Mater. Res., 1995, 29:65–72.

34. H. M. Kim, F. Miyaji, T. Kokubo, and T. Nakamura, Preparation of bioactive Ti and its alloys via simple chemical surface treatment, J. Biomed. Mater. Res., 1996, 32:409–417.

35. Y. Mu, T. Kobayashi, M. Sumita, A. Yamamoto, and T. Hanawa, Metal ion release from titanium with active oxygen species generated by rat macrophages *in vitro*, J. Biomed. Mater. Res., 2000, 49:238–243.

36. P. Tengvall, I. Lundstrom, L. Sjoqvist, H. Elwing, and L. M. Bjursten, Titanium-hydrogen peroxide interaction: model studies of the influence of the inflammatory response on titanium implants, Biomaterials, 1989, 10:166–175.

37. C. Ohtsuki, H. Iida, S. Hayakawa, and A. Osaka, Bioactivity of titanium treated with hydrogen peroxide solutions containing metal chlorides, J. Biomed. Mater. Res., 1997, 35:39–47.

38. T. Hanawa, M. Kon, H. Ukai, K. Murakami, Y. Miyamoto, and K. Asaoka, Surface modification of titanium in calcium-ion-containing solutions, J. Biomed. Mater. Res., 1997, 34:273–278.

39. K. Hamada, M. Kon, T. Hanawa, K. Yokoyama, Y. Miyamoto, and K. Asaoka, Hydrothermal modification of titanium surface in calcium solutions, Biomaterials, 2002, 23:2265–2272.

40. T. Hanawa, S. Kihara, and M. Murakami, Calcium phosphate precipitation on calcium-ion-implanted titanium in electrolyte, in Characterization and performance of calcium phosphate coatings for implants, eds. E. Horowitz and J. E. Parr, (American Society for Testing and Materials, Philadelphia) ASTM STP 1196, pp:170–184.

41. T. Hanawa, Y. Nodasaka, H. Ukai, K. Murakami, and K. Asaoka, Cell compatibility of calcium-ion-implanted titanium, J. Jpn. Soc. Biomater., 1994, 12:209–216.

42. T. Hanawa, Y. Kamiura, S. Yamamoto, T. Kohgo, A. Amemiya, H. Ukai, K. Murakami, and K. Asaoka, Early bone formation around calcium-ion-implanted titanium inserted into rat tibia, J. Biomed. Mater. Res., 1997, 36:131–136.

43. T. Hanawa, H. Ukai, and K. Murakami, X-ray photoelectron spectroscopy of calcium-ion-implanted titanium, J. Electron Spectrosc., 1993, 63:347–354.

44. T. Hanawa, M. Kon, H. Doi, H. Ukai, K. Murakami, H. Hamanaka, and K. Asaoka, Amount of hydroxyl radical on calcium-ion-implanted titanium and point of zero charge of constituent oxide of the surface-modified layer, J. Mater. Sci. Mater. Med., 1998, 9:89–92.

45. T. Hanawa, K. Asami, and K. Asaoka, Microdissolution of calcium ions from calcium-ion-implanted titanium, Corros. Sci., 1996, 38:1579–1594.

46. T. Hanawa, K. Asami, and K. Asaoka, AES studies on the dissolution of surface oxide from calcium-ion-implanted titanium in nitric acid and buffered solutions, Corros. Sci., 1996, 38:2061–2067.

47. C. Viornery, H. L. Guenther, B. O. Arronson, P. Pechy, P. Descouts, and M. Gratzel, Osteoblast culture on polished titanium disks modified with phosphonic acids, J. Biomed. Mater. Res., 2002, 62:149–155.

48. D. A. Puleo, R. A. Kissling, and M. S. Sheu, A technique to immobilize bioactive proteins, including bone morphogenetic protein–4 (BMP–4), on titanium alloy, Biomaterials, 2002, 23:2079–2087.

49. A. Nanci, J. D. Wuest, L. Peru, P. Brunet, V. Sharma, S. Zalzal, and M. D. McKee, Chemical modification of titanium surfaces for covalent attachment of biological molecules, J. Biomed. Mater. Res., 1998, 40:324–335.

50. N. P. Huang, R. Michel, J. Vörös, M. Textor, R. Hofer, A. Rossi, D. L. Dlbert, J. A. Hubbell, and N. D. Spencer, Poly(L–lysine)–g–poly(ethylene glycol) layers on metal oxide surfaces: surface analytical characterization and resistance to serum and fibrinogen adsorption, Langmuir, 2001, 17:489–498.

51. S. J. Xiao, M. Textor, N. D. Spencer, and H. Sigrist, Covalent attachment of cell-adhesive, (Arg–Gly–Asp)-containing peptides to titanium surfaces, Langmuir, 1998, 114:5507–5516.
52. F. Zhang, E. T. Kang, K. G. Neoh, P. Wang, and K. L. Tan, Surface modification of stainless steel by grafting of poly(ethylene glycol) for reduction in protein adsorption, Biomaterials, 2001, 22:1541–1548.
53. M. Textor, L. Ruiz, R. Hofer, A. Rossi, K. Feldman, G. Hähner, and N. D. Spencer, Structural chemistry of self-assembled monolayers of octadecylphosphoric acid on tantalum oxide surfaces, Langmuir, 2000, 16:3257–3271.
54. R. D. Bloebaum, K. N. Bachus, N. G. Momberger, and A. A. Hoffman, Mineral apposition rates of human cancellous bone at the interface of porous-coated implants, J. Biomed. Mater. Res., 1994, 28:537–544.
55. J. W. M. Vehof, A. E. de Ruijter, P. H. M. Spauwen, and J. A. Jansen, Influence of rh BMP–2 on rat bone marrow stromal cells cultured on titanium fiber mesh, Tissue Eng., 2001, 7:373–383.

CHAPTER 5

BIORESTORATIVE MATERIALS IN DENTISTRY

Adrian U Jin Yap

Department of Restorative Dentistry
Faculty of Dentistry, National University of Singapore
E-mail: rsdyapuj@nus.edu.sg

Dentistry is a science and art concerned with the prevention, diagnosis, and treatment of diseases of the teeth and adjacent tissues, and the restoration of missing dental and maxillo-facial structures. Every dental restorative procedure requires the use of materials. This chapter introduces the restorative materials used in clinical dentistry. Dental biomaterials can be broadly classified into ceramics, polymers, and metals. Many restorative materials are fixed permanently into the patient's mouth or are removed only occasionally for cleaning. The materials have to withstand the effects of a most hostile environment. Temperature variations, wide variations in acidity or alkalinity, and high stresses all have an effect on the durability of restorative materials. Most restorative materials are managed entirely by clinicians and their assistants. Some are, however, associated with the work of the dental technologists. Successful restorative dentistry is dependent on the correct selection of material for a given application and the ability to carry out manipulative procedures to arrive at the optimum properties of the material.

5.1   Introduction

Dentistry is a science and art concerned with the prevention, diagnosis, and treatment of diseases of the teeth and adjacent tissues, and the restoration of missing dental and maxillo-facial structures. Every dental restorative procedure requires the use of materials. As the former makes up the bulk of clinical work, a dentist spends much of his/her professional career handling materials. The success or failure of restorative treatment depends upon the "correct choice of material for a given application" and the "ability to carry out manipulative procedures to arrive at the optimum properties" of that material [1]. Restorative materials in dentistry can be broadly classified into ceramics, polymers, and metals (Figure 5–1). As many of these materials are fixed permanently into the patient's mouth or are removed only occasionally for cleaning, they have to withstand the effects of a most hostile environment. Normal mouth temperature varies between 32°C and 37°C. Intake of hot or cold drink or food extends this temperature range from 0 to 70°C. The pH of oral fluids ranges from 4 to 8.5 and extends from pH 2 to 11 with the consumption of acidic juices and alkaline medications [2]. The load on tooth and restorations can reach levels as high as 170 N — signifying a demanding mechanical property required of some biorestorative materials [3].

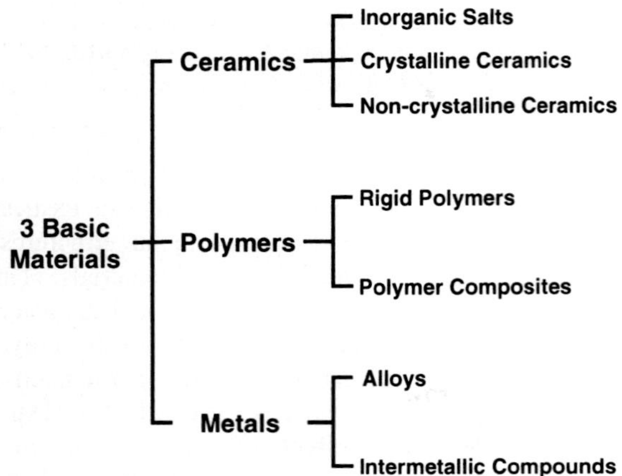

Figure 5–1 The three basic materials used in restorative dentistry

Although many restorative materials are managed entirely by the dentist and his assistant, others are generally associated with the dental technologists. A third group of materials links the dental surgery to the laboratory, e.g., impression material. This group of materials is beyond the scope of this chapter and will not be considered. This chapter serves to introduce the restorative materials used in clinical dentistry with special emphasis on materials science, engineering, and processing.

5.2   Ceramics

5.2.1 Inorganic Salts (Dental Cements)

Dental cements are typically formulated as powders and liquids. The powders are basic (proton acceptors) in nature while the liquids are acidic (proton donors). A viscous paste is formed when the powder and liquid are mixed. This subsequently hardens to a solid mass. The equation for the cement forming reaction [1] can be simplified as:

$$\mathbf{XO} \quad + \quad \mathbf{H_2A} \quad \rightarrow \quad \mathbf{XA} + \mathbf{H_2O}$$

$$\text{Proton acceptor} \qquad \text{Proton donor} \qquad\qquad \text{Gel-salt}$$

As only part of the powder reacts with the liquids, the set cement is heterogeneous, composing of unreacted powder particles surrounded by a matrix of gel-salt (reaction product). Five main types of acid-base cement can be derived from two types of powder (Figure 5–2).

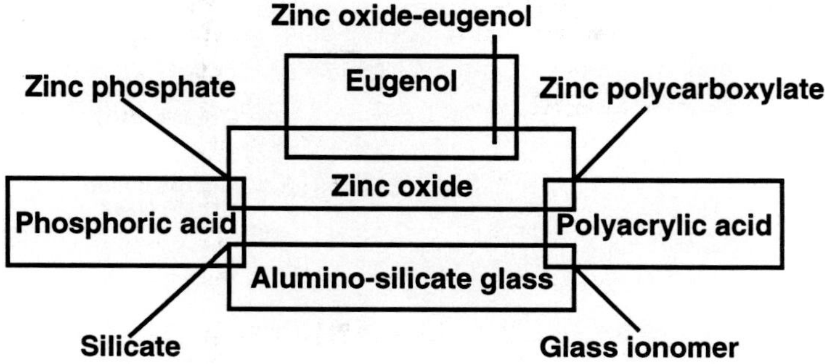

Figure 5–2 Five main types of dental cement

Clinical usage of these cements includes temporary and permanent restoration of teeth:
- Cementing of inlays, crowns, bridges, and orthodontic brackets;
- Lining of cavities; and
- Filling of root canals.

Amongst the various inorganic salts, the glass ionomer cements are worthy to be highlighted. They are derived from aqueous polymeric acid and a glass component, which is usually a fluoroalumino silicate (Figure 5–3). The glass is obtained by fusing silica, alumina, and calcium fluoride at high temperature, followed by fine grinding the shocked-cooled molten mass. They have the dual advantages of chemical adhesion to teeth (hydroxyapatite) and sustained fluoride release. The lack of exotherm during setting, the absence of monomer as well as the improved release of incorporated therapeutic agents have led to the development of glass ionomer cements for biomedical applications. They have been successfully used to stabilize implanted devices and bony fragments, and likewise in the reconstruction/obliteration of bony defects in osteological and reconstructive surgery [4]. In order to improve biocompatibility and biomechanically match glass ionomers to bone, HAIonomer (Hydroxyapatite-Ionomer) cements are currently being developed [5].

5.2.2 Crystalline and Non-crystalline Ceramics

Crystalline ceramics like silica and alumina are used to reinforce polymers and porcelain. Dental porcelain is essentially a non-crystalline ceramic (glass) prepared from high-purity feldspar. Ceramics are inherently brittle and must not be subjected to large tensile stresses. The latter can lead to catastrophic failures.

One method of reducing the influence of the brittleness of ceramics is to fuse them to a material of higher toughness (e.g., metal), as with porcelain-fused-to-metal prostheses (Figure 5–4). Ceramics can also be reinforced with dispersions of alumina or a core of pure alumina.

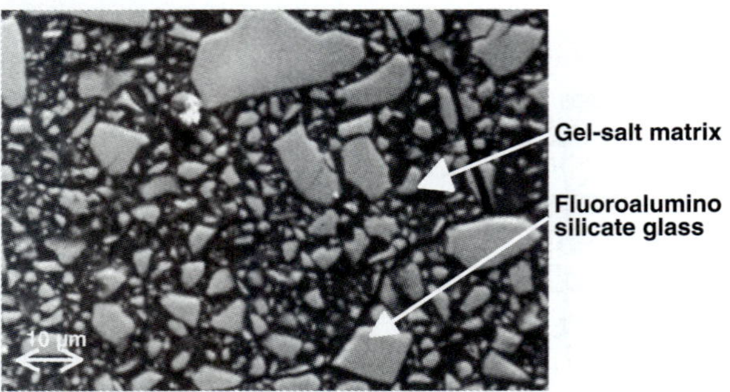

Figure 5-3 SEM of a typical glass ionomer

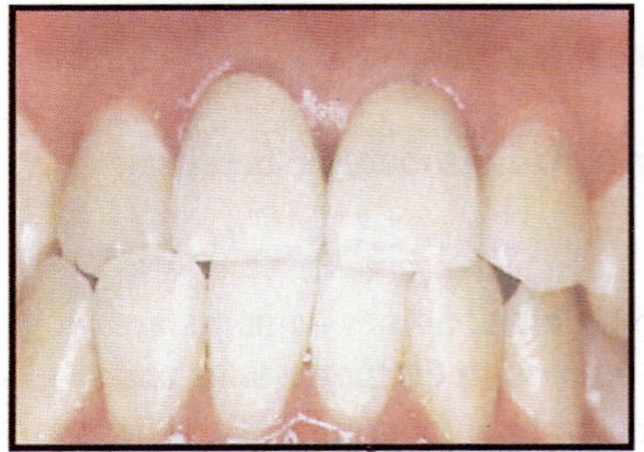
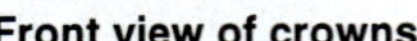
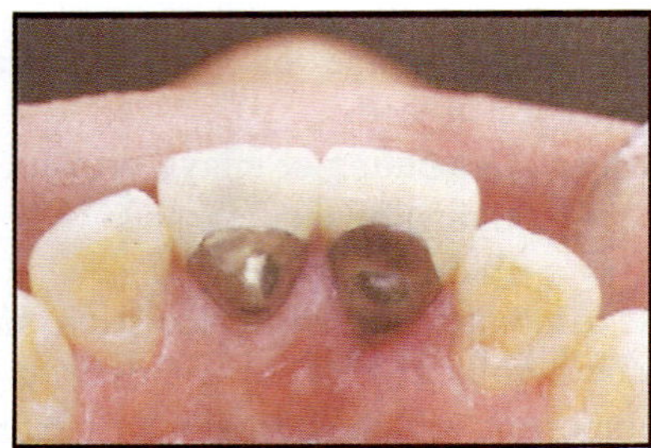

Figure 5–4 Porcelain-fused-to-metal (PFM) crowns

In addition to traditional firing, ceramic restorations can now be processed in several other ways. These include pressing, casting, machining, and CAD/CAM (Computer Aided Design/Machining) [6]. All these are made possible due to advances in processing technology. Both injection and pressed ceramic systems (Figure 5–5) involve the use of "loss-wax" technique. The restorations are modeled in wax, mounted on a sprue before investment and injecting/pressing.

With the machined ceramic system, a resin prototype restoration is first modeled. The restoration is then reproduced via milling of non-porous, high-density ceramic blocks using a copy-milling device (Figure 5–6).

All the aforementioned techniques for processing ceramic restorations require human work, which implies room for error. A logical objective of the pioneers of CAD/CAM systems was to "simplify, make more profitable, and standardize the production" of ceramic restorations [6]. A number of devices have been developed. They range from fully integrated CAD/CAM devices

(Figure 5–7) that allow for chairside production of restorations to systems that consist of several modules with, at least, distinctive CAD and CAM stations. The two key modules may be used in one of the following ways:

a) CAD and CAM stations are located in the dental office and operated successively for chairside restoration manufacturing;

b) Optical or traditional impression is taken in the dental office where the CAD operation is carried out. Data is transmitted to a central CAM station for restoration fabrication;

c) Optical or traditional impression is taken in the dental office, and collected information is then transmitted to a central station where CAD and CAM modules operate.

While laboratory-fabricated metal restorations are retained principally by means of macro-mechanical retention and friction provided by cements, ceramic restorations are retained by micro-mechanical or chemical adhesion between resin cements, dental tissues, and restorative material. This makes luting procedures a very important step of the whole treatment. It includes restoration try-in, rubber dam isolation, etching of tooth tissues with phosphoric acid, etching of ceramic restoration with hydrofluoric-based acid, silanization of ceramic restoration, application of resin cement to tooth/restoration and light-polymerization of the resin cement (Figure 5–8).

5.3   Polymers

5.3.1 Rigid Polymers

Polymers are long chain molecules derived from many repeating units called monomers. Two types of chemical polymerization reaction, Condensation and Addition, are used to make dental polymers. Condensation is the reaction between two molecules to form a larger molecule, with the elimination of a smaller molecule. Examples of polymers derived from this reaction include polycarbonates used for provisional crowns. Addition is the reaction which occurs between two molecules to give a larger molecule without the elimination of a smaller molecule. This type of reaction takes place for vinyl compounds, which are reactive organic compounds containing carbon–carbon double bonds. Examples include acrylic acids and methyl methacrylate monomers, which respectively form poly(acrylic acid) and poly(methyl methacrylate) or acrylic. The latter (acrylic) is the most widely used rigid polymeric material. Its applications include the fabrication of denture bases, provisional crowns, and bridges.

Acrylic materials can be heat- or self-cured. The composition of self-cured materials is similar to heat-cured materials except that activators, such as dimethyl–p–toluidine, are present in the liquid component. Self-cured acrylics are also called autopolymerizing or cold-curing materials. They have lower molecular weights, higher residual monomer contents, poorer rheological properties, poorer color stability, and greater porosity, and are weaker than heat-cured acrylics. Although acrylic prostheses (e.g., dentures and dental splints) can theoretically be processed by a number of techniques including compression and injection molding, the most commonly used one is the dough technique. In this technique, a dough is formed from a mixture of the monomer (liquid) and polymer (powder). This is subsequently packed into a mold and polymerized under the appropriate conditions to give a solid prosthesis (Figures 5–9 and 5–10). For heat-cured acrylics, two alternative heating techniques are used: (a) Heat at 72°C for at least 16 hours, or (b) Heat at 72°C for two hours followed by continued heating at 100°C for a further two hours [1]. The latter heating technique enables prosthesis to be produced in a shorter time but increases the likelihood of warpage. Microwave curing techniques are now currently being suggested. The free radical addition polymerization reactions in light-cured acrylic materials are initiated by visible light via tungsten halogen lamps with a light wavelength of 400 to 500 nm.

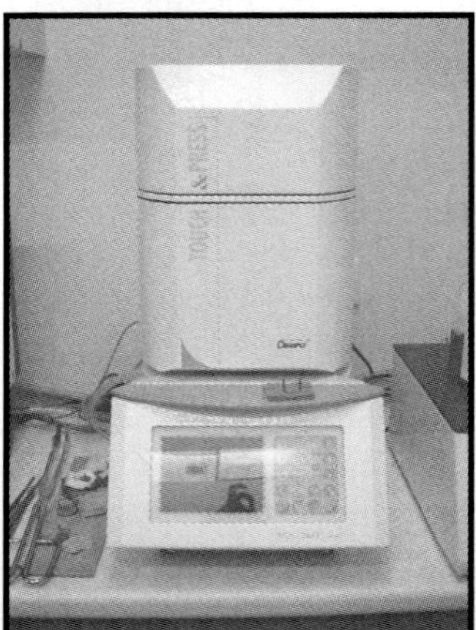

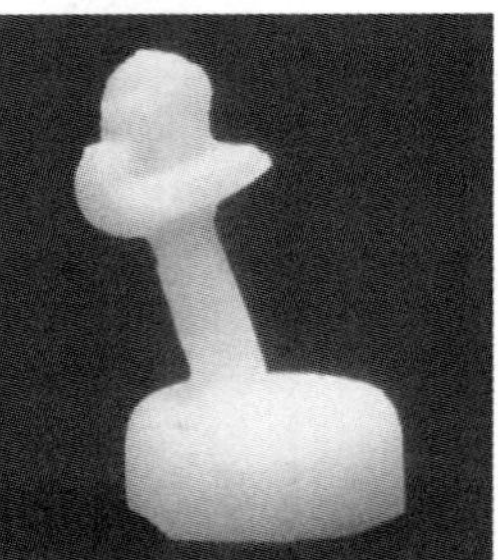

Figure 5–5 Injection and pressed ceramic systems involve the use of "loss-wax" technique

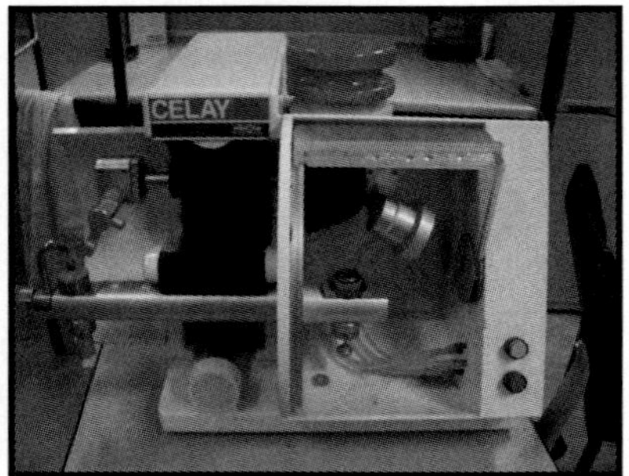

Figure 5–6 The Celay copy-milling system

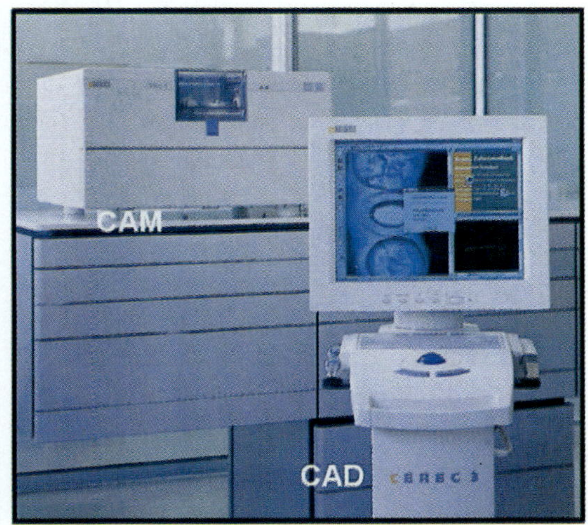

Figure 5–7 Computer-aided restoration design with the fully integrated CAD/CAM Sirona dental system (Courtesy of Siemens Pte Ltd, Singapore)

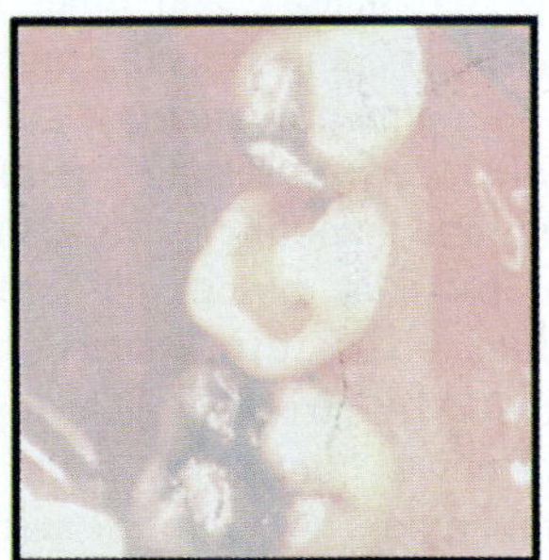

Cavity preparation

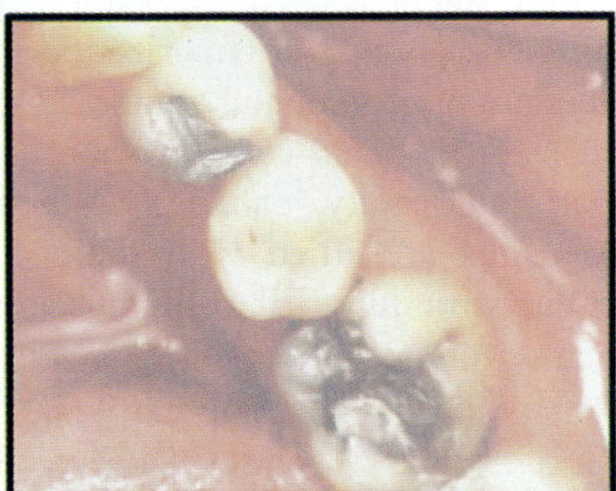

Ceramic restoration after luting

Figure 5–8 Ceramic restoration after luting

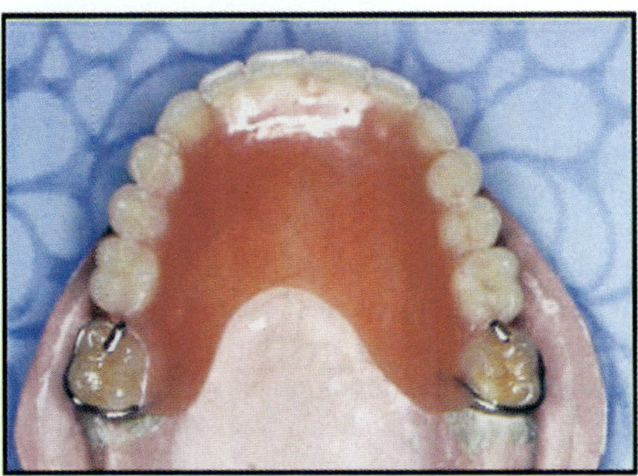

Figure 5–9 Acrylic dentures on cast

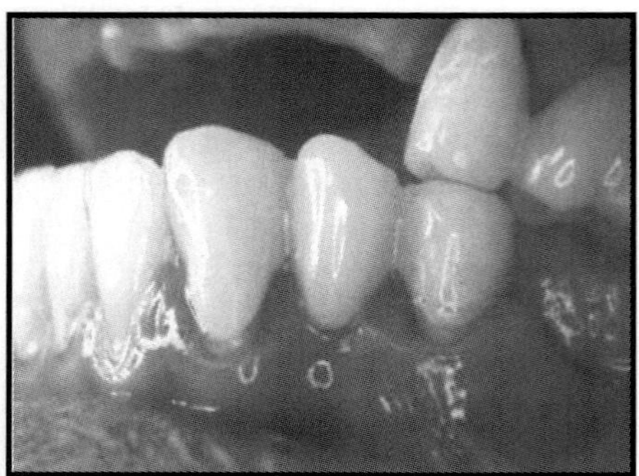

Figure 5–10 Acrylic provisional bridge in patient

5.3.2 *Polymer Composites*

Composites can be defined as three-dimensional combinations of at least two chemically different materials with a distinct interface. Dental composites (Figure 5–11) essentially comprise a resin matrix (organic phase), a filler-matrix coupling agent (interface), filler particles (dispersed phase), and other minor additions including polymerization initiators, stabilizers, and coloring pigments. Fillers are used in dental composites to provide strengthening, increase stiffness, reduce dimensional change when heated or cooled, reduce setting contraction, impart radiopacity, enhance aesthetics, and improve handling. Most current composites are filled with radiopaque silicate particles based on oxides of barium, strontium, zinc, aluminum, or zirconium. The resin matrix usually contains dimethacrylate monomers of which BisGMA (Bisphenol A–glycidyl methacrylate) is most popular. The hardening of dental composites is the result of a chemical reaction between the resin monomers. A rigid and well cross-linked polymer network which surrounds the inert fillers is produced. The degree of cure is influenced by many parameters, which include [7]:

- Addition of polymerization promoters and inhibitors;
- Chemical structure of the monomers;
- Chemical or light energy imparted to activate the reactions;
- Filler composition; and
- Composite shade.

Due to the well-recognized anticariogenic effects of fluoride, fluoride-releasing and polyacid-modified composites (compomers) are developed. These composites contain either one or both essential components of glass ionomer cements. The components, however, do not react as part of the setting process — they undergo an acid-base reaction only after hydration. Three different approaches to the development of fluoride-releasing composites have been reported. These approaches involve the addition of water-soluble fluoride salts, matrix-bound fluoride, or fluoride-releasing fillers [8]. The first approach is not ideal because soluble fluoride salts are easily washed out, resulting in a porous structure. This can compromise the physio-mechanical properties of the composite. The second group of materials has been intensely investigated, and fluoride-releasing resin systems are currently used in some commercial composites. The fluoride-releasing filler system approach has been adopted by most commercially available fluoride-releasing composites.

Composite restorative techniques may be categorized into three groups:

- Direct techniques which consist of only intraoral procedures and require only one appointment (Figure 5–12);
- Semi-direct techniques which include both intraoral and extraoral procedures to produce luted restorations; and
- Indirect techniques which require several appointments and the support of a dental laboratory.

In both semi-direct and indirect techniques, composites are subjected to photothermic treatment in special ovens. This procedure allows for optimal resin conversions, which results in increased hardness and wear resistance [9,10].

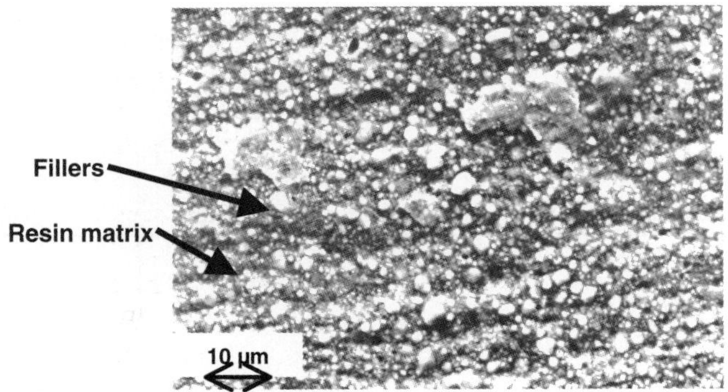

Figure 5–11 Microstructure of a dental composite

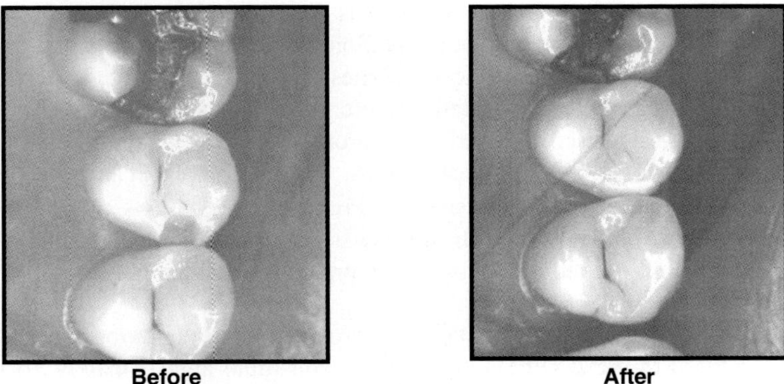

Figure 5–12 Direct restorative technique for dental composites

Fiber reinforced composites have been introduced for the laboratory and chairside fabrication of bridges. Different types of reinforcing fiber are used including glass, polyethylene, and carbon. The fibers may be arranged in various configurations. Unidirectional, long continuous, and parallel fibers are the most popular, followed by woven and braided fibers. Typically the fibers are about 7 to 10 μm in width and span the length of the prosthesis or appliance.

Table 5–1 shows the differences between composite and ceramic restorations. Both are bonded to tooth via micro-mechanical retention, and both involve the acid-etching of tooth tissues followed by the application of resin primers and/or adhesives.

Table 5–1 Differences between ceramic and composite restorations

Evaluation Parameters	Ceramics	Composites
Ease of clinical procedures	Satisfactory	Good
Ease of laboratory procedures	Satisfactory	Good
Intraoral repair	Poor	Excellent
Aesthetics	Excellent	Good
Surface polish	Good	Excellent
Wear resistance	Excellent	Good
Brittleness	Satisfactory	Good
Intraoral chemical stability	Excellent	Satisfactory

5.4 Metals

5.4.1 Alloys

Since the introduction of investment casting to dentistry in the early 1900s, alloys have been used for different types of prosthesis including crowns, bridges, dentures, and implants. An alloy is a mixture of two or more metallic elements. The constituents can be a metalloid or a non-metal, provided that the resultant mixture exhibits metallic properties. Dental alloys for fabrication of crowns/bridges can be broadly divided into precious metal casting alloys and alloys for porcelain-fused-to-metal restorations. Precious or high-gold-content alloys are used for inlays, full-cast crowns, and partial-veneer crowns (Figure 5–13) as they are soft and burnishable. Precious metal alloys contain mainly gold, palladium, platinum (which are classified as noble metals), and silver. They also contain limited amounts of non-precious alloying elements like iron, tin, and indium.

Due to aesthetic requirements, most crowns and bridge works are of the porcelain-fused-to-metal (PFM) type. They constitute approximately 70 to 80 percent of all cast restorations used clinically. Alloys intended for use in PFM restorations have several special requirements, such as:

- Melting temperatures must be above that of porcelain application;
- Close matching of thermal properties to those of porcelain;
- High modulus of elasticity; and
- Good corrosion resistance.

Two groups of alloy are used for PFM applications: noble metal alloys and base metal alloys (Figure 5–14).

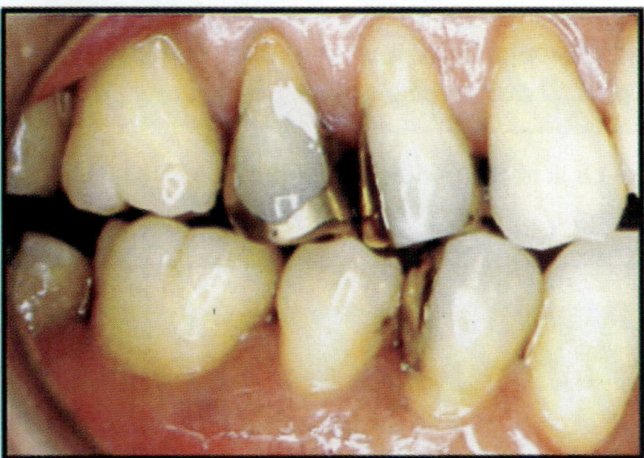

Figure 5–13 Gold inlay and partial-veneer restorations

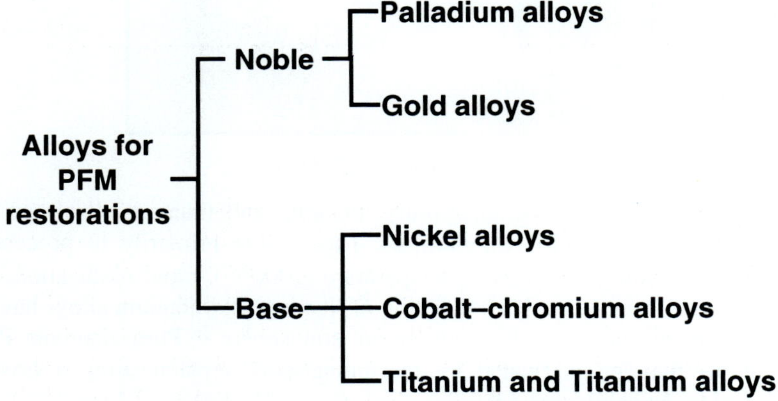

Figure 5–14 Classification of Porcelain-Fused-to-Metal alloys

Ni–Cr–Be alloys are not popular as nickel is allergenic and beryllium is toxic. The processing of these alloys in the laboratory may be hazardous. They are also difficult to cast because of their low density and high shrinkage on cooling, and are difficult to finish because of their hardness. Amongst the base metal alloys, Co–Cr (cobalt–chromium) alloys are most popular. They are used for the fabrication of acid-etch bridges (bridges bonded by composite resins to etched enamel) and denture frameworks (Figures 5–15 and 5–16).

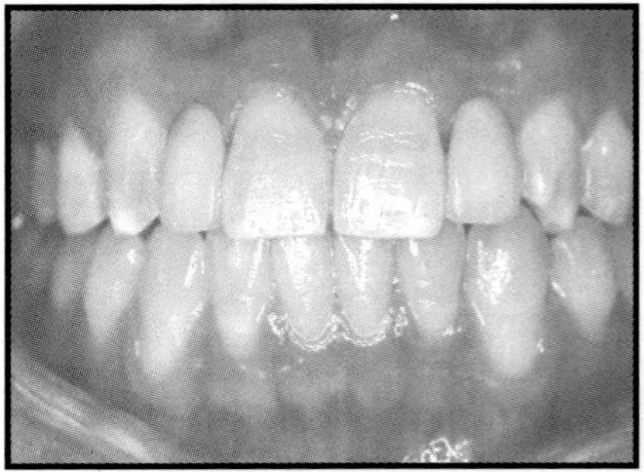

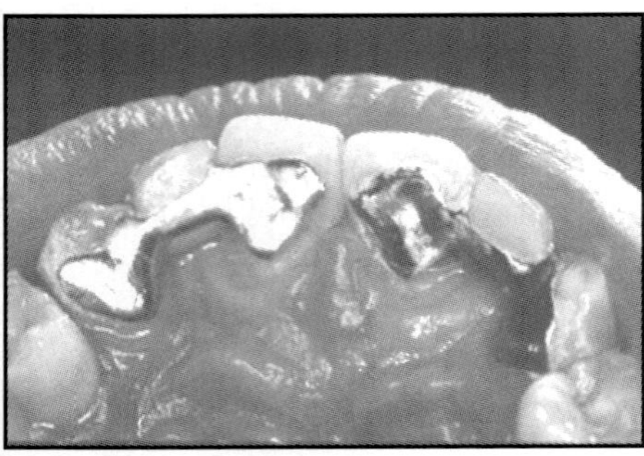

Figure 5–15(a) Co–Cr acid-etch bridges (front view)

Figure 5–15(b) Co–Cr acid-etch bridges (back view)

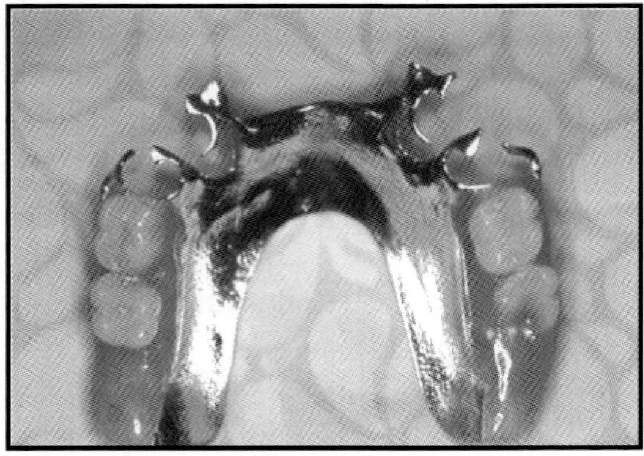

Figure 5–16 Co–Cr denture

Despite their high biocompatibility, titanium and titanium alloys are not commonly used for PFM restorations. This is due primarily to processing difficulties including high casting temperature (2000°C), rapid oxidization, and reactions with investments [11]. Melting of titanium and titanium alloys have to be done in special furnaces with argon atmosphere. Pure titanium PFM restorations may be fabricated by machining/spark erosion using a process developed by Nobelpharma AB.

The most common use of titanium and titanium alloys is for dental implants. In general dental implants are classified as endosseous, subperiosteal, or transosteal. Root-form endosseous implants are the most commonly used implants in clinical practice (Figure 5–17). This class of implants is the only one for which good long-term clinical data are available. Success rates for implants in the lower jaw are approximately 96 percent, 94 percent and 86 percent at 5, 10 and 15 years respectively. For the upper jaw, success rates are 88 percent, 82 percent and 78 percent at the same time intervals [12]. Clinician's expertise and surgical techniques are two important factors that determine clicnical outcome. They are significantly more important than the specific implant itself. Due to the need to develop a stable interface prior to biomechanical loading, bioceramic coatings and surface roughening have been used to accelerate tissue apposition to implant surfaces. The general requirement for the use of dental implants is available bone to support the implant. Bone augmentation materials (*i.e.*, bone grafts or bone graft substitutes) are used to replace bone deficits and defects.

Noble metals (Figure 5–18) are defined on the basis of their resistance to oxidation and attack by acids. Three noble metals are widely used in dental alloys. They are gold, palladium, and platinum. High-gold alloys (80–90% Au) bond well to porcelain, but creep of alloy may occur during porcelain firing due to their comparatively low melting range. As their moduli are low, a minimum alloy thickness of 0.5 mm is required. Gold–palladium alloys have better creep properties than high-gold alloys and are more economical. Palladium–silver alloys have similar mechanical properties to high-gold alloys but have high shrinkage and are difficult to cast. They may also have problems with discolouration (greening) when used with certain procelains. The observed bond between gold alloys and porcelain is believed to result from a combination of the following factors:

- Mechanical bonding between fused porcelain and small irregularities on the metal surface;
- Chemical bonding between surface film of oxide and procelain if tin or indium is present;
- Compressive bonding resulting from the contraction of porcelain.

While bonding between gold alloys and porcelain is multi-faceted, bonding between base metals is predominantly chemical in nature.

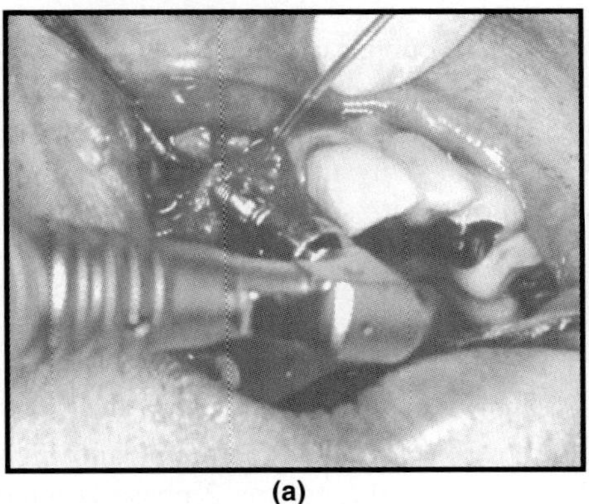
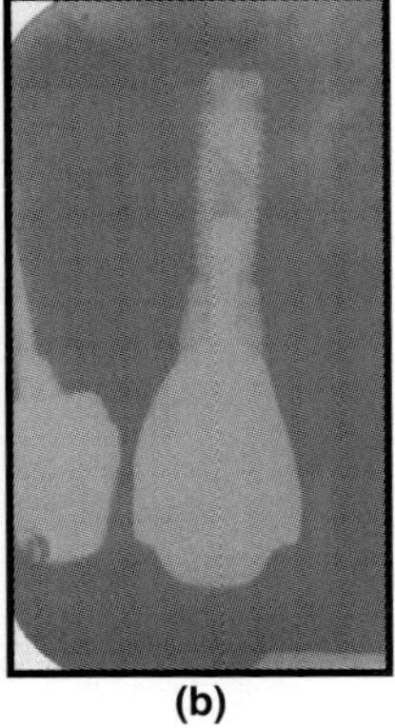

(a) **(b)**

Figure 5–17 (a) Surgical placement of dental implant; (b) radiograph of implant after restoration with a PFM crown (Courtesy of Dr. Keson BC Tan)

5.4.2 Intermetallic Compounds

Metals with chemical affinity for each other can form intermetallic compounds. The most well known intermetallic compound in dentistry is probably dental amalgam. Amalgam was the material of choice for direct posterior restorations for more than 150 years. The reason for its popularity lies in its ease of manipulation, relatively low cost, and long clinical service. Recently, biological and environmental concerns have arisen due to the mercury it contains. It is, however, presently believed that amalgam presents an acceptable risk-to-benefit ratio when properly used. An exception to this position has been taken in several parts of Europe where concerns have been raised regarding their use in populations thought to be more susceptible to mercury exposure. The latter includes children as well as pregnant women.

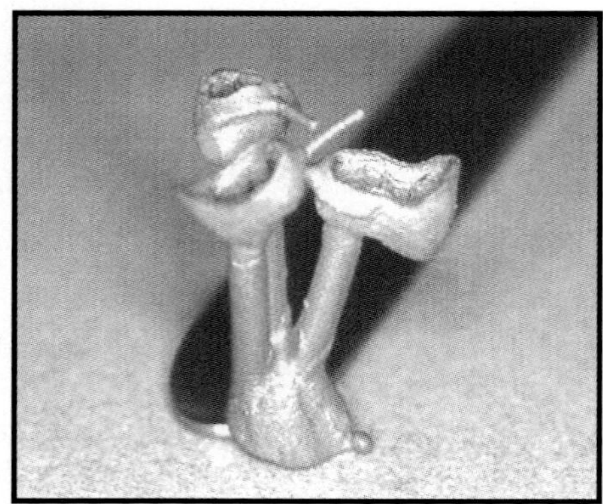

Figure 5–18 Noble metal crowns after casting and prior to addition of porcelain

Contemporary amalgams have high copper contents (Figure 5–19) and are classified into lathe cut, spherical and admixed types. Lathe cut alloy particles are milled from a cast ingot and sifted to the appropriate particle size distribution. Spherical alloys are created by means of an atomizing process where a spray of tiny drops is allowed to solidify in an inert atmosphere. Admixed alloys are a mix of lathe cut and spherical powders. The amalgamation reaction of traditional amalgam alloys can be represented as follows:

$$Ag_3Sn \quad + \quad Hg \quad \rightarrow \quad Ag_2Hg_3 \quad + \quad Sn_7Hg \quad + \quad Ag_3Sn$$
$$\text{gamma} \quad + \quad \text{mercury} \quad \rightarrow \quad \text{gamma 1} \quad + \quad \text{gamma 2} \quad + \quad \text{gamma (unreacted)}$$

In high-copper blended compositions (where traditional and high-copper phases are mechanically blended together), the gamma 2 phase is removed via the following reaction:

$$Sn_7Hg \quad + \quad AgCu \quad \rightarrow \quad Cu_6Sn_5 \quad + \quad Ag_2Hg_3$$
$$\text{gamma 2} \quad + \quad AgCu \quad \rightarrow \quad \text{eta prime phase} \quad + \quad \text{gamma 1}$$

In single-composition systems (where components are melted together), the eta prime phase is also formed during the amalgamation reaction. The reaction is, however, thought to be $2Cu_3Sn + 3Sn \rightarrow Cu_6Sn_5$ as the source of copper is in the epsilon phase. Absence of the weak gamma 2 phase improves corrosion, strength and creep properties as well as the marginal durability of amalgam restorations.

In an attempt to circumvent the problems with mercury, gallium alloys (Figure 5–19) were introduced. The melting temperature of gallium can be kept below room temperature with the addition of indium and tin. This liquid can be triturated with spherical silver–tin–copper alloy powder as with other amalgam alloys [11]. Palladium has been added to the alloy powder to improve corrosion properties. Clinical data pertaining to the long-term performance of gallium alloys are currently not available. Significant changes in luster and surface roughness have, however, been reported as early as four months after placement [13].

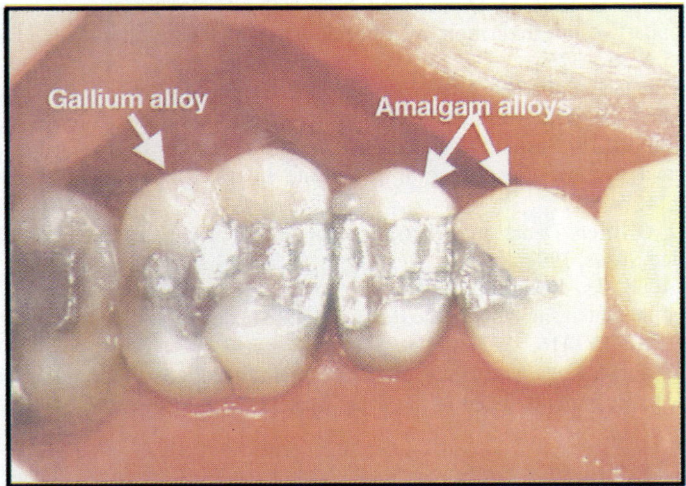

Figure 5–19 Amalgam and gallium alloy restorations (Courtesy of Dr. Jennifer CL Neo)

5.5 Conclusions

An overview of the biorestorative materials used in clinical dentistry has been presented. Dental biomaterials can be broadly classified into ceramics, polymers, and metals. The success of these restorations is dependent on the correct selection of materials for a given application and the ability to carry out manipulative procedures to arrive at the optimum properties of the material.

References

1. E. C. Combe, Notes on Dental Materials (Longman, Singapore, 1992).
2. J. F. McCabe, Applied Dental Materials (Blackwell Science Publications, Oxford, 1994).
3. H. W. Fields, W. R. Proffit, J. C. Case, and K. W. L. Vig., Variables affecting measurement of vertical occlusal forces, J. Dent. Res., 1986, 65:135–138.
4. I. M. Brook and P. V. Hatton, Glass ionomers: bioactive implant materials, Biomaterials, 1998, 19:565–571.
5. A. U. J. Yap, Y. S. Pek, R. A. Kumar, P. Cheang, and K. A. Khor, Experimental studies on a new bioactive material: HAIonomer cements, Biomaterials, 2002, 23:955–962.
6. D. Dietschi and R. Spreafico, Adhesive metal-free restorations: current concepts for esthetic treatment of posterior teeth (Quintessence Publishing Co., Germany, 1997) pp:139–184.
7. J. L. Ferracane, Current trends in dental composite, Crit. Rev. Oral. Biol. Med., 1995, 6:302–318.
8. J. Arends, G. E. H. M. Dijkma, and A. G. Dijkman, Review of fluoride release and secondary caries reduction by fluoride-releasing composites, Adv. Dent. Res., 1995, 9:367–376.
9. A. J. de Gee, P. Pallav, A. Werner, and C. L. Davidson, Annealing as a mechanism of increasing wear resistance of composites, Dent. Mat., 1990, 6:266–270.
10. K. Shinkai, S. Susuki, K. F. Leinfelder, and Y. Katoh, How heat treatment and thermal cycling affect wear of composite inlays, J. Am. Dent. Assoc., 1994, 125:1467–1472.
11. W. J. O'Brien, Dental materials and their selection (Quintessence Publishing Co., United States, 1997).
12. R. Adell, U. Lekholm, B. Rockler, and P. Branemark, A 15-year study of osseointegrated implants in the treatment of the edentulous jaw, Int. J. Oral. Surg., 1981, 10:387–416.
13. T. Sakai, M. Kaga, and H. Oguchi, Two-year clinical observation of gallium alloy in pediatric patients, Trans. Acad. Dent. Mat., 1993:P–053.

CHAPTER 6

BIOCERAMICS: AN INTRODUCTION

Besim Ben-Nissan[1] and Giuseppe Pezzotti[2]

[1]*Department of Chemistry, Materials and Forensic Science, University of Technology, Sydney, PO BOX 123 Broadway, 2007 NSW Australia,*
E-mail: B.Ben-Nissan@uts.edu.au

[2]*Department of Materials, Kyoto Institute of Technology, Sakyo-ku, Matsugasaki, Kyoto, 606-8585, Japan,*
E-mail: pezzotti@ipc.kit.ac.jp

An improved understanding of currently used bioceramics in human implants and bone replacement materials could contribute significantly to the design of new-generation prostheses and post-operative patient management strategies. Overall, the benefits of advanced ceramic materials in biomedical applications have been universally appreciated — specifically in terms of their strength, biocompatibility, and wear resistance. However, the amount of supporting data is not large. Against this background, continuous development of new methods is pertinent — if not imperative — for better understanding of the microstructure-properties relationship as well as obtaining new directives to further improve ceramics as biomaterials. This chapter gives an overview of and re-examines key issues which concern both the processing and applications of ceramics as biomaterials.

6.1   Introduction

Trauma, degeneration, and diseases often make surgical repair or replacement necessary. When a person suffers from joint pain, the main priorities are the relief of pain and prompt return to a healthy and functional life style. These concerns usually require replacement of skeletal parts that include knees, hips, finger joints, elbows, vertebrae, teeth, and repair of the mandible. The worldwide biomaterials market is valued at close to US\$24,000M. Orthopedic and dental applications represent approximately 55 percent of the total biomaterials market. Orthopedics products worldwide exceeded US\$13 billion in year 2000 — an increase of 12 percent over 1999 revenues. Expansion in these areas is expected to continue due to a number of factors. These include an aging population, increasing preference by younger- to middle-aged candidates to undertake surgery, improvements in technology and lifestyle, better understanding of body functionality, availability of improved aesthetics, and need for better function [1].

Biomaterial, by definition, is "a non-drug substance suitable for inclusion in systems which augment or replace the function of bodily tissues or organs". As early as a century ago artificial materials and devices had been developed to a point where they could replace various components of the human body. These materials were capable of being in contact with bodily fluids and tissues for prolonged periods of time, whilst eliciting little — if any — adverse reaction [2].

Some of the earliest biomaterial applications were as far back as ancient Phoenicia where loose teeth were bound together with gold wires to tie artificial ones to neighboring teeth. In the early 1900s bone plates were successfully implemented to stabilize bone fractures and accelerate their healing. By the time of the 1950s to 1960s, blood vessel replacements were in clinical trials and artificial heart valves and hip joints were in development.

Even in the preliminary stages of this field, surgeons and engineers identified materials and design problems that resulted in premature loss of implant function — such as through mechanical failure, corrosion, or inadequate biocompatibility of the component. Key factors in a biomaterial usage are its biocompatibility, biofunctionality, as well as availability (to a lesser extent). Ceramics are ideal candidates with respect to all the above criteria, except for their brittle behavior.

In this chapter, we shall revisit the presently available and currently investigated bioceramics, their preparation methods, properties, and their applications in comparison to biogenic, metallic and polymeric biomaterials.

6.2   General Concepts in Bioceramics

It has been accepted that no foreign materials placed within a living body can be completely compatible. The only substances that conform completely are those manufactured by the body itself (autogenous). Any other substance that is recognized as foreign initiates some kind of reaction (host-tissue response). Figure 6–1 shows four response types of bioceramics. Each response type then determines the means of attaching the implant to the muscular skeletal system.

When a man-made material is placed within the human body, tissue reacts towards the implant in a variety of ways depending on the material type. The mechanism of tissue interaction (if any) depends on the tissue response to the implant surface. In general, tissue responses to a biomaterial may be described or classified as bioinert, bioresorbable, or bioactive. These responses have been well covered in a range of excellent review papers [3–5].

1. **Bioinert** refers to any material that once placed within the human body has minimal interaction with its surrounding tissue.   Examples of bioinert

materials are stainless steel, titanium, alumina, partially stabilized zirconia, and ultra high molecular weight polyethylene. Generally a fibrous capsule forms around a bioinert implant. Hence the implant's biofunctionality relies on tissue integration through the capsule (Figure 6–1(a)).

2. **Bioactive** refers to a material, which upon being placed within the human body interacts with the surrounding bone and in some cases, even with the soft tissue. This occurs through a time-dependent kinetic modification of the surface, triggered by its implantation within the living bone. An ion exchange reaction between the bioactive implant and surrounding body fluids results in the formation of a biologically active carbonate apatite (CHAp) layer on the implant that is chemically and crystallographically equivalent to the mineral phase of bone. Prime examples of bioactive materials are synthetic hydroxyapatite [6,7] $[Ca_{10}(PO_4)_6(OH)_2]$, glass-ceramic A–W [8,9], and Bioglass$^{®}$ [10] (Figure 6–1(b,c)).

3. **Bioresorbable** refers to a material that upon placement within the human body starts to dissolve (resorbed) and is slowly replaced by advancing tissue (such as bone). Common examples of bioresorbable materials are tricalcium phosphate $[Ca_3(PO_4)_2]$ and polylactic–polyglycolic acid copolymers. Calcium oxide, calcium carbonate (coral), and gypsum are other common materials that have been used during the last three decades (Figure 6–1(d)).

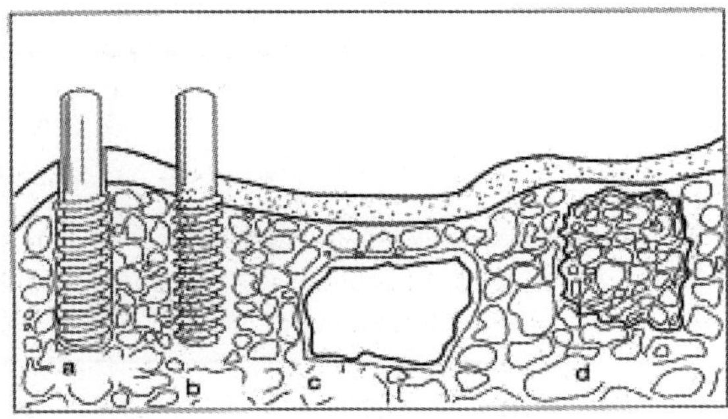

Figure 6–1 Classification of bioceramics according to their responses at the bone-implant interface: (a) bioinert alumina dental implant; (b) bioactive hydroxyapatite $(Ca_{10}(PO_4)_2(OH)_2)$ coating on a metallic dental implant; (c) surface active bioglass; (d) bioresorbable tricalcium phosphate implant $(Ca_3(PO_4)_2)$

6.3   Bioceramics and Production Methods

In clinical practice, four basic classes of material are used for biomedical implants and devices. They are bioceramics, bio-metals (metals that could be used as biomaterials), bio-polymers, and composites. Each material class has combinations of properties determined by material composition and production methods used, while each set of properties has its own benefits and limitations. Recently a fifth group of inorganic-organic composites is introduced. They are appropriately named as hybrids since some natural materials are used.

Ceramics are the hardest of solids. Table 6–1 gives some of the mechanical properties of natural and synthetic biomaterials.

Table 6–1   Mechanical properties of biomaterials (modified from Lutton and Ben-Nissan [1])

	Young's Modulus GPa	Compressive Strength MPa	Tensile Strength MPa	Density g/cm^3	Fracture Toughness MPam$^{1/2}$
METALS					
Titanium (Ti–6Al–4V)	114	450–1850	900–1172	4.43	44–66
Cr–Co–Mo	210	480–600	400–1030	8.3	120–160
Stainless Steel (316L)	193	-	515–620	8.0	20–95
CERAMICS					
Alumina	420	4400	282–551	3.98	3–5.4
Zirconia (TZP)	210	1990	800–1500	5.74–6.08	6.4–10.9
Silicon Nitride (HPSN)	304	3700	700–1000	3.3	3.7–5.5
Hydroxyapatite (3% porosity)	7–13	350–450	38–48	-	3.05–3.15
HUMAN TISSUE					
Cortical Bone	3.8–11.7	88–164	82–114	1.7–2.0	2–12
Cancellous Bone	0.2–0.5	23	10–20	-	-
Cartilage	0.002–0.01	-	5–25	-	-
OTHERS					
Bone Cement (PMMA)	2.24–3.25	80	48–72	-	1.19
UHMWHD Polyethylene	0.69	20	38–48	0.94	-

When a material yields under load such as in a mechanical testing, line defects (dislocations) move through its structure. Metals are intrinsically soft and ductile due to their appropriate slip systems which allow yielding and metallic bonding, and where electrons are free to move around the ion cores. Metals can be shaped easily by machining or by casting from molten state without any major difficulties. However most ceramics are intrinsically hard due to their ionic, covalent and/or mixed bonding which presents an enormous lattice resistance to the motion of dislocations. Hence ceramics cannot be shaped by melting and casting. These properties of hardness and strength of ceramics are exploited in areas where wear resistance is required.

In general, crack-tip plasticity gives metals their high toughness. Energy is absorbed in the plastic zone, generating a tortuous path that makes crack propagation much more difficult. Although some plasticity can occur at the tip of a crack in a ceramic too, the energy absorption is relatively small and fracture toughness is low. As a result (with the exception of partially stabilized zirconia (PSZ)), most ceramics have values of fracture toughness (K_{IC}) roughly one-fiftieth of those of ductile materials.

Due to their strong bonding, ceramics have very high melting — or more appropriately, dissociation — temperatures. Hence, ceramics can be produced only through high temperature sintering. Sintering is a process of densification where powders are heated up usually to two-third of their melting temperature, and with the aid of a driving force such as diffusion, they consolidate (Figure 6–2). During densification particles bond together to form necks between the particles, thereby causing the surface area to reduce and the powders to consolidate.

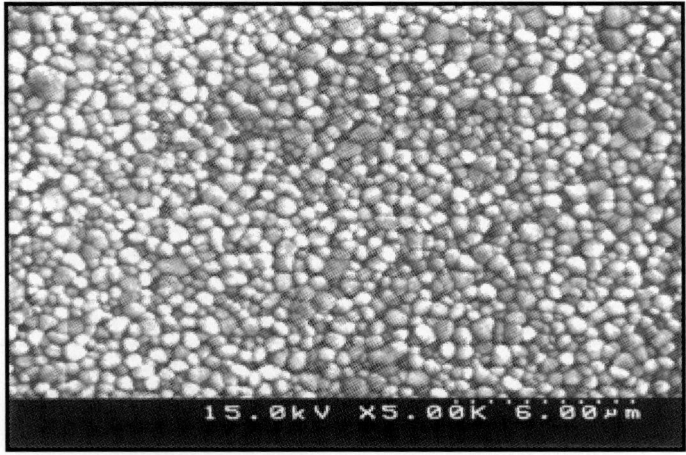

Figure 6–2 SEM of a sintered bioceramic

Full density is not achieved in normal pressureless sintering without the incorporation of sintering additives. Some porosity is usually retained in the sintered final products. Higher densities and small grain structures required by bioceramics can be achieved by hot pressing (HP) where temperature and uni-axial pressure are applied simultaneously, or by hot isostatic pressing (HIP) where the powder is isostatically pressurized within a gaseous environment and heated to a high temperature (Figure 6–3).

Sintering rate is controlled by diffusion. However large driving force shortens the sintering time and increases the final density. Various methods used in producing advanced ceramics are given in Table 6–2. Hot isostatic pressing is most commonly used.

In sintering of engineering-advanced ceramics, the density could be further improved by adding sintering aids. However for bioceramics where high purity is important, additives need to be kept to a minimum or must be totally avoided.

To produce high-purity alumina ceramic, the raw materials are bauxite and native corundum. However, alumina can be easily prepared by calcining alumina trihydrate. Alumina is commercially available either as a raw powder (up to purities > 99.99%) or as tabular sintered bodies that have been sintered without adding permanent binders. Sintering temperatures depend on the processes used.

Single-crystals of alumina (*i.e.*, sapphire rods) can be prepared by feeding fine alumina powders onto the surface of a seed crystal — which is slowly withdrawn from an electric arc or oxyhydrogen flame — as the fused powder builds up. Alumina single-crystals up to 100 mm in diameter have been grown by this method. Since late 1970s alumina single crystals named Bioceram® produced by Kyocera, Japan, have been used as sapphire dental implants.

Table 6–2 Some common bioceramic production methods

PRESSING	CASTING
Uniaxial	Slip Casting
Cold Isostatic Pressing (CIP)	Thixotropic Casting
Hot Pressing (HP)	Gel Casting
Hot Isostatic Pressing (HIP)	Soluble Mold Casting

PLASTIC FORMING	COATINGS
	Sol-Gel Coating
Extrusion	Electrodeposition
Injection Molding	Flame / Plasma Spray
Compression Molding	SBF
	PVD / CVD

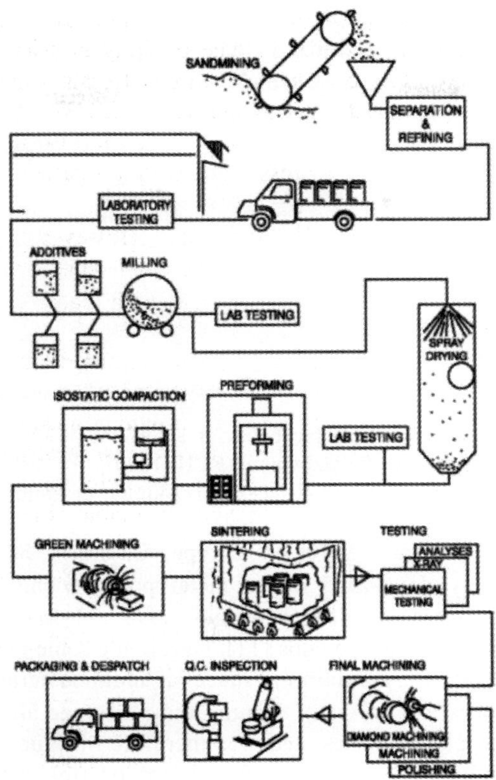

Figure 6–3 Schematic representation of one of the high-density bioceramic oxide fabrication steps

6.4 Bioinert Ceramics in Articulation

Ceramics are considered hard, brittle materials with relatively poor tensile properties. Other characteristics include excellent compressive strength, high resistance to wear, and favorably low frictional property in articulation. The low frictional property is enhanced by the fact that ceramics are hydrophilic with good wettability (Figure 6–4). They can be highly polished, thus providing a superior load bearing surface with itself or against polymeric materials in physiologic environment. Bioceramics used singularly or with additional natural, organic, or polymeric materials are amongst the most promising of all biomaterials for hard and soft tissue applications.

Interest in ceramics for biomedical applications has increased over the last 30 years. Ceramics that are used in implantation and clinical purposes include aluminum oxide (alumina), partially stabilized zirconia (PSZ) (both yittria [Y–TZP] and magnesia stabilized [Mg–PSZ]), Bioglass®, glass-ceramics, calcium phosphates (hydroxyapatite and β-tricalcium phosphate), and crystalline or glassy forms of carbon and its compounds.

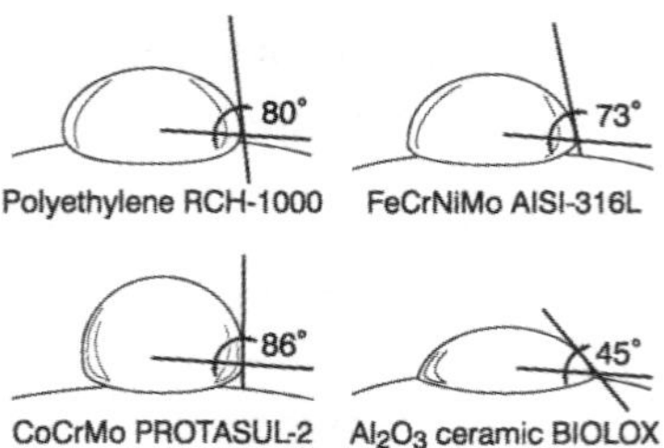

Figure 6–4 Hydrophilic/hydrophobic behavior shown by wetting angles of different orthopedic biomaterials: (a) Polyethylene (RCH–1000); (b) FeCrNiMo, AISI–316L stainless steel; (c) CoCrMo alloy (Protasul–2); (d) Alumina ceramic (Biolox)

During the 1960s and 1970s in Europe, Charnley, Scales, McKee, and Muller had already developed either metal–polyethylene (M–PE) bearings for total hip replacements (THR) or all metal (M–M) cobalt–chromium–molybdenum (CoCr) heads and cups [11]. During the same period an alternative concept was introduced by Boutin in France: an alumina ceramic cup combined with alumina femoral head (A–A). Boutin was concerned about tissue reactions to both metal and plastic debris, and was therefore intrigued by the reputation of alumina ceramic as a highly wear-resistant bearing surface for extreme conditions.

Sir John Charnley proposed employing metal on plastic total hip replacement (THR) in 1962. Most total joint prostheses consist of an articulation of a metal alloy on UHMWPE. The latter material does not have the strength required by the stem of weight-bearing joint replacements, or for intermedullary nails or bone plates. Both cobalt–chrome alloy and stainless steel are used for the bearing surface of joints. They can likewise be used for the entire femoral component of hips and knees, as well as for other joints such as the shoulder and the ankle. Metal-on-metal articulation in a total joint prosthesis has a high coefficient of friction and poor wear resistance — unless it has a very high surface finish. A good example of the use of HDPE is the total hip replacement carried out in 1962 by Charnley, where HDPE was used for the acetabular cup [11]. This particular design has continued, and in early 1970s a metal alloy stem was employed with an alumina femoral head on a UHMWPE acetabular cup. For the last 25 years, this design has reportedly reduced wear rates by as much as 10 to 20 times as compared to wear rates of metal-on-metal alone. UHMWPE and recently developed Highly Cross Linked Poly Ethylene (HCPE) are at present the preferred materials for use in conjunction with a metal or ceramic prosthesis. Creep in the PE remains a problem. Wear of the polyethylene component of these prostheses does occur, and these wear particles can sometimes cause a severe tissue reaction and eventual loosening of the implant. UHMWPE is being improved in both strength and wear characteristics. It is essential that the bearing surface in contact with the polyethylene be very highly polished. The quality of the bearing surface finish is critical to the wear characteristics of UHMWPE. HCPE has proved to be a better material for articulating surfaces.

Alumina and to a lesser extent, zirconia ceramics and recently their composites are currently used in THR as the femoral head and liners. As a result, wear particles from ultra high molecular weight polyethylene used in various other combinations are greatly reduced [12].

6.4.1 Alumina Ceramics

High-purity alumina bioceramics have been developed as an alternative to surgical metal alloys for total hip prostheses and tooth implants. The high hardness, low friction coefficient and excellent corrosion resistance of alumina offers a very low wear rate as the articulating surface in orthopedic applications. Medical grade alumina has a very low concentration of sintering additives (< 0.5 wt%), relatively small grain size (< 7 μm) and a narrow grain-size distribution. Such a microstructure is capable of inhibiting static fatigue and slowing crack growth while the ceramic is under load. The average grain size of current medical grade aluminas is 1.4 μm, and surface finish is usually controlled to a roughness of less than 0.02 μm. However, unless its surface is modified or used directly in articulating areas, alumina has a fundamental limitation as an implant material in that, like other "inert" biomaterials, a non-adherent fibrous membrane may develop at the interface. In certain circumstances interfacial failure can occur, leading to loosening — as was observed in some dental implant designs.

Currently alumina is used for orthopedic and dental implants, and which can be polished to a high surface finish and high hardness. It has been used in wear bearing environments [13], such as in total hip arthroplasties (THA) as the femoral head to help reduce wear particles from ultra high molecular weight polyethylene (UHMWPE). Other applications for alumina include porous coatings for femoral stems or as porous alumina spacers (Huckstep nails) in revision surgeries. In the past, alumina — in polycrystalline and single crystal forms — was also used in tooth implants in dental applications [3,14–16].

The mechanical behavior of alumina ceramics in simulated physiological environments has led to long-term survival predictions for these materials when they were subjected to sub critical stresses. At 112 MPa stress level, the probability for medical grade alumina to survive 50 years is 99.9 percent. Considering the tensile stresses encountered in many implants (such as in a ceramic hip joint ball), alumina ceramics can therefore be reliably employed. In a recent work by Oonishi *et al.* [17], hip simulator tests and clinical studies indicated that wear on alumina/UHMWPE THA was decreased by 25–30 percent when compared to that of metal/UHMWPE. Wear on THR of alumina/alumina was observed to be near zero in a similar hip simulator test. In knee simulator tests, UHMWPE wear against alumina decreased to one-tenth of that against metal. They further reported that during the last 23 years, no revisions were required due to PE or other wear problems. In retrieved cases, the UHMWPE surface against alumina was very smooth. However, in a comparative study on UHMWPE surface against metal, many fibrils and scratches were found — hence illustrating the extremely good performance of alumina ceramics against UHMWPE. Recently, several *in vitro* and *in vivo* studies using larger than 28 mm femoral heads demonstrated the advantage of using alumina–alumina pairing in young patients or patients with high-demand bodily function [17–19].

6.4.2 *Partially Stabilized Zirconia (PSZ)*

Compared to alumina, PSZ has high Weibull modulus — hence better reliability, higher flexural strength and fracture toughness, lower Young's modulus (Table 6–1), and the ability to be polished to a superior surface finish [20,21]. The higher fracture toughness is of particular importance in femoral heads due to the tensile stresses induced by the taper fit onto the femoral stem.

Following the production of particulate wear debris from implant materials, the consequential osteolysis has been pinpointed as the major cause of long-term failure in total hip replacements. The basic strategy to address the osteolysis problem is to reduce the number of polyethylene particles generated. This is done by improving the material at the articulating surface. For young active patients, the ceramic femoral head is strongly advocated because it produces less polyethylene wear compared to a conventional metal femoral head. On the other hand, attempts were also made to eliminate the use of polyethylene through metal-on-metal or ceramic-on-ceramic couples [17].

Partially stabilized zirconia femoral heads make up about 25 percent of the total number of operations per year in Europe, and eight percent of the hip implant procedures in USA. It has been reported that over 400,000 zirconia hip joint femoral heads have been implanted since 1985 until 2001. Most of the zirconia femoral heads (tetragonal zirconia polycrystal, TZP) consist of $97mol\%ZrO_2$ and $3mol\%Y_2O_3$.

Although not quite as hard as alumina, PSZ still possesses excellent wear resistance and has been used for similar orthopedic applications as alumina. Wear rates of UHMWPE against partially stabilized zirconia have been found to be low enough such that tribological debris would not be a problem in clinical applications [21,22]. Preliminary results indicate that a ceramic-on-ceramic femoral head/acetabular cup system is preferred over ceramic/UHMWPE systems as polymeric wear debris is avoided [23]. In fact, Chevalier and co-workers in 1997 [24] reported that not only was the friction coefficient between an alumina cup and zirconia head much lower than that of ceramic against UHMWPE, the resultant wear between the two components was almost zero. Clarke *et al.* (2000) conducted a recent study [21,22,25] on the articulation of the femoral head in total hip replacement (THR), using hip simulators with alpha-calf serum as a lubricant. In this study, wear rates of alumina/alumina, zirconia/alumina, and zirconia/zirconia couples were investigated. Results revealed that wear rates using zirconia/zirconia exhibit a mild run-in phase, as compared to a more evident run-in phase for alumina/alumina articulation.

Following the run-in phase, weight changes of all couple samples were observed. Zirconia/zirconia wear offered little observable weight change. Alumina/alumina wear (although very low) revealed a steady weight loss trend after the run-in phase. In the case of zirconia/alumina (where the head was made of zirconia and the liner made of alumina), the zirconia head showed little weight loss but the alumina liner revealed a typical run-in phase followed by a steady state weight loss. The study thus revealed promise for hard-on-hard THR systems where wear rates were three times less in order of magnitude when compared to PE cups. The study had employed alpha-calf serum at 50% concentration, while most other studies published were carried out using either water or saline solution — which can be quite detrimental to the performance of the zirconia ceramics.

Zirconia ceramic implants have had a somewhat controversial history regarding their longevity, phase-metastability, tetragonal to monoclinic transformations, degradation in water lubricant in simulation studies, and the influence of lubricants on their frictional and wear properties. At a Japanese orthopedic meeting in 1988, the orthopedic group from Bologna, Italy, reported that the wear of zirconia-on-zirconia is 5,000 times worse than that of alumina-on-alumina. While the zirconia samples used in these studies came from four different sources, the common denominator in these studies appeared to be the use of water as the test lubricant.

It has been shown that when evaluating total hip joint replacements (THR), the lubricant used in these laboratory evaluations significantly influences the wear results. Various studies have been conducted successfully when alumina-on-alumina bearings were lubricated using water, saline, and serum. However, zirconia-on-zirconia tests in water have consistently shown catastrophic results while those in serum have demonstrated good results. One such study by Oonishi and co-workers [13] showed that Y−TZP balls transformed from tetragonal to monoclinic phase when tested with saline in a hip simulator.

Widely available is a number of clinical studies which showed excellent short-term results when zirconia balls were combined with alumina cups [24]. However, contemporary clinical studies of zirconia on polyethylene have shown mixed results. Given these somewhat contradictory results between laboratory and clinical studies, Clarke *et al.* studied [22,25] the wear of zirconia-on-zirconia bearings in both water and serum. The debris and zirconia implants were then analyzed using Raman Microprobe Spectroscopy. The water lubrication test resulted in a wear about 10,000 times greater than with serum lubrication. The wear of both zirconia femoral head and cup in water lubrication showed a high weight loss of 28 mg after only 6,100 cycles. In contrast, the zirconia wear with serum lubrication had a weight loss of only 0.74 mg after 20 million cycles. This difference between the two lubricants was also distinct in the micro-wear of the ball surfaces. With serum, there were still some original machine tracks to be seen; with water there was total surface deterioration (Figure 6–5).

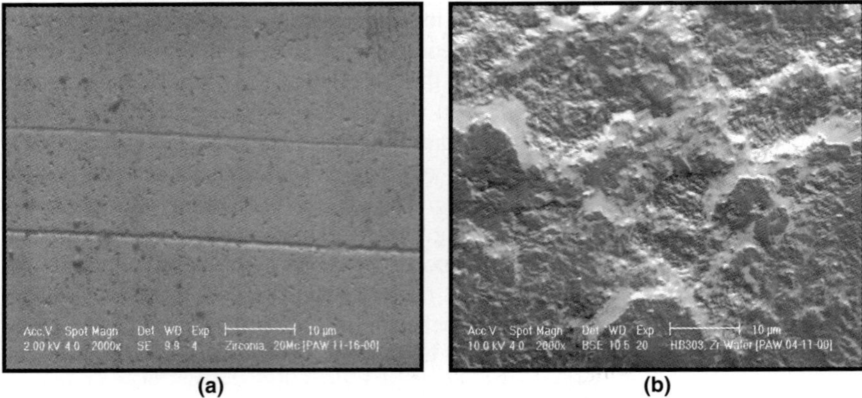

(a)   (b)

Figure 6–5 SEM images of zirconia (TZP) femoral head deterioration in hip simulator studies showing comparative wear surfaces: (a) zirconia with serum lubrication; (b) zirconia with water lubrication (after Williams *et al.* [26])

Size of the wear debris ranged from 0.38 to 16.78 microns, averaging at 1.80 microns. Analysis of the debris by Raman spectroscopy showed that the debris was almost exclusively monoclinic phase [26]. Therefore it was proposed that the simulator with water lubrication created extensive zirconia transformation. However under serum lubricant conditions, this transformation did not occur — hence the wear surface showed very little wear evidence even at 20 Mc. This phenomenon illustrated that an appropriate joint analogue fluid was of paramount importance for satisfactory wear tests. The metastability of Y–TZP ceramic is greatly affected by moisture and high temperature, and it can also be stress-activated. Based on this difference in lubricant performance, Clarke *et al.* [25] postulated that the serum proteins either formed an effective solid lubricant film between the zirconia surfaces, or acted to trap an adequate supply of moisture that effectively reduced the friction between opposing zirconia surfaces. Their study revealed the dramatic effect that serum proteins had at the bearing surface, thus greatly reducing the wear rate of zirconia.

It has been widely accepted that to improve THA longevity, it is also necessary to solve the late complications associated with implant fixation and polyethylene wear. It was reported by Woolson *et al.* [27] that the average wear rate of polyethylene against 28 mm Co–Cr head was 0.14 mm/year at the mean follow-up of 5.7 years in cementless THA (Harris–Galante prostheses) [28]. Although the present wear rate (0.139 mm/year) is almost equal to the reported value, the present zirconia-on-polyethylene combination is in effect more superior to the CoCr-on-polyethylene one in terms of volumetric wear because of the different head size used. Since the wear rate of metal-backed polyethylene tends to be influenced greatly by the polyethylene creep in the acetabular metal shell (particularly at the short follow-up duration), the present wear rate may become lower at a longer follow-up duration.

Despite these promising results, concerns remain regarding the above-mentioned degradation phenomenon — which is associated with the tetragonal-to-monoclinic phase transformation — when under long-term aqueous conditions such as an *in vivo* environment. One of the current zirconia femoral head manufacturers has improved the conventional zirconia, leading to increased strength and high resistance against the phase transformation. In addition, it was reported that in hip simulator testing, polyethylene wear against the improved zirconia head was lower than that against the Co–Cr head. When articulated with highly cross-linked polyethylene, not only zirconia heads but likewise Co–Cr heads showed very low wear rates. However, because zirconia is more scratch-resistant than Co–Cr, the former is a more suitable implant material for long-term clinical use [29].

Yttrium stabilized tetragonal polycrystalline zirconia (Y–TZP) has a fine grain size and offers the best mechanical properties. Low temperature degradation of TZP is known to occur due to the spontaneous phase transformation of tetragonal zirconia to monoclinic phase, and which occurs during aging at 130–300°C and possibly within water environment. It has been reported that this degradation leads to a decrease in strength, because alongside phase transformation microcracks are formed.

6.4.3 New Modified Zirconia Implants

Recently, new degradation-free zirconia–alumina composites have been reported: TZP/alumina composite (80%TZP of [90mol%ZrO$_2$–6mol%Y$_2$O$_3$–4mol%Nb$_2$O$_5$ composition] and 20%Al$_2$O$_3$) [12]. Another potential composite — which comprises 70vol%TZP (stabilized with 10mol%CeO$_2$) and 30vol%Al$_2$O$_3$, and 0.05mol5TiO$_2$ — is currently being investigated in Japan.

Implant stability is critical in ensuring good long-term success of total joint replacements. Loss of either biological or cement fixation can lead to accelerated wear, pain, loss of function, or even fracture of the implant — each of which could potentially necessitate revision surgery. Fixation strength can be improved by using macrotextured (porous or textured) surface, which enhances the potential for mechanical interlock at the implant-bone interface.

Oxidized zirconium, a material recently introduced for orthopedic bearing applications (Oxinium™, Smith & Nephew Inc., Memphis, TN), is reported to have beneficial wear and abrasion resistance [30,31]. However, it cannot be easily processed using traditional coating techniques. Therefore an alternative chemical surface texturing method was used. Chemical texturing process has been used clinically on Ti–6Al–4V total hip replacement components to create a surface morphology suitable for bone ingrowth [32].

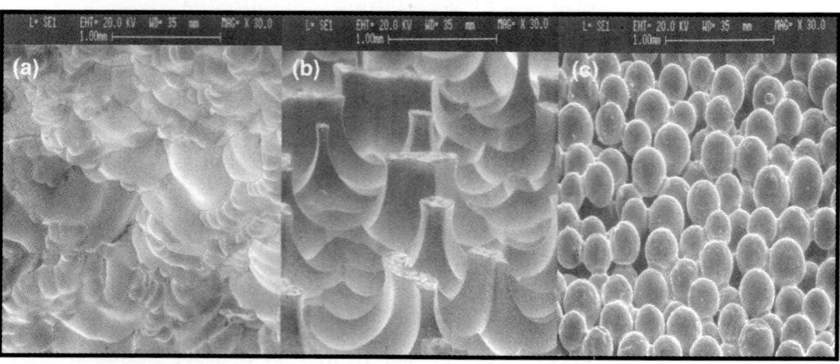

Figure 6–6 Surface texture SEM images of: (a) ChemTex® textured (CT) surface; (b) Tecotex® textured (TT) surface; and (c) porous sintered bead (SB) coating (30x) (after Heuer *et al.* [33])

This texturing method (known commercially as ChemTex® 5–5–5 (CYCAM Inc., Houston, PA)) and a newly developed chemical texturing process (known commercially as Tecotex® I–103 (Tecomet, Woburn, MA)) were used to produce macrotextured surfaces ($R_{max} > 0.4$ mm) on a zirconium alloy (Zr–2.5Nb). These textured surfaces are subsequently oxidized to form a hard ceramic layer uniformly about 5 μm thick over the entire surface, which consists predominantly of monoclinic zirconia (Figure 6–6) [33].

6.5 Bioresorbable and Bioactive Ceramics

6.5.1 Calcium Phosphates for Bone Replacement Applications

In 1926, De Jong initiated the first x-ray diffraction study of the bone [34]. In this study, apatite was identified as the only recognizable mineral phase. He also reported marked broadening of the diffraction lines of bone apatite, which he attributed to small crystal size. Following this study, numerous other studies have suggested the existence of other mineral phases in the bone. These include amorphous calcium phosphate (ACP), brushite, and octacalcium phosphate (OCP). The presence of substantial amounts of ACP or brushite has not been yet experimentally proved, and nuclear magnetic resonance studies support the conclusion that bone is composed essentially of carbonate-substituted hydroxyapatite (CHAp).

It was not until the 1970s that synthetic hydroxyapatite [$Ca_{10}(PO_4)_2(OH)_2$] was accepted as a potential biomaterial. Synthetic hydroxyapatite forms a strong chemical bond with bone *in vivo*, and it is also able to remain stable under the harsh conditions encountered in the physiologic environment.

Bone-like carbonated apatite $Ca_{(10-x)}$ $(PO_4)_{6-y}$ $(OH)_{2-z}$ $A_xB_yC_z$ (where A, B, and C are substitutional elements) is a non-stoichiometric mineral found in hard tissues of all mammals. Synthetic hydroxyapatite $Ca_{10}(PO_4)_6(OH)_2$ has been an attractive material for chromatographic separation catalysis, ion exchange, bone and tooth implants [35]. Since its inception, two common and easy methods have been used to produce synthetic HAp:

- Solid state reaction between Ca^{2+}- and PO_4^{3-}-bearing compounds; or
- When under solution conditions, powders are sintered to a dense polycrystalline body by firing.

It must be noted that parameters which control the bioactivity of HAp include Ca/P ratio, purity, grain size, and secondary compounds that could be formed during production.

Albee and Morrison [36] proposed the use of calcium phosphate ceramics for biomedical applications, after observing accelerated bone growth when tricalcium phosphate was injected into bone defects. Pure tricalcium phosphate (TCP) $Ca_3(PO_4)_2$ is more soluble in physiological environment than other phosphate ceramics (bioresorbable). Consequently, it can be used in situations where accelerated bone growth is desired. β-tricalcium phosphates have been used successfully as fillers for bone defects to stimulate new bone formation [37]. Their study also showed that after a 12-month period, β-tricalcium phosphate was totally absorbed. It was targeted that these materials will be used to fill voids in bone structure since they will dissolve over a period of time. It was also targeted that while the dissolution takes place, bone regrowth or advancement takes place at a similar rate.

Dissolution rates of some materials under simulated physiological conditions have been investigated, with particular emphasis on hydroxyapatite, β-tricalcium phosphate, and tetracalcium phosphate. Under *in vitro* conditions, the solubility of these materials has been shown to decrease in the following order [4,38]:

Tetracalcium phosphate > β-Tricalcium Phosphate > Hydroxyapatite

It has been stated that hydroxyapatite is "scarcely resorbable", hence justifying the use of hydroxyapatite for osseous implants [39–40].

It was proposed by various investigators that the initial formation of an amorphous calcium phosphate (ACP) at high pH could be followed by its transformation to hydroxyapatite (HA). The latter transformation could be via the formation of a precursor in the form of octacalcium phosphate (OCP). This chain of reactions has been proposed to be one of the templates that forms HA. It has also been stated that as the pH decreases, other precursor phases such as dicalcium phosphate dihydrate (DCPD) may form [35]. Therefore it has been accepted that other calcium phosphate phases (Table 6–3) could actively participate in the crystallization reaction of biological (biogenic) apatites.

Table 6–3 Calcium phosphate phases (modified from Ben-Nissan *et al.* [35])

Calcium phosphate phases	Mineral	Empirical formulas	Ca/P ratio	JCPDS
Dicalcium phosphate dihydrate	Brushite	$CaHPO_4.2H_2O$	1.00	11–293
Dicalcium phosphate	Monetite	$CaHPO_4$	1.00	
Octacalcium phosphate		$Ca_8H_2(PO_4)_6.5H_2O$	1.33	26–1056
β-Tricalcium phosphate	Whitlockite	β-$Ca_3(PO_4)_2$	1.50	9–169
Hydroxyapatite		$Ca_{10}(PO_4)_6(OH)_2$	1.67	9–432
Tetracalcium phosphate monoxide		$Ca_4(PO_4)_2O$	2.00	25–1137
Defect apatites		$Ca_{10-x}(HPO_4)_x(PO_4)_{6-x}(OH)_{2-x}$ $0 < x < 2$	$(10-x):6$	

Hydroxyapatite powders can be synthesized using a range of production methods [35]. However, one of the most commonly used methods [7,41,42] is from an aqueous solution of $Ca(NO_3)_2$ and NaH_2PO_4. After filtering and drying in this method, the product is calcined for about three hours at 1173 K to promote crystallization. Upon cold-press forming, the desired shape can be obtained by sintering for about one hour at about 1500 K to obtain a full densification. Once sintering reaches above 1523 K, hydroxyapatite shows a second-phase precipitation along grain boundaries and at multiple-grain junctions with formation of grain-boundary microcracks — indicating significant degradation of mechanical properties.

6.5.2 Simulated Body Fluid (SBF)

Introduced by Kokubo and co-workers [43–44], the simulated body fluid (SBF) is welcomed as a promising method in bioceramics production. This synthetic body fluid is highly supersaturated in calcium and phosphate — in relationship to apatite formation — even under normal conditions. Therefore if a material has a functional group effective for apatite nucleation on its surface, apatite can be formed spontaneously. For an artificial material to bond to the living bone, it is widely accepted that a bone-like apatite layer must form on its surface. Formation of the bone-like apatite layer on bioactive materials can be produced in a simulated body fluid (SBF) which has ion concentrations almost equal to those of the human blood plasma. Currently most bioceramics research studies use this solution to measure an artificial material's bioactivity by examining the apatite-forming ability on its surface when immersed in SBF.

Hydroxyapatite layers can be easily produced on various organic or inorganic substrates in SBF. Kokubo *et al.* in 1989 showed that after immersion in SBF, a wide range of biomaterial surfaces showed very fine crystallites of carbonate ion containing apatite [43]. Osteoblasts have also been shown to proliferate and differentiate on this apatite layer.

SBF is a metastable solution. If an apatite-nucleating functional group is present on a substrate which is immersed in the fluid, the apatite spontaneously nucleates. It has been reported that this nucleation rate increases whenever excessive amounts of Ca^{2+} ions, PO_4H_2, and Si–OH, Ti–OH, Zr–OH, Ta–OH, Nb–OH or similar functional groups are present [44]. For example, it has been shown that highly porous gels of SiO_2, TiO_2, ZrO_2, Nb_2O_5, and Ta_2O_5 could form apatite layers on their surfaces in SBF. All these observations indicate that the above-mentioned functional groups with a specific structure are effective for apatite nucleation in the body environment [44].

6.5.3 Coralline Apatites

Coralline apatites can be derived from the sea coral. Coral is composed of calcium carbonate in the form of aragonite. As coral is a naturally occurring structure, it has optimal strength and structural characteristics. The pore structure of coralline calcium phosphate produced by certain species is similar to human cancellous bone, making it a suitable material for bone graft applications (Figure 6–7). Coral and converted coralline hydroxyapatite have been used as bone grafts and orbital implants since the 1980s. This is because the porous nature of the structure allows ingrowth of blood vessels to supply blood for bone, which eventually infiltrates the implant.

Size and interconnectivity of pores are of utmost importance when hard and soft tissue ingrowth is required. Kühne *et al.* [45] showed that implants with average pore size of around 260 μm had the most successful ingrowth as compared to no implants (that is, simply leaving the segment empty). It was further reported that the interaction of the primary osteons between the pores via the interconnections allows propagation of osteoblasts.

The hydrothermal method was first used by Roy and Linnehan [46] in 1974 to form hydroxyapatite directly from corals. It was reported that complete replacement of aragonite ($CaCO_3$) by phosphatic material — via the hydrothermal process — was achieved using less than 533 K and 103 MPa. In 1996, HAp derived from Indian coral using the hydrothermal process was reported [47]. However the resultant material was in powder form and it required further forming and sintering.

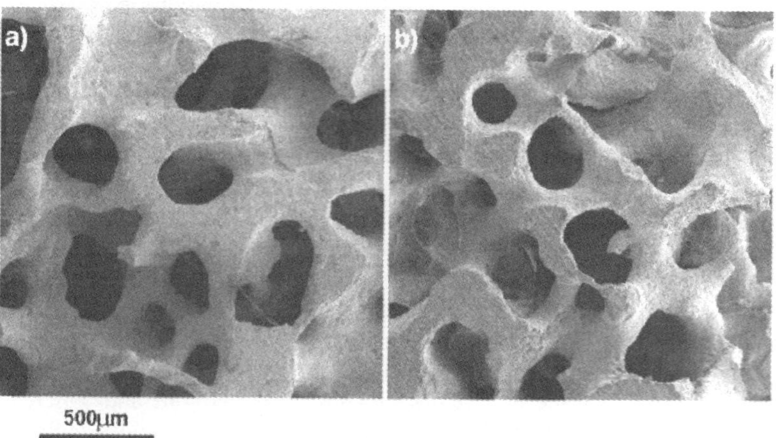

Figure 6–7 Comparison of the Australian coral: (a) in original state; and (b) after hydrothermal conversion

During the hydrothermal treatment, hydroxyapatite replaces the aragonite whilst preserving the porous structure. The following exchange takes place:

$$10CaCO_3 + 6(NH_4)_2HPO_4 + 2H_2O \rightarrow Ca_{10}(PO_4)_6(OH)_2 + 6(NH_4)_2CO_3 + 4H_3CO_3 \tag{1}$$

The resulting material is known as coralline hydroxyapatite, be it in the porous coralline structure or in powdered form.

Alternatively, aragonite can be converted to carbonate hydroxyapatite using microwave processing technique. Higher extends of conversion were reported [48].

Hu *et al.* [49] succeeded in converting a high-strength Australian coral (Porites) to monophasic hydroxyapatite using a two-stage process where the hydrothermal method was followed by a patented hydroxyapatite sol-gel coating process based on alkoxide chemistry. They reported 120% increase in the biaxial strength of the double-treated coral as compared to the one that is merely converted.

6.5.4 Calcium Phosphate Coatings

Due to its unfavorable mechanical properties, it has been accepted that porous hydroxyapatite cannot be used under load bearing conditions. Instead hydroxyapatite has been used as thin film coatings on metallic alloys. Of the metallic alloys investigated, titanium-based alloys have shown to be the preferred material for thin film coatings [50]. Being lightweight and with high strength-to-weight ratios, titanium alloys possess good mechanical strength and fatigue resistance under load bearing conditions.

Of the coating techniques utilized, thermal spraying (plasma, and to a lower extend flame spraying) tends to be the most commonly used and analyzed. This technique has been faced with the challenge of producing a controllable resorption response in clinical situations. While striving towards this target, thermally sprayed coatings are being improved continuously by using different compositions and post-heat treatments which convert amorphous phases to crystalline calcium phosphates. Currently plasma coating of macrotextured orthopedic implants is used commercially, and other techniques involving less soluble fluorapatite compositions are also being investigated. Techniques that are capable of producing thin coatings include pulsed-laser deposition [51] and sputtering [52] which, like thermal spraying, involve high-temperature processing. Other techniques such as electrodeposition [53,54] and sol-gel [55] use lower temperatures and avoid the challenge associated with the structural instability of hydroxyapatite at elevated temperatures [56].

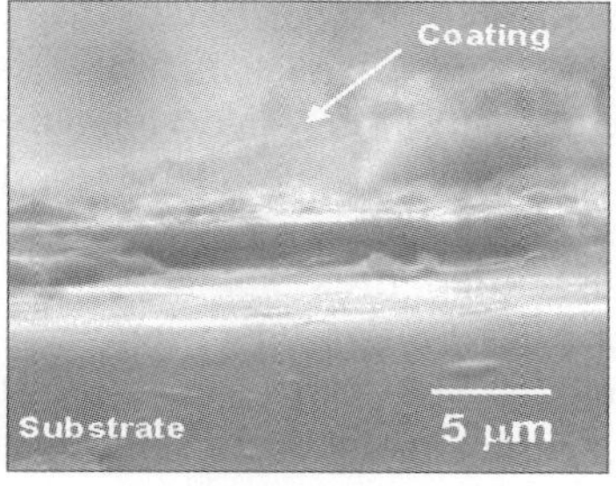

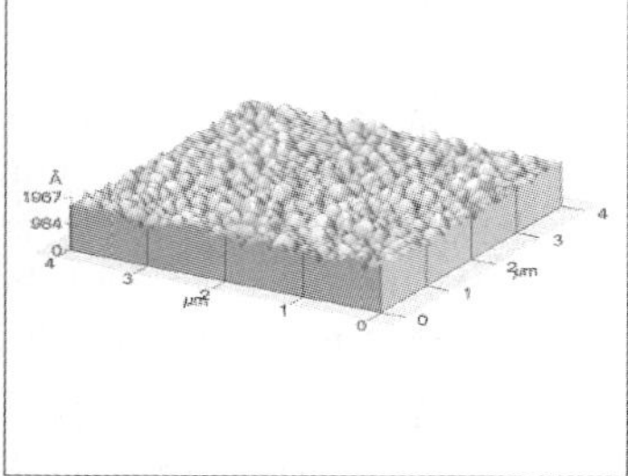

Figure 6–8 SEM and AFM images of sol-gel (alkoxide) derived hydroxyapatite coatings

The advantages of sol-gel technique are numerous, namely:

- It results in a stoichiometric, homogeneous, and pure coating due to mixing on a molecular scale;
- Firing temperatures are reduced due to small particle sizes with high surface areas;
- It is able to produce uniform fine-grained structures (Figure 6–8);
- It uses different chemical routes (alkoxide or aqueous based);
- It is easy to be applied to complex shapes using a range of coating techniques such as dip, spin, and spray coating;
- Due to its lower processing temperature, it avoids the phase transition (~1156 K) observed in titanium-based alloys used for biomedical devices.

6.5.5 *Synthetic Bone Graft Ceramics*

Bone grafting is currently used in orthopedic and maxillofacial surgeries for these treatments: diaphyseal defects bridging, non-union, metaphyseal defects filling, and mandibular reconstruction.

Autogeneous bone graft has the following characteristics:

- Osteogenic (that is, able to form bone due to living cells such as osteocytes or osteoblasts);
- Osteoconductive (that is, no capacity to induce or form bone but provides an inert scaffold upon which osseous tissue can regenerate bone);
- Osteoinductive (that is, able to stimulate cells to undergo phenotypic conversion to osteoprogenitor cell types capable of bone formation).

There are no substitutes for autogenous bone; there are, however, synthetic alternatives. Allografts have been used as an alternative. However this alternative offers low or no osteogenicity, increases immunogenicity, and resorbs more rapidly than autogenous bone. In clinical practice, fresh allografts are rarely used because of unfavorable immune response and the risk of disease transmission. The frozen and freeze-dried types are osteoconductive but are considered, at best, to be only weakly osteoinductive. Freeze-drying diminishes the structural strength of the allograft and renders it unsuitable for use in situations where structural support is required. Allograft bone is a useful material for patients who require bone grafting of a non-union but have inadequate autograft bone. Bulk allografts can be utilized to treat segmental bone defects [57]. Their use in reconstruction after bone tumors resection is well documented. However they are not commonly used in post-trauma reconstruction in which bone lengthening and transport are usually required.

Calcium sulfate (plaster of Paris) or its composites are one of the oldest osteoconductive materials available. They have been used to fill bony defects.

However its main drawback is the chemical reaction that occurs during setting, which results in non-homogeneous structure with anisotropic properties.

Demineralized bone matrix (DBM) was first observed by Urist in 1965 to induce heterotopic bone [58]. The active components of DBM are a series of glycoproteins which belong to a group of transforming growth factor family (TGF–β). The members of this group are responsible for the morphogenic events involved in tissues and organs development. Urist also isolated a protein from the bone matrix, which was termed as bone morphogenic protein (BMP) [58]. DBM is commercially available and is used in management of non-union of fractures. They are not suitable where structural support is required. To date, the main delay in developing clinical products has been the need to find a suitable carrier to deliver BMP to the site where its action is required. New-generation ceramic composites/hybrids could fill this gap. Experimentally, BMP–2 and OP–1® (BMP–7) have been shown to stimulate new bone formation in diaphyseal defects in the rat, rabbit, dog, sheep, and non-human primates [59]. The use of BMPs as well as collagen with new calcium phosphate derivatives or composites could be used for bone remodeling where bone regeneration is required (such as therapeutic applications in osteoporosis).

Bovine collagen mixed with hydroxyapatite is marketed as a bone graft substitute, which can be combined with bone marrow aspirated from the fracture site. Although no disease transmissions have been recorded, its use will continue to be a source of concern. This material is osteogenic, osteoinductive, and osteoconductive, but it lacks the structural strength required.

6.5.6 *Bioglasses and Glass-Ceramics*

Since Hench and Wilson [60] discovered the bioglasses which bond to living tissue (Bioglass®), various kinds of bioactive glasses and glass-ceramics with different functions — such as high mechanical strength, high machinability, and fast setting ability — have been developed. The glasses that have been investigated for implantation are primarily based on silica (SiO_2) which may contain small amounts of other crystalline phases. The most prominent and successful application of this is Bioglass® which can be found in detail in various comprehensive reviews [5,9,61,62]. Bioactive glass compositions lie in the $CaO–P_2O_5–SiO_2$ system. The first development of such a bioglass began in 1971 when 45S5 Bioglass® was proposed with a composition of 45%SiO_2, 24.5%CaO, 24.5%NaO_2, and 6%P_2O_5 by weight [10]. Hench [5] and Vrouwenvelder *et al.* [63] suggested that 45S5 Bioglass® has greater osteoblastic activity as compared to hydroxyapatite. The reasoning behind this was due to a rapid exchange of alkali ions at the surface, which then leads to the formation of a silica-rich layer over a period of time. This paves way for Ca^{2+} and PO_4^{3-} ions to migrate to the silica-rich surface where they combine with soluble calcium and phosphate ions from the solution, eventually forming an amorphous $CaO-P_2O_5$ layer. This layer undergoes crystallization upon interacting with OH^-, CO_2^{3-}, and F^- from the solution. Similar phenomenon has been observed by other researchers of bioglass with similar compositions [64]. Li *et al.* [65] prepared glass-ceramics from a similar composition with different degrees of crystallinity. They found that the amount of remaining glassy phase directly influenced apatite layer formation, and that total inhibition occurred when the glassy phase constituted less than about 5 wt%.

Due to the surface-active response of these materials, they have been accepted as bioactive (or surface-active) biomaterials and have been used in middle ear and other non-load bearing applications. Bioglasses[®] has been used successfully in clinical applications as artificial middle ear bone and in alveolar ridge maintenance implants [60].

Bioglass[®], when subjected to heat treatment, will result in reduced alkaline oxide content and precipitated crystalline apatite in the glass. The resultant glass-ceramic is named Ceravital[®], which exhibits fairly high mechanical strength but lower bioactivity than Bioglass[®].

Kokubo *et al.* in 1982 [8] produced a glass-ceramic which contained oxyfluorapatite $Ca_{10}(PO_4)_6(OH,F_2)$ and wollastonite $(CaO.SiO_2)$ in a $MgO-CaO-SiO_2$ glassy matrix. It was named A–W glass-ceramic. It was reported that this A–W glass-ceramic spontaneously bonds to living bone without forming any fibrous tissue around them.

A bioactive and machinable glass-ceramic named Bioverit[®] has also been developed. It contains apatite and phlogophite $(Na,K)Mg_3(AlSi_3O_{10})(F)_2$, and is used in clinical applications as artificial vertebra.

6.6   Nano-bioceramics, Composites and Hybrids

6.6.1 Nanoapatite-polymer Fiber Composites

Bone is a composite in which nanosized apatite platelets are deposited on organic collagen fibers. If three-dimensional synthetic organic fibers can be fabricated into a composite structure and then modified with functional groups effective for apatite nucleation, morphologically similar bone structures could perhaps be prepared in such a manner. The resultant composite could be expected to exhibit bioactivity as well as mechanical properties analogous to those of the living bone.

Quite recently ethylene–vinyl alcohol copolymer (EVOH) fibers constituting two-dimensional fabrics were subjected to a silane coupling treatment and subsequent soaking in a calcium silicate solution with a molar ratio of $Si(OC_2H_5)_4/H_2O/C_2H_5OH/Ca(NO_3)_2$ of 1.0/4.0/4.0/0.014/0.2. In this investigation, Kim *et al.* [66] and Kokubo *et al.* [67] have shown that after soaking in SBF for two days, nanosized apatite particles could be deposited uniformly on individual fibers constituting a fabric. The same fibers were also modified with a anatase-type titania on their surfaces after silane coupling treatment. This was done by soaking the fibers in a titania solution $Ti(OiC_3H_7)_4/H_2O/C_2H_5OH/HNO_3$ with a molar ratio of 1.0/1.0/9.25/0.1, followed by soaking them in 0.1M-HCl solution at 80°C for eight days.

These pioneering works thus show that if these techniques were to be successfully applied to three-dimensional fabrics, then bioactive materials somehow similar to those of the living hard and soft tissues could possibly be produced.

6.6.2 Bioceramics in In Situ Radiotherapy and Hyperthermia

One of the most common approaches in cancer treatment is the removal of the diseased parts. Unfortunately recovery of or return to full function is seldom achieved. Non-invasive treatment techniques — where only the cancer cells are destroyed — were introduced in mid 1980s. In 1987, microspheres of $17Y_2O_3-19Al_2O_3-64SiO_2$ (mol%) glass, 20–30 µm in diameter were shown to be effective for *in situ* radiotherapy of liver cancer [68,69]. ^{89}Yttrium in this glass is non-radioactive but can be activated by neutron bombardment to become ^{90}Y — which is a β-emitter with half-life of 64.1 hours. The glass microspheres are usually injected into diseased liver through the hepatic artery. Once entrapped in small blood vessels, they block the blood supply to the cancer and directly irradiate the cancer with β-rays. Since the β-ray transmission is only 2.5 mm in diameter on living tissue, and since the glass microspheres have high chemical durability the surrounding normal tissue is hardly damaged by the β-rays.

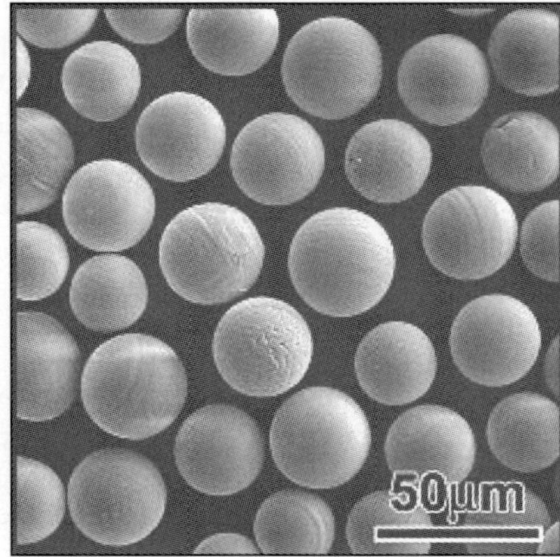

Figure 6–9 SEM image of Y_2O_3 microspheres for radiotherapy applications (after Kokubo *et al.* [67])

These glass microspheres are already used clinically in Australia, Canada, and U.S.A. The content of Y_2O_3 in the microspheres is, however, limited to only 17 mole% as they are prepared by conventional glass melting techniques. Recently, Kokubo *et al.* successfully prepared pure Y_2O_3 polycrystalline microspheres — which are 20 to 30 μm in diameter — by high-frequency induction thermal plasma melting technique [70] (Figure 6–9). It was reported that they observed higher chemical durability than the Y_2O_3-containing glass microspheres. It was further reported that these ceramic microspheres are more effective for *in situ* radiotherapy of cancer.

Oxygen is known to be poorly supplied to cancer cells to produce lactic acid. Hence cancer cells can be destroyed at around 43°C, whereas normal living cells are kept alive even at 48°C. If ferri- or ferromagnetic materials are implanted around cancer cells and placed under an alternating magnetic field, it is expected that through magnetic hysteresis loss of the ferri- or ferromagnetic materials, cancer cells locally heated can be destroyed.

Kokubo and co-workers prepared ferrimagnetic glass-ceramic compositions containing 36 wt% of 200nm-sized magnetite (Fe_3O_4) within a CaO–SiO$_2$ matrix. It was reported that cancer cells in medullary canal of rabbit tibia were completely destroyed when this glass-ceramic was inserted into the tibia and placed under alternating magnetic field of 300 Oe with 100 kHz [71]. This kind of invasive treatment, however, cannot be applied to humans since cancer cells metastasize. In the case of humans, ferri- or ferromagnetic material must be injected to the cancer in microspheric form of 20 to 30 μm in diameter through blood vessels — an approach similar to that used for radioactive microspheres. For this purpose, heat generating efficiency of the ferrimagnetic material must be further increased. Recently microspheres of 20 to 30 μm in diameter, with magnetite particles of 50 nm in size, were deposited on silica microspheres of 12 μm in diameter. The technique involved first of all, deposition of FeO(OH) from a solution, followed by its transformation into Fe_3O_4 by a specific heat treatment at 600°C under CO_2–H_2 gas atmosphere [72]. It was reported that the heat generating efficiency of this material was about four times that of the glass-ceramic described above.

6.6.3 Bone Cement Composites

During the last five years, bone cement materials have grown in popularity and are slated to be the osteoconductive substitutes for bone graft. They are prepared like acrylic cements, where a range of powders such as monocalcium phosphate, tricalcium phosphate, and calcium carbonate is mixed in a sodium phosphate solution. These cements are produced without polymerization, and the reaction is nearly non-exothermic. The final compounds are reported to have strength of 10–100 MPa in compression. However the strength is only 1–10 MPa in tension, and very weak under shear forces. These composites are currently used in orthopedics for fractures management. It has been suggested that these materials could improve the compressive strength of vertebral bodies in osteoporosis. Injection of calcium phosphate cement has been shown to be feasible and effective: the cement indeed improved their compressive strength [73].

Attempts have been made to prepare hydroxyapatite/ceramic composites by adding various ceramic reinforcements: metal fibers [74], Si_3N_4 or hydroxyapatite whiskers [75], Al_2O_3 platelets [76], and ZrO_2 particles [77]. In many cases, the composites could not be successfully prepared due to problems related to poor densification.

Hydroxyapatite/metal and hydroxyapatite/polymer composites are two typical classes of materials which have been examined for improving the toughness characteristics of synthetic hydroxyapatite. In both cases, improvement in toughness can be detected by studying the crack-face bridging mechanism in operation during plastic stretching of metallic or polymeric ligaments. Zhang *et al.* [78] proposed a toughened composite consisting of hydroxyapatite dispersed with silver particles. This material was obtained by a conventional sintering method. It was reported that the toughness of these composites increased to 2.45 MPa m$^{1/2}$ upon loading the mixture with 30 vol% of silver. Silver is used not only because of its ductility in terms of fracture toughness, but also because it is inert and has antibacterial properties [79]. Attempts to supersede metal alloys by carbon-fiber reinforced plastics and various composites to stabilize fractures have met with limited success. To date, the only exception is a new titanium metal core-composite hip implant which has been clinically assessed in Europe with promising results [76,77].

6.6.4 *Biomimetic Hybrid Composites*

The conventional way to synthesize an inorganic material-based composite is to subject one of the mixture constituents to a specifically designed heat treatment. This process is also commonly used to produce biomaterials. However, conceptually, it is far from the biomineralization process which occurs in nature. The natural process produces fine hybrid structures which are hardly reproducible by classic consolidation processes. Traditional sintering route is not directly applicable to produce ceramic/polymer composites because no polymers will withstand the densification temperature of any ceramic material. Hydroxyapatite/polyethylene (HAp/PE) composites have been obtained by loading the polymeric matrix with an inorganic filler. In recent years, several research groups have demonstrated the feasibility of *in vitro* techniques to synthesize biomimetic material structures [43,77–83]. Currently a range of HAp/PE-based composites are produced and marketed by an UK based company. The sophistication of the biomimetic route has not been paired yet and these techniques, so far, have not proved to be fully applicable for clinical applications [82].   It can be easily predicted that more and more dense bioceramics-based hybrid materials will be introduced, thus opening up new horizons in biomaterials production and application methods.

A new alternative route has been proposed recently [79]. It is based on an *in situ* polymerization process carried out in an inorganic scaffold (which has submicrometer-sized open porosity). This is an intermediate method between conventional sintering and *in vitro* biomineralization, because it still employs sintering for the preparation of the inorganic scaffold; however, the subsequent hybridization of the scaffold with organic phase is carried out through a chemical route. While this method is targeted at relatively complex structural designs, it enables the synthesis of biomimetic (hybrid) inorganic/organic composites in rather simple and easily reproducible ways. A schematic representation of this efficient synthesis route is given in Figure 6–10.

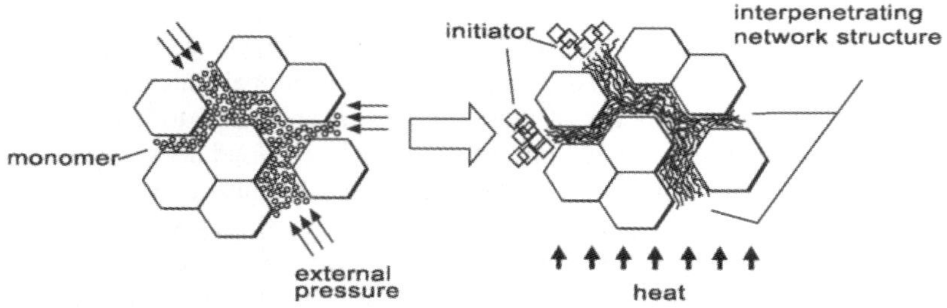

Figure 6–10 Schematic representation of the *in situ* polymerization synthesis route of new-generation hybrid materials

A common characteristic of natural biomaterials — such as bone, nacre, sea urchin tooth, and other tough hybrid materials in nature — is the strong microscopic interaction between the inorganic and organic phases. This characteristic allows the organic phase to act as a plastic energy-dissipating network, where stretching (bridging) ligaments are formed across the surfaces of a propagating crack on a nanoscale level. Such complexity has led to the common perception that, to mimic the natural designs, *in situ* synthesis techniques should be adopted. Precipitation of calcium carbonate or hydroxyapatite into a polymeric matrix, for example, has been proposed as a novel synthetic route to biomimetic composites [81–84]. Despite significant advances in understanding biological mineralization and developing new fabrication processes, the composites to-date obtained by these methods are by far in embryonic stage for actual biomedical applications due to their low structural performance.

Fracture tests were carried out on two natural biomaterials, bovine femur and Japanese nacre (*Crassostrea Nippona*). Their results were then compared with a synthetic hydroxyapatite/nylon–6 composite obtained by *in situ* polymerization of caprolactam infiltrated into a porous apatite scaffold. The comparison showed that the level of fracture incurred was about two orders of magnitude higher than that of monolithic hydroxyapatite, and it is due to stretching of protein or polymeric ligaments across the crack faces during fracture propagation [79].

Nanoscale modeling of synthetically manufactured hybrids and composites is still in infancy. However, mimicking natural microstructures by using strong synthetic molecules may lead to new-generation biomaterials, whose toughness characteristics will be comparable with those of the materials available in nature. A formidable challenge remains on the optimization of morphology and bioactivity in these novel hybrid composites.

6.7 Design with Bioceramics

Five important factors should be considered in any implantation work:

1. Production method of the material used;
2. Biocompatibility, tissue-implant interface reactions, and choice of the material used;
3. Applied stresses and biomechanics of the joint;
4. Physical well-being and age of the patient; and
5. Surgical technique.

Various criteria exist when selecting a biomaterial for a particular biomedical application. After biocompatibility, mechanical properties are the second decisive criterion when it comes to selecting a material for a particular orthopedic or maxillofacial application. Selected mechanical properties of a range of synthetic and natural biomaterials are shown in Table 6–1.

In the context of mechanical properties, an important criterion involves a scrutiny of the modulus of elasticity and Poisson's ratio. These are intrinsic material constants that describe a material's deformability, and which therefore influence the stiffness of any structure made from this material. At a bone-implant load carrying interface, the greater the stiffness of the implant material, the more load it will carry while less will be carried by the surrounding tissue. However, this issue can be detrimental due to stress shielding and resultant bone resorption.

For example, evaluation of plate stiffness is crucial when it comes to choosing a material for fracture plate. Woo [85] has experimentally verified this by comparing a rigid Co–Cr alloy and a flexible composite plate made of graphite, carbon fibers, and polymethylmetacrylate resin (GFMM). The latter material has an elastic modulus approximately 1/10(10–40 GPa) that of Co–Cr alloy (250 GPa). Four-point bending tests were performed on cortical bone adjacent to the fracture plate. These specimens were removed post-operatively after one-year implantation in dog femurs. The tests showed that the strength of the bone adjacent to less rigid GFMM-plated bone was much greater than that of the Co–Cr-plated bone. Although stiffness is not the only determining factor of this increase, its importance is nevertheless highlighted here.

Material failure can occur in tensile, compressive, and shear modes. Metals tend to have tensile and compressive strengths that do not differ greatly; ceramics tend to be weak in tension and strong in compression. The lack of crystallographic slip systems in ceramics and glasses prevents dislocation motion and generation, resulting in a material that is hard and brittle. To determine if a class of materials is appropriate for a particular application, it is mandatory to carefully assess the nature of loading that this application demands. For example, if an application requires the selected material to withstand tensile stress, then the material's tensile strength must be improved by making surface layers compressive relative to the interior. After all, applied force should overcome the compressive force before tensile force takes over. Depending on the bioceramics used, surface compression can be introduced by various surface modification techniques such as ion exchange, quenching, and surface crystallization. The ion exchange in glass and glass-ceramics can be accomplished by diffusion or electrical-migration techniques. Larger ions are exchanged with smaller ions (e.g., K^+ for Na^+), making the surface compressive due to lattice straining.

As for a material's resistance to fracture, it is determined by an extrinsic property named fracture toughness. This tends to be high for metals and low for ceramics. This is an important parameter because it more appropriately reflects a material's performance than its tensile strength data. Fracture toughness data of ceramics and metals show that resistance to crack propagation and failure is much higher for metals — which means that tensile failure would occur more readily in ceramics.

Strength and fracture toughness testing procedures usually involve short-term assessments and are prone to statistical scatter. In addition, they neglect the effects of dynamic fatigue on metals or static fatigue (slow crack growth) on ceramics. Therefore results from these assessments can be considered only as upper limits to a material's performance. Given the complex overlapping of various degradation phenomena, mechanical analyses have to be carefully performed according to case-by-case testing procedures. For example, the fatigue behavior of a vapor-deposited pyrolytic carbon film of about 500 nm in thickness onto a stainless steel substrate showed that the film did not break until the substrate underwent plastic deformation (deformation of 0.0013 strain after 10^6 cyclic loading) [86]. This case illustrated that fracture of thin films strongly depends on the behavior of the substrates used.

Microhardness and nanohardness indicate a material's ability to resist wear and impact. Wear performance is a very important consideration in the selection of an implant material, as wear results from the removal and relocation of matter through the contact of two surfaces. However, both plastic and elastic deformations involve many different types of wear.

- Corrosive wear is due to chemical activity on one of the sliding materials. The sliding action promotes the removal of corrosion products (that otherwise protect the surface from further corrosive attack), resulting in faster corrosion rates.

- Surface fatigue wear is due to the formation of subsurface microcracks followed by breaking off of large chunks under repeated loading and sliding cycles.

- Abrasive wear is a process in which particles are pulled off from one surface and adhere to the other during sliding. This type of wear is the most important process in biomaterials and can be minimized with particular care on smoothing the sliding surfaces.

- Wear related to phase transformation is a kind of wear process peculiar to zirconia implants. It arises from the metastability of some polycrystalline zirconia materials and from the tendency of the tetragonal phase to transform into the monoclinic polymorph. Since the tetragonal-to-monoclinic transformation occurs with volume expansion, hard monoclinic particles tend to detach from the sliding surface and, being trapped in between the sliding surfaces, strongly accelerate surface degradation. The resistance to transformation wear of a zirconia material is remarkably affected by the kind of lubricant between the sliding surfaces as explained in previous sections [17].

In summary, mechanical properties data of any potential implant material must be considered with care because many extrinsic factors dominate the properties — particularly in the case of bioceramics. A material's microstructure and testing environment are the main controlling factors among the variables. In all cases, published data can be considered only as guidelines for the behavior of materials in use.

6.8   Future of Bioceramics

As discussed in this chapter, the properties of bioceramics are strongly influenced by these factors: raw materials selected for preparation, method used to fabricate, processes used to consolidate, and the final machining processes. All these factors contribute to their final structure and hence to their long-term performance as bioceramics. The optimization of bioceramics in medical applications can be achieved by further studies of the effects of processing conditions on their structures and hence their long-term properties.

In particular, the nature and effect of additives — whether to improve biological performance or to ease processing — on the local and systemic responses need further investigation. Sometimes, improvement of one property could be detrimental to the other properties.

In the early 1970s bioceramics were employed to perform singular, biologically inert roles, such as to provide parts for bone replacement. The realization that cells and tissues in the body perform many other vital regulatory and metabolic roles has highlighted the limitations of synthetic materials as tissue substitutes. Demands of bioceramics have changed from maintaining an essentially physical function without eliciting a host response, to providing a more integrated interaction with the host. This is accompanied by increasing demands for medical devices to improve the quality of life, as well as extend its duration. Bioceramics potentially can be used as body interactive materials — helping the body to heal or promoting regeneration of tissues, thus restoring physiological functions. This approach is being explored in the development of a range of new-generation bioceramics which incorporates biogenic materials with a widened selection of applications.

Recently tissue engineering has been directed to take advantage of the combined use of living cells with tri-dimensional ceramic scaffolds to deliver vital cells to the damaged site in a patient. To date, strategies that combine a relatively traditional approach (such as bioceramic implants) with the acquired knowledge have been found to be feasible and productive when applied to the fields of cell growth and differentiation of osteogenic cells. A stem cell is a cell from the embryo, fetus, or adult that has the ability to reproduce for long periods. It also can give rise to specialized cells that make up the tissues and organs of the body. An adult stem cell is an undifferentiated (unspecialized) cell that occurs in a differentiated (specialized) tissue. It is able to renew itself and become specialized to yield all of the specialized cell types of the tissue from which it originates. Cultured bone marrow cells can be regarded as a mesenchymal precursor cell population derived from adult cells. They can differentiate into different lineages (osteoblasts, chondrocytes, adipocytes, and myocytes) and undergo limited mitotic divisions without expressing any telomerase activity. When implanted onto immuno-deficient mice, these cells can combine with mineralized tri-dimensional scaffolds to form a highly vascularized bone tissue. Cultured-cells/bioceramic composites can be used to treat full-thickness gaps of bone diaphysis with excellent integration of the ceramic scaffold with bone and good functional recovery. Excellent innovative work is in progress, and clinical applications are becoming quite common.

Ultimately the field of bioceramics is fundamental to advances in the performance and function of medical devices, and is a critical part of medicine and surgery. Bioceramics science is truly interdisciplinary. Therefore the development of improved bioceramics hinges on the outcome of advances in materials, physical and biological sciences, engineering, and medicine. The correlations between materials property and biological performance will be useful in the design of improved bioceramics, particularly to overcome the problems of implant rejection and related infections.

The challenge remains to provide safe and efficacious bioceramics with the required properties and an acceptable biocompatibility level. As the field of biomaterials finds increasing applications in cellular and tissue engineering, it will continue to be used in new ways as part of the most innovative therapeutic strategies.

References

1. P. P. Lutton and B. Ben-Nissan, Biomaterials in the marketplace: Focus on orthopedic and dental applications, Materials Technology, 1997, 12(3–4):121–126.
2. R. H. Doremus, Review — Bioceramics, J. Mater. Sci., 1992, 27:285–297.
3. J. W. Boretos, Advances in bioceramics, Adv. Ceram. Mater., 1987, 2:15–24.
4. R. Z. LeGeros, Calcium phosphate materials in restorative dentistry: a review, Adv. Dent. Res., 1988, 2:164–183.
5. L. L. Hench, Molecular design of bioactive glasses and ceramics for implants, in Ceramics: Towards the 21st Century, eds. W. Soga and A. Kato, (Ceram. Soc. of Japan, 1991) pp:519–534.
6. H. Aoki, $CaO–P_2O_5$ Apatite, Japanese Patent JP 78110999 (1978).
7. M. Jarcho, C. H. Bolen, M. B. Thomas, J. F. Bobick, J. F. Kay, and R. H. Doremus, J. Mater. Sci., 1976, 11:2027–2035.
8. T. Kokubo, M. Shigematsu, Y. Nagashima, M. Tashiro, T. Nakamura, T. Yamamuro, and S. Higashi, Apatite–Wollastonite containing glass-ceramic for prosthetic application, in Bulletin of Institute for Chemical Research, (Kyoto University, 1982) 60:260–268.
9. T. Kokubo, Novel biomaterials derived from glasses, in Ceramics: Towards the 21st Century, eds. W. Soga and A. Kato, (J. Ceramic. Soc. Japan, 1991) pp:500–518.
10. L. L Hench, R. J. Splinter, W. C. Allen, and T. K. Greenlee, Bonding mechanisms at the interface of ceramic prosthetic materials, J. Biomed. Mater. Res. Symp., 1972, 2:117–141.
11. I. C. Clarke, Role of ceramic implants – design and clinical success with total hip prosthetic ceramic-to-ceramic bearings, Clinical Orthopedics and Related Research, 1992, 282:19–30.
12. D. J. Kim, D. Y. Lee, and J. S. Han, Low temperature stability of zirconia/alumina hip joint heads, in Key Engineering Materials, 240–242, in Bioceramics 15, eds. B. Ben-Nissan, D. Sher, and W. Walsh, (Trans. Tech. Publications, Switzerland, 2003) pp:831–834.
13. H. Oonishi, Y. Takayaka, I. C. Clarke, and H. Jung, Comparative wear studies of 28-mm ceramic and stainless steel total hip joints over two to seven year period, J. Long-Term Effects Med. Implants, 1992, 2:37–47.
14. S. F. Hulbert, J. C. Bokros, L. L. Hench, J. Wilson, and G. Heimke, Ceramics in clinical applications: past, present and future, in Ceramics in Clinical Applications, ed. P. Vincenzini, (Elsevier Sci. Publ., Amsterdam, 1997) pp:3–27.

15.   K. Hayashi, N. Matsuguchi, K. Uenoyama, T. Kanemaru, and Y. Sugioka, Evaluation of metal implants coated with several types of ceramics as biomaterials, J. Biomed. Mater. Res., 1989, 23:1247–1259.

16.   R. L. Huckstep and P. P. Lutton, New concepts in stabilization and replacement of bones and joints, Mater. Forum, 1991, 15:253–260.

17.   H. Oonishi, I. C. Clarke, V. Good, H. Amino, M. Ueno, S. Masuda, K. Oomamiuda, H. Ishimaru, M. Yamamoto, and E. Tsuji, Needs of bioceramics to longevity of total joint arthroplasty, in Key Engineering Materials, 240–242, in Bioceramics 15, eds. B. Ben-Nissan, D. Sher, and W. Walsh, (Trans. Tech. Publications, Switzerland, 2003) pp:735–754.

18.   L. Sedel, Tribology and clinical experience of alumina–alumina articulations, in Proceeding of the 66th Annual Meeting of the American Academy of Orthopedic Surgeons, (USA, 1999) pp:120.

19.   G. Willmann, The evolution of ceramics in total hip arthroplasty, Hip International, 2000, 10:193–203.

20.   O. C. Standard, K. Schindhelm, B. K. Milthorpe, C. R. Howlett, and C. C. Sorrell, Biocompatibility of zirconia ceramics, in Proc. of Int. Ceram. Conf. Austceram, 92, Vol. 2, ed. M. J. Bannister, (CSIRO Pub., Melbourne, Australia, 1992) pp:611–616.

21.   V. Saikko, Wear of polyethylene acetabular cups against zirconia femoral heads studied with a hip joint simulator, Wear, 1994, 176:207–212.

22.   I. C. Clarke, V. Good, P. Williams, D. Schroeder, L. Anissian, A. Stark, H. Oonishi, J. Schuldies, and G. Gustafson, Ultra-low wear rates for rigid-on-rigid bearings in total hip replacements, in Proc. Inst. Mech. Engrs., 2000, Vol. 214, Part H:331–347.

23.   A. Pizzoferrato, S. Stea, and G. Ciapetti, Alternative articulating surfaces for total hip replacement, Current Opinion in Orthop., 1995, 6:42–47.

24.   J. Chevalier, B. Cales, J. M. Drouin, and Y. Stefani, Ceramic–Ceramic bearing systems compared on different testing configurations, in Bioceramics 10, eds. L. Sekel and C. Rey, (University Press, Cambridge, UK, 1997) pp:271–274.

25.   I. C. Clarke, Clinical and tribological perspectives of wear in alumina–alumina THR, in Key Engineering Materials, 240–242, Bioceramics 15, eds. B. Ben-Nissan, D. Sher, and W. Walsh, (Trans. Tech. Publications, Switzerland, 2003), pp:755–764.

26.   P. A. Williams, I. C. Clarke, G. Pezzotti, D. D. Green, and B. Ben-Nissan, Water lubrication effects on zirconia debris production in hip-joint simulators, in Key Engineering Materials, 240–242, Bioceramics 15, eds. B. Ben-Nissan, D. Sher, and W. Walsh, (Trans. Tech. Publications, Switzerland, 2003) pp:835–838.

27.   S. T. Woolson and M. G. Murphy, Wear of the polyethylene of Harris–Galante acetabular components inserted without cement, J. Bone Joint Surg., 1995, 77(9):1311–1314.

28.   K. Tanaka, J. Tamura, K. Kawanabe, M. Shimizu, and T. Nakamura, Effect of alumina femoral heads on polyethylene wear in cemented total hip arthroplasty: old versus current alumina, J. Bone Joint Surg. Br., 2002, 85B(5):655–660.

29. T. Nakamura, Novel zirconia/alumina composites for TJR, in Key Engineering Materials, 240–242, Bioceramics 15, eds. B. Ben-Nissan, D. Sher, and W. Walsh, (Trans. Tech. Publications, Switzerland, 2003) pp:765–768.

30. M. Spector, M. D. Ries, R. B. Bourne, W. S. Sauer, M. Long, and G. Hunter, Wear performance of Ultra High Molecular Weight Polyethylene on oxidized zirconium total knee femoral components, J. Bone Joint Surg. AM, 2001, 83A, Supp. 2, Part 2:80–86.

31. G. Hunter and M. Long, Abrasive wear of oxidized Zr–2.5Nb, CoCrMo and Ti–6Al–4V against bone cement, in Trans. of 6th Biomater. Congress, (Soc. Biomat., Hawaii, 2000), p.835.

32. D. D. D'Lima, S. M. Lemperle, P. C. Chen, R. E. Holmes, and C. W. Colwell, Bone response to implant surface morphology, J. Arthrop., 1998, 13(8):928–934.

33. D. Heuer, A. Harrison, H. Y. Gupta, and G. Hunter, Chemically textured and oxidized zirconium surfaces for implant fixation, in Key Engineering Materials, 240–242, Bioceramics 15, eds. B. Ben-Nissan, D. Sher, and W. Walsh, (Trans. Tech. Publications, Switzerland, 2003) pp:789–792.

34. W. F. De Jong, La Substance Material darts lesos, Rec. Tav. Chim., 1997, 45:415–448.

35. B. Ben-Nissan, C. Chai, and L. Evans, Crystallographic and spectroscopic characterization and morphology of biogenic and synthetic Apatites, in Encyclopedic Handbook of Biomaterials and Bioengineering Vol. 1, Part B: Applications, eds. D. L. Wise, D. J. Trantolo, D. E. Altobelli, M. J. Yaszemski, J. D. Gresser, and E.R. Schwartz, (Marcel Dekker Inc., New York, 1995) pp:191–221.

36. F. H. Albee and H. F.Morrison, Bone graft surgery, Ann. Surg., 1920 (reprinted in Clin. Orthro. & Rel. Res., 1996, 324:5–12) 71:32–39.

37. A. M. Gatti, D. Zaffe, and G. P. Poli, Behavior of tricalcium phosphate and hydroxyapatite granules in sheep bone defects, Biomaterials, 1990, 11:513–517.

38. C. P. A. T. Klein, A. A. Driessens, and K. de Groot, Relationship between the degradation behavior of calcium phosphate ceramics and their physical chemical characteristics and ultrastructural geometry, Biomaterials, 1984, 5:157–160.

39. W. Den Hollander, P. Patka, C. P. A. T. Klein, and G. A. K. Heidendal, Macroporous calcium phosphate ceramics for bone substitution: a tracer study on biodegradation with ^{45}Ca tracer, Biomaterials, 1991, 12:569–573.

40. M. M. A. Ramselaar, F. C. M. Driessens, W. Kalk, J. R. de Wijn, and P. J. van Mullen, Biodegradation of four calcium phosphate ceramics; *in vivo* rates and tissue interactions, J. Mater. Sci.: Mater. Med., 1991, 2:63–70.

41. E. Hayek and H. Newesely, Pentacalcium Monohydroxyorthophosphate, Inorg. Synth., 1963, 7:63–65.

42. D. J. Greenfield and E. D. Eanes, Formation chemistry of amorphous calcium phosphates prepared from carbonate-containing solutions, Calcif. Tissue Res., 1972, 9:152–162.

43. T. Kokubo, H. Kushitani, Y. Ebisawa, T. Kitsugi, S. Kotani, K. Ohura, and T. Yamamuro, Apatite formation on bioactive ceramics in body environment, in Bioceramics Vol. 1, eds. H. Oonishi, H. Aoki, and K. Sawai, (Ishiyaku Euro America, 1989) pp:157–162.

44. T. Kokubo, H. M. Kim, M. Kawashita, and T. Nakamura, Novel ceramics for biomedical applications, J. Aust. Ceram. Soc., 2000, 36(1):37–46.

45. J. H. Kuhne, R. Bartl, B. Frisch, C. Hammer, V. Jannson, and M. Zimmer, Bone formation in coralline hydroxyapatite — effects of pore size studied in rabbits, Acta Orthopedica Scandinava, 1994, 65(3):246–252.

46. D. M. Roy and S. K. Linnehan, Hydroxyapatite formed from coral skeletal carbonate by hydrothermal exchange, Nature, 1974, 247:220–222.

47. M. Sivakumar, T. S. Kumar, K. L. Shantra, and K. P. Rao, Development of hydroxyapatite derived from Indian coral, Biomaterials, 1996, 17:1709–1714.

48. J. Pena, R. Z. Le Geros, R. Rohanizadeh, and J. P. Leros, $CaCO_3$/Ca–P biphasic materials prepared by microwave processing of natural aragonite and calcite, in Key Engineering Materials, 192–195, Bioceramics 13, eds. S. Giannini and A. Moroni, (Trans Tech Publications, Switzerland, 2001) pp:267–270.

49. J. Hu, J. J. Russell, B. Ben-Nissan, and R. Vago, Production and analysis of hydroxyapatite from Australian corals via hydrothermal process, J. Mater. Sci. Letters, 2001, 20:85–87.

50. C. S. Chai and B. Ben-Nissan, Interfacial reactions between hydroxyapatite and titanium, J. Aust. Ceram. Soc., 1993, 29:81–90.

51. C. M. Cottel, D. B. Chrisey, K. S. Grabowski, J. A. Sprague, and C. R. Rossett, Pulsed laser deposition of hydroxyapatite thin films on Ti–6Al–4V, J. Appl. Biomater., 1992, 3:87–93.

52. J. L. Ong, L. C. Lucas, W. R. Lacefield, and E. D. Rigney, Structure, solubility and bond strength of thin calcium phosphate coatings produced by ion beam sputter deposition, Biomaterials, 1992, 13(4):249–254.

53. P. Ducheyne, W. van Raemdock, J. C. Heughebaert, and M. Heughebaert, Structural analysis of hydroxyapatite coatings on titanium, Biomaterials, 1986, 7:97–103.

54. I. Zhitomirsky and L. Gal-Or, Electrophoretic deposition of hydroxyapatite, J. Biomed. Mater. Res., 1997, 21:1375–1381.

55. B. Ben-Nissan, D. D. Green, G. S. K. Kannangara, and A. Milev, ^{31}P NMR studies of diethyl phosphite derived nanocrystalline hydroxyapatite, J. Sol-Gel Sci. Tech., 2001, 21:27–37.

56. W. Van Raemdonck, P. Ducheyne, and P. DeMeester, Calcium phosphate ceramics, in Metal and Ceramic Biomaterials Vol. II, eds. P. Ducheyne and G. W. Hastings, (CRC Press, 1984) pp:143–162.

57. G. E. Friedlaender, D. M. Strong, W. W. Tomford, and H. J. Mankin, Long term follow-up of patients with osteochondral allografts: a correlation between immunogenic responses and clinical outcome, Orthop. Clin. North. Am., 1999, 30:583–585.

58. M. R. Urist, Bone: Formation by autoinduction, Science, 1965, 12:893–899.

59. S. D. Cook, M. W. Wolfe, S. L. Salkeld, and D. C. Rueger, Effect of recombinant human osteogenic Protein–1 on healing of segmental defects in non-human primates, J. Bone Joint Surg., 1996, 77–A:734–750.

60. L. L. Hench and J. Wilson, Surface active materials, Science, 1984, 226:630–636.

61. L. L. Hench, Bioactive ceramics, in Bioceramics: Materials Characteristics vs. *in vivo* Behavior, Vol. 523, eds. P. Ducheyne and J. E. Lemons, (Ann. of the New York Academy of Science, New York, 1988) pp:54–71.

62. T. Kokubo, Recent progress in glass-based materials for biomedical applications, J. Ceramic. Soc. Japan, 1991, 99:965–973.

63. W. C. A. Vrouwenvelder, C. G. Groot, and K. de Groot, Histological and biochemical evaluation of osteoblasts cultured on bioactive glass, hydroxyapatite, titanium alloy, and stainless steel, J. Biomed. Mater. Res., 1993, 27:465–475.

64. O. H. Andersson and I. Kangasniemi, Calcium phosphate formation at the surface of bioactive glass *in vitro*, J. Biomed. Mat. Res., 1991, 25:1019–1030.

65. P. Li, Q. Yang, F. Zhang, and T. Kokubo, The effect of residual glassy phase in a bioctive glass-ceramic on the gormation of its surface apatite layer *in vitro*, J. Mater. Sci.: Mater. Med., 1992, 3:452–456.

66. H. M. Kim, Y. Sasaki, J. Suzuki, S. Fujibayashi, T. Kokubo, T. Matsushita, and T. Nakamura, Mechanical properties of bioactive titanium metal prepared by chemical treatment, in Key Engineering Materials, 192–195, Bioceramics 13, eds. S. Giannini and A. Moroni, (Trans. Tech. Pub., Switzerland, 2000) pp:227–230.

67. T. Kokubo, Novel inorganic materials for biomedical applications, in Key Engineering Materials, 240–242, Bioceramics 15, eds. B. Ben-Nissan, D. Sher, and W. Walsh, (Trans. Tech. Publications, Switzerland, 2003) pp:523–528.

68. H. M. Kim, F. Miyaji, T. Kokubo, S. Nishiguchi, and T. Nakamura, Graded surfaces structure of bioactive titanium prepared by chemical treatment, J. Biomed. Mater. Res., 1999, 45(2):100–107.

69. G. J. Ehrhardt and D. E. Day, Therapeutic use of ^{90}Y microspheres, Int. J. Radiation Appl. & Inst., Part B, Nucl. Med. & Biol., 1987, 14(3):233–242.

70. M. Kawashita, T. Kokubo, and Y. Inoue, Preparation of Y_2O_3 microspheres for *in situ* radiotherapy of cancer, in Bioceramics Vol. 12, eds. H. Ohgushi, G. W. Hastings, and T. Yoshikawa, (World Scientific, Singapore, 1999) pp:555–558.

71. M. Ikenaga, K. Ohura, T. Yamamuro, Y. Kotoura, M. Oka, and T. Kokubo, Localized hyperthermic treatment of experimental bone tumors with ferromagnetic ceramics, J. Orthop. Res., 1993, 11(6):849–855.

72. M. Kawashita, M. Tanaka, T. Kokubo, T. Yao, S. Hamada, and T. Shinjo, Preparation of magnetite microspheres for hyperthermia of cancer, in Key Engineering Materials, 218–220, Bioceramics 14, eds. S. Brown, I. Clarke, and P. Williams, (Trans Tech Pub., Switzerland, 2002) pp:645–648.

73. K. D. Kuhn, Bone cements, (Springer, New York, 2000).

74. A. J. Ruys, K. A. Zeigler, A. Brandwood, B. K. Milthorpe, S. Morrey, and C. C. Sorrell, Reinforcement of hydroxyapatite with ceramic and metal fibers, in Bioceramics Vol. 4, eds. W. Bonfield, G. W. Hastings, and K. E. Tanner, (Butterworth–Heinemenn Ltd, London, UK, 1991) pp:281–286.

75. K. Ioku, T. Noma, N. Ishizawa, and M. Yoshimura, Hydrothermal synthesis and sintering of hydroxyapatite powders dispersed with Si_3N_4 whiskers, J. Ceram. Soc. Jpn. Int. Ed., 1990, 98:48–53.

76. S. Gautier, E. Champion, and D. Bernache-Assollant, Effect of processing on the characteristics of a $20vol\%Al_2O_3$ platelet reinforced hydroxyapatite composite, in Bioceramics Vol .10, eds. L. Sedel and C. Rey, (University Press, Cambridge, UK, 1997) pp:549–552.

77. W. Bonfield, M. D. Grynpas, A. E. Tully, J. Bowman, and J. Abram, Hydroxyapatite reinforced polyethylene: a mechanically compatible implant material for bone replacement, Biomaterials, 1981, 2:185–186.

78. X. Zhang, G. H. M. Gubbels, R. A. Terpstra, and R. Metselaar, Toughening of calcium hydroxyapatite with silver particles, J. Mater. Sci., 1997, 32:235–243.

79. G. Pezzotti and S. M. F. Asmus, Fracture behavior of hydroxyapatite/polymer interpenetrating network composites prepared by *in situ* polymerization process, Mater. Sci. Eng., 2001, 316:231–237.

80. M. Sarikaya, J. Liu, and I. A. Aksay, Nacre: Properties, Crystallography, and formation, in Biomimetics: Design and Processing of Materials, eds. M. Sarikaya and I. A. Aksay, (American Institute of Physics, New York, 1995) pp:34–90.

81. P. Calvert and S. Mann, Review: Synthetic and biological composites formed by *in situ* precipitation, J. Mater. Sci., 1988, 23:3801–3806.

82. N. H. Ladizesky, I. Ward, and W. Bonfield, Hydrostatic extrusion of polyethylene filled with hydroxyapatite, Polymers Adv. Tech., 1997, 8:496–504.

83. R. L. Reis, A. M. Cunha, and M. J. Bevis, Load bearing and ductile hydroxyapatite polyethylene composites for bone replacement, in Bioceramics Vol. 10, eds. L. Sedel and C. Rey, (University Press, Cambridge, UK, 1997) pp:515–518.

84. N. Almqvist, N. H. Thomson, B. L. Smith, G. D. Stucky, D. E. Morse, and P. K. Hansma, Methods for fabricating and characterizing a new generation of biomimetic materials, Mater. Sci. Eng., 1999, C7:37–43.

85. S. L. Y. Woo, The relationships of changes in stress levels on long bone remodeling, in Mechanical Properties of Bone, ed. S. C. Cowin, (American Society of Mechanical Engineers, New York, 1981) pp:107–129.

86. J. C. Bokros, Deposition structure and properties of pyrolytic carbon, in Chemistry and Physics of Carbon Vol. 5, ed. P. L. Walker, (Marcel Dekker Inc., New York, 1969) pp:70–81.

CHAPTER 7

POLYMERIC HYDROGELS

Jun Li

Division of Bioengineering, Faculty of Engineering
National University of Singapore, Lower Kent Ridge Road, Singapore 119260;
Institute of Materials Research and Engineering, Singapore 117602
E-mail: bielj@nus.edu.sg; jun-li@imre.a-star.edu.sg

Polymeric hydrogels are of special importance in polymeric biomaterials because of their favorable biocompatibility. Hydrogels are cross-linked macromolecular networks formed by hydrophilic polymers swollen in water or biological fluids. The cross-links can be formed by either covalent bonds or physical cohesion forces that exist between the polymer segments. Polymeric hydrogels are primarily classified into chemical and physical hydrogels (based on the bonding type of the cross-links), though they can also be classified in many other ways. Chemical hydrogels can be prepared by copolymerization of a monomer with cross-linker, or by cross-linking of water-soluble polymers. Physical hydrogels can be made of natural biopolymers, thermo-sensitive synthetic polymers, amphiphilic triblock copolymers or many other copolymers. Further, polyelectrolyte complexes and polymer-cyclodextrin inclusion complexes can likewise form hydrogels. All chemical and physical hydrogels described in this chapter are of biomedical significance. Their biomedical applications in drug delivery and tissue engineering are hence discussed.

7.1 Introduction

Of many polymeric biomaterials, hydrogels are of special interest because of their favorable biocompatibility and a host of unique advantages that accompany them. For example, hydrogels play an important role in controlled drug delivery: they are able to deliver delicate bioactive agents such as proteins and peptides. In addition, hydrogels have also been reported to promote tissue repair and regeneration. In this chapter, a general overview of polymeric hydrogels — in terms of their definition and classification — is first presented. This is followed by discussion of both chemical and physical hydrogels with biomedical significance — in terms of their structures and preparation methods. On the note of biomedical significance, the biomedical applications of different types of hydrogel — such as controlled drug delivery and tissue engineering — are also discussed.

7.2   Definition and Classification of Hydrogels

7.2.1 Definition of Hydrogels

Hydrogels are cross-linked macromolecular networks formed by hydrophilic polymers swollen in water or biological fluids [1]. Their three-dimensional networks can retain large volumes of water in the cross-linked structures. The extent of swelling and the content of water retained depend on two factors: the hydrophilicity of the polymer chains and the cross-linking density. The cross-links can be formed by covalent bonds. Alternatively, they can be formed by physical cohesion forces that exist between the polymer segments — such as ionic bonding, hydrogen bonding, van der Waals forces, or forces that arise due to hydrophobic interactions (Figure 7–1) [2].

Hydrogels can also be described in a rheological way [3]. Aqueous solutions of hydrophilic polymers without cross-linking at low concentration (where no significant chain entanglements occur) normally show Newtonian behavior. However, the cross-linked polymer networks — either chemically or physically — show visco-elastic and sometimes pure elastic behavior upon swelling in water.

7.2.2 Classification of Hydrogels

Polymeric hydrogels can be classified in two different ways as follows [4]:
- Based on the bonding type of the cross-links, hydrogels are divided into chemical and physical hydrogels (Figure 7–2).
- Based on the sources of the polymers, hydrogels are classified into natural hydrogels, synthetic hydrogels, and natural and synthetic combination hydrogels (Figure 7–3).

In addition to the above classifications, Figures 7–4 to 7–6 show other forms of classification based on polymer structures, physical properties, and biodegradability. (Examples for each hydrogel type are also given in Figures 7–2 to 7–6.)

7.3   Chemical Hydrogels and Their Biomedical Applications

Hydrogels are cross-linked macromolecular networks formed by hydrophilic polymers swollen in water or biological fluids [1]. Their three-dimensional networks can retain large volumes of water in the cross-linked structures. The extent of swelling and the content of water retained depend on two factors: the hydrophilicity of the polymer chains and the cross-linking density. The cross-links can be formed by covalent bonds. Alternatively, they can be formed by physical cohesion forces that exist between the polymer segments — such as ionic bonding, hydrogen bonding, van der Waals forces, or forces that arise due to hydrophobic interactions (Figure 7–1) [2].

Polymer networks of chemical hydrogels are formed by chemical cross-linking through covalent bonding. Chemical hydrogels are also called permanent hydrogels. They cannot be dissolved in water or other solvents unless the covalent cross-links are cleaved. Chemical hydrogels are mainly prepared using one of these approaches [1,2,4]:

- Copolymerization of a monomer with cross-linker;
- Cross-linking of water-soluble polymers with cross-linker;
- Cross-linking of water-soluble polymers with irradiation.

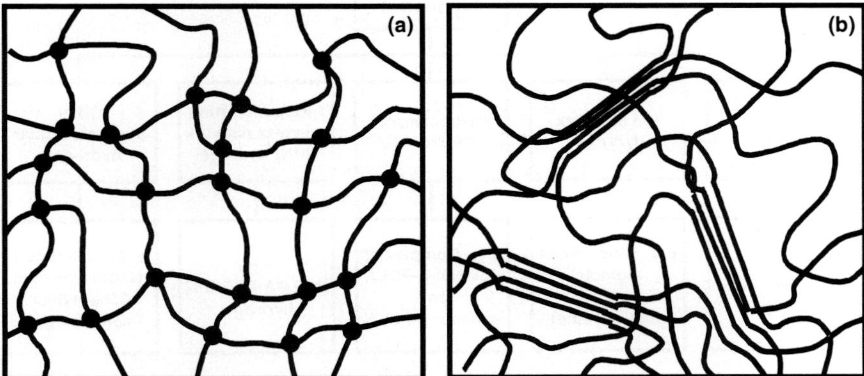

Figure 7–1 Schematic presentation of (a) chemically cross-linked hydrogel; and (b) physical hydrogel with multiple interaction zones (Reprinted from reference [6] with permission)

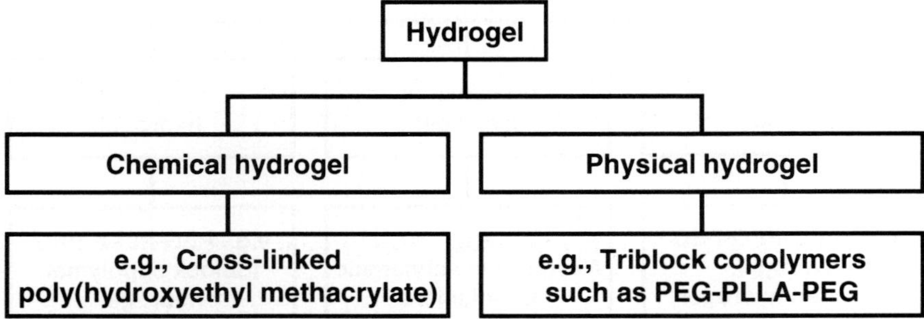

Figure 7–2 Classification of polymeric hydrogels based on the bonding type of the cross-links

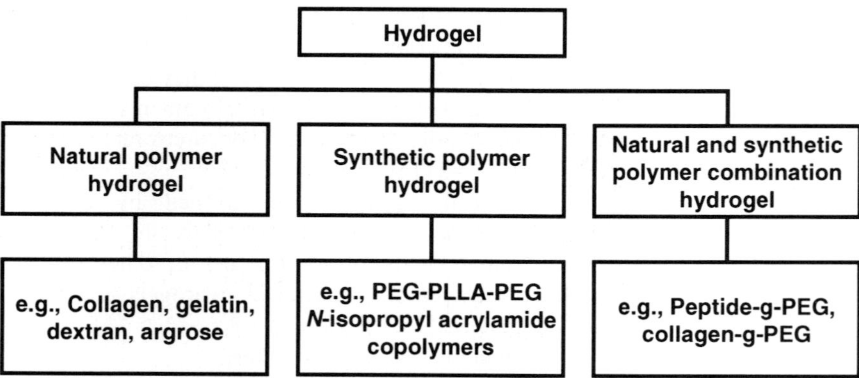

Figure 7–3 Classification of polymeric hydrogels based on the sources of the polymers

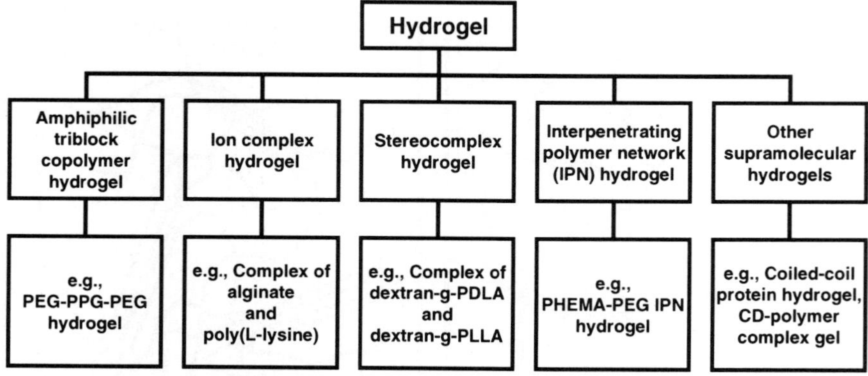

Figure 7–4 Classification of polymeric hydrogels based on the chemical and higher structures of the polymer

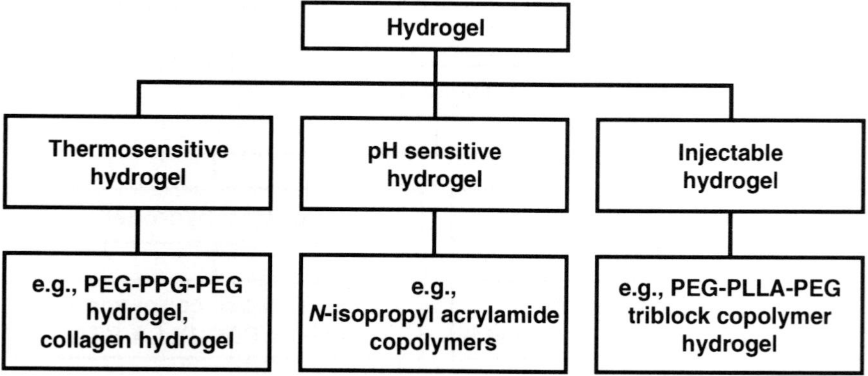

Figure 7–5 Classification of polymeric hydrogels based on the physical properties of the polymer

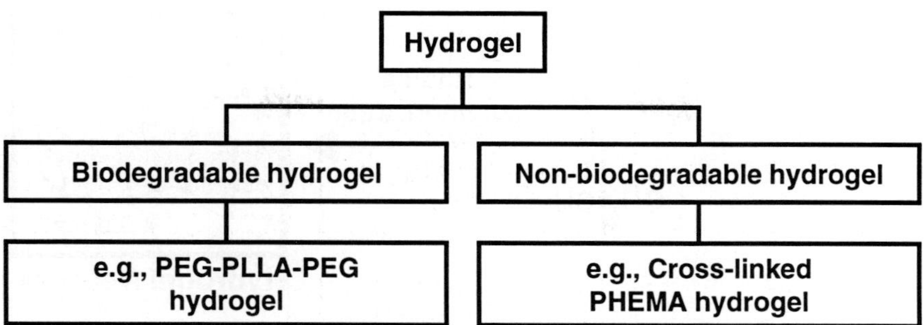

Figure 7–6 Classification of polymeric hydrogels based on the biodegradability of the polymer

7.3.1 Copolymerization of Monomer with Cross-linker

Free radical polymerization of water-soluble monomers in the presence of cross-linker results in chemical cross-linked hydrogels (Figure 7–7) [4]. An example is shown in Figure 7–8(a), where hydrogels based on copolymers of *N*–(2–hydroxypropyl)–methacrylamide (HPMA) and *N,O*–dimethacrylayhydroxylamine (DMHA) were synthesized [5]. The hydrolytic stability of these hydrogels was studied in buffers with pH range of 2 to 8. The hydrogels were stable at acidic pH (below 5), but were hydrolyzed at neutral and mildly alkaline pH (Figure 7–8(b)). This study showed that although the hydrogels were chemically cross-linked, they were biodegradable because the cross-linker could be hydrolyzed under physiological conditions.

For controlled release of anticancer drug, doxorubincin was chemically bonded to the water-soluble poly(HPMA) segments. Release rate examination of the anticancer drug was then carried out (Figure 7–9). It was found that the rate at which Dox-polymer conjugate was released from the hydrogel depended on the pH of the incubation medium.

- At pH 5.0, conjugate release could occur only by diffusion since the hydrogel matrix remained stable at this pH, and the drug was released slowly.
- At pH 6.5, the conjugate was released faster: the rate of release being controlled both by its rate of diffusion and the rate of matrix degradation.
- At pH 7.4 and 8.0, conjugate release rates ranked the highest: the release rate was comparable to that of gel degradation, which meant that conjugate release was controlled mainly by the rate of matrix degradation.

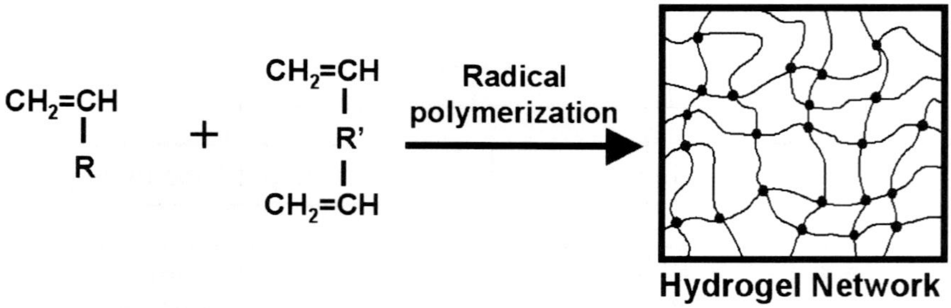

                                          J. Li

Figure 7–7 Formation of chemical hydrogel by copolymerization of a monomer with cross-linker

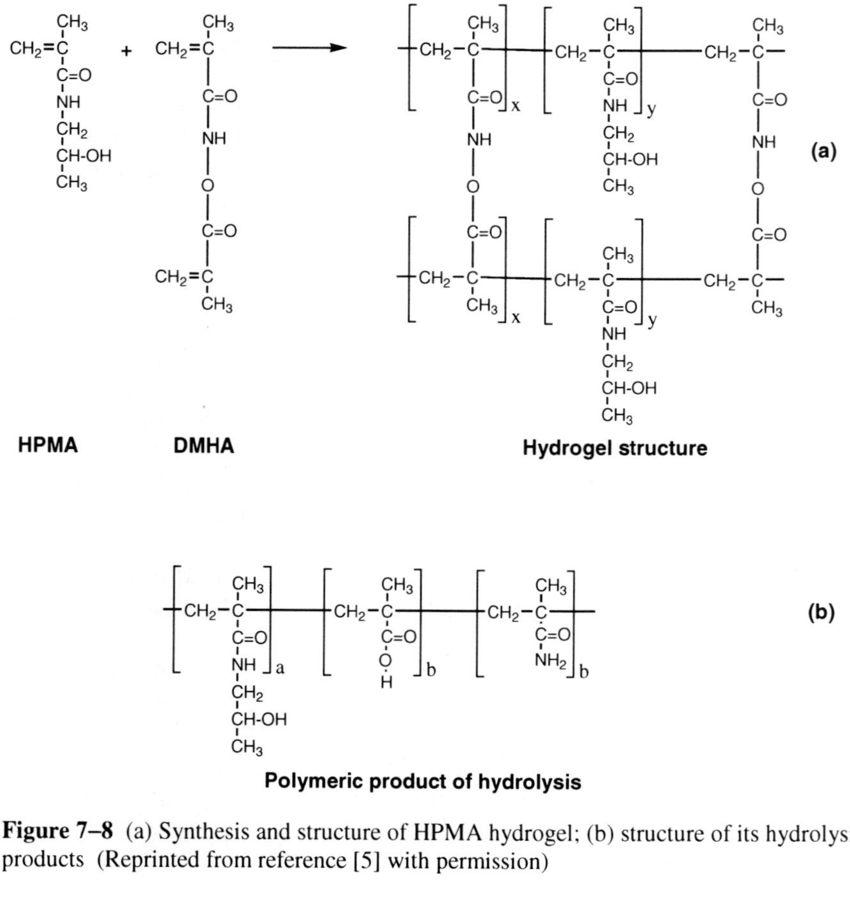

Figure 7–8 (a) Synthesis and structure of HPMA hydrogel; (b) structure of its hydrolysis products (Reprinted from reference [5] with permission)

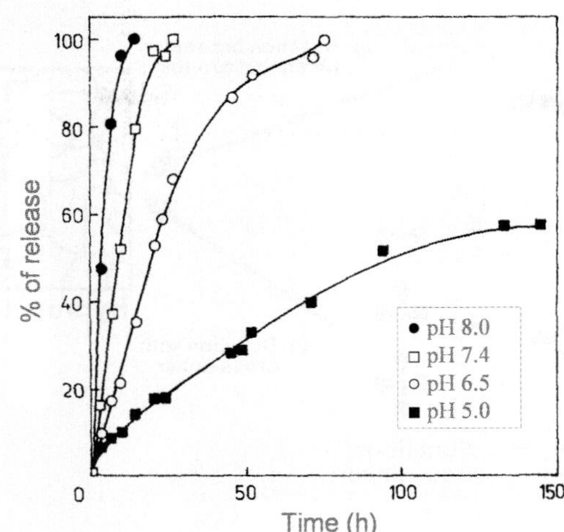

Figure 7–9 *In vitro* release of Dox-polymer conjugate from HPMA–DMHA hydrogel in phosphate at pH 5.0, 6.5, 7.4, and 8.0 (Reprinted from reference [5] with permission)

7.3.2 Cross-Linking of Water-Soluble Polymers

Cross-linking of water-soluble multifunctional polymers by reaction between the functional groups results in chemical hydrogels (Figure 7–10(a)). Besides this approach, cross-linking of water-soluble multifunctional polymers by addition of bifunctional or multifunctional reagents also results in chemical hydrogels (Figure 7–10(b)). Figure 7–11 shows some examples of the cross-linking reactions.

- In Figure 7–11(a), water-soluble polymers modified with vinyl groups can be polymerized to produce hydrogels once the radical reaction is started by chemical initiation or UV-/γ-irradiation. Polysaccharides such as dextran have been cross-linked in this way (Figure 7–12) [6].
- In Figure 7–11(b), water-soluble polymers having amino groups are cross-linked by bisepoxy compounds. Many natural biopolymers such as collagen and gelatin have been cross-linked in this way to produce chemical hydrogels [7,8].

The release of proteins from the dextran hydrogel represented in Figure 7–12 was studied. It was found that the release rate depended on and could be manipulated by the initial water content and cross-linking density of the gel. By incorporating dextranase, degradation systems were obtained: degradation rate of the gel was dependent on the concentration of dextranase in the gel and the cross-linking density of the gel.

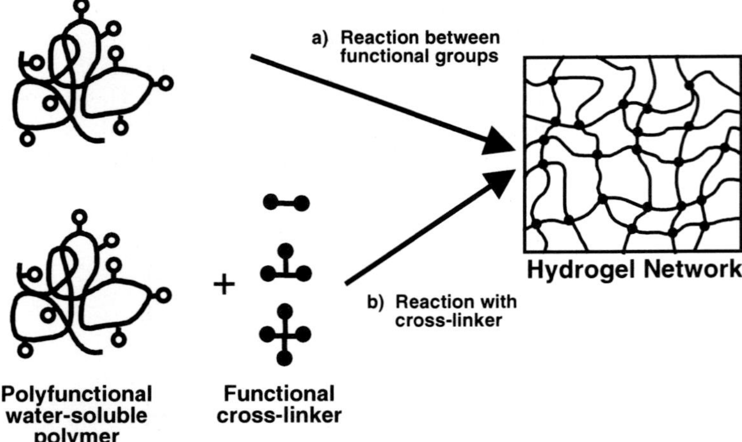

Figure 7–10   Preparation of hydrogel by cross-linking of water-soluble polymers: (a) reaction between functional groups; (b) reaction with cross-linker

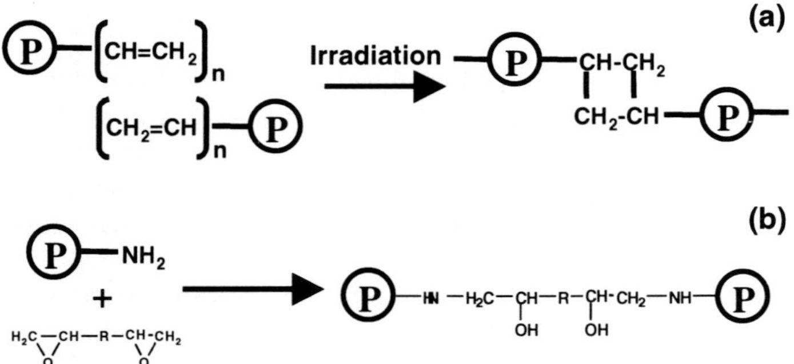

Figure 7–11 Examples of cross-linking reaction to prepare hydrogels from water-soluble polymers: (a) addition reaction of vinyl groups; (b) reaction of amino groups with bisepoxy compounds (Reprinted from reference [2] with permission)

7.4   Physical Hydrogels and Their Biomedical Applications

Physical hydrogels are continuous, disordered, and three-dimensional hydrophilic polymer networks formed by cohesion forces capable of constituting non-covalent cross-links [2]. The cohesion forces include ionic bonding, hydrogen bonding, van der Waals forces, as well as forces that arise due to hydrophobic interaction, stereocomplexation, crystallization, and other weak interactions. Since physical hydrogels are not covalently cross-linked, the formation of the physical cross-links is largely dependent on the thermodynamic parameters of the medium such as temperature, pH, salt type, and ionic strength. This also means that the formation is reversible upon change in any of these thermodynamic parameters — which renders a physical hydrogel as an *in situ* gelation system in water without any chemical reaction. This property thus makes it feasible to utilize physical hydrogels in macromolecular drug delivery and tissue engineering applications because of their simplicity and safety in *in vivo* situations.

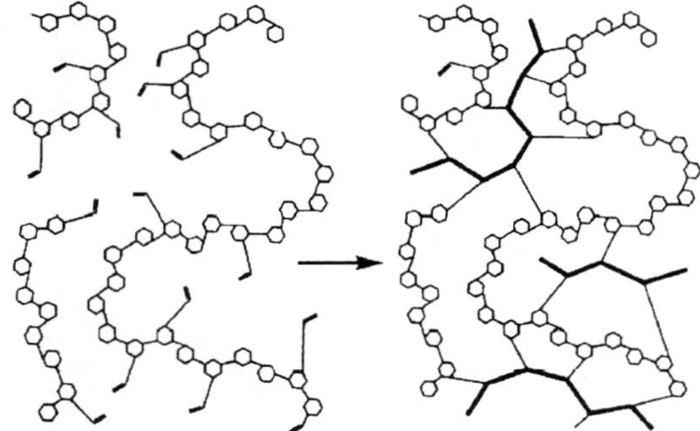

Figure 7–12 Schematic representation of the formation of dextran hydrogel by radical addition reaction (Reprinted from reference [6] with permission)

7.4.1 Natural Biopolymer Hydrogels

Typical natural biopolymers that form physical hydrogels include proteins such as collagen and gelatin, and polysaccharaides such as agarose, amylose, and cellulose derivatives [9]. Renaturation to the triple helical conformation in the proteins and double helical conformation in polysaccharides induces physical cross-linking during gel formation [2,9].

As an example, type I collagen is predominant in higher order animals especially in the skin, tendon, and bone where extreme forces are transmitted [10]. Figure 7–13 shows the chemical, secondary, tertiary, and quaternary structures of type I collagen. A helix formation followed by aggregation of the helices results in a junction point, which acts as physical cross-linking for the gelation of the biopolymer aqueous solution (Figure 7–14).

The attractiveness of collagen and gelatin as biomaterials stems from the view that they are natural materials of low immunogenicity. As such, they are perceived by the body as normal constituents rather than foreign matters [10]. Against this background, collagen and gelatin hydrogels have been proposed for controlled release of protein drugs based on polyion complexation [11]. Figure 7–15 shows a conceptual scheme of the release system. A positively charged protein drug is electrostatically complexed with negatively charged polymer chains, constituting a carrier matrix. If an environmental change — such as increased ionic strength — occurs, the complexed drug will be released from the drug-carrier complex. Even if such an environmental change does not take place, degradation of the polymer carrier itself will also lead to drug release. Since the latter is more likely to happen *in vivo* than the former, it is preferable that the drug carrier is prepared from biodegradable polymers. Biodegradation behavior of the carrier then shapes the drug release profile in this drug-carrier system.

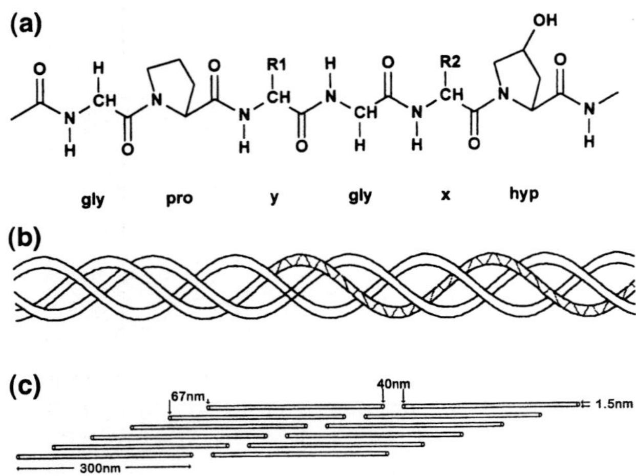

Figure 7–13 Chemical structure of type I collagen: (a) primary amino acid sequence; (b) secondary left-handed helix and tertiary right-handed triple-helix structure; (c) staggered quaternary structure (Reprinted from reference [10] with permission)

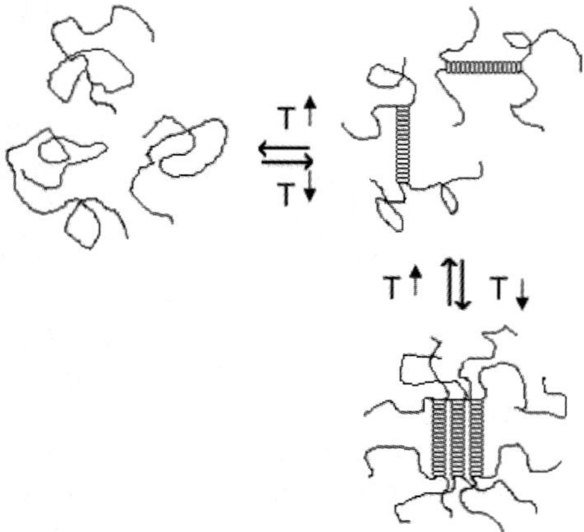

Figure 7–14 Gelation mechanism of biopolymers in water: random coils become helices, which subsequently aggregate to form the junction zones of a gel (Reprinted from reference [9] with permission)

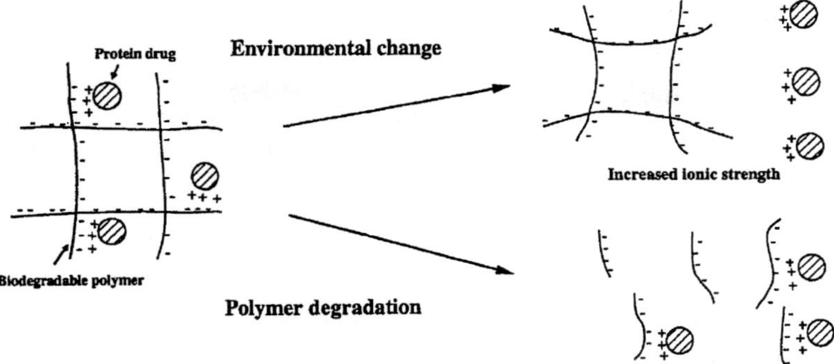

Figure 7–15 Release of protein drug from biodegradable polymer carrier on the basis of polyion complexation (Reprinted from reference [11] with permission)

7.4.2 Thermo-shrinking Hydrogels

Aqueous solutions of some polymers, such as poly(N–isopropylacrylamide) (poly(NiPAAM) as shown in Figure 7–16), undergo precipitation upon temperature increase. The temperature at which a polymer solution undergoes precipitation is called low critical temperature (LCST). Below LCST, the enthalpy term — which is mostly contributed by the hydrogen bonding between polymer polar groups and water molecules — leads to dissolution of the polymer. Hydrogels made of such polymers or their copolymers accordingly undergo shrinking upon temperature increase. Hence they are known as thermo-shrinking hydrogels. Thermo-shrinking hydrogels undergo thermally reversible swelling and deswelling [2,9].

It was found that an aqueous solution of high-molecular-weight NiPAAM/acrylic acid copolymer (2–5 mol%) showed reversible gelation above a critical concentration (~4 wt%), without noticeable hysteresis at around 32°C [9]. This resulted in an opaque, loose gel that was deformable under shear stress. It was proposed that such properties could be used for the design of a refillable macrocapsule-type biohybrid artificial pancreas. Isolated islets of Langerhans suspended in the polymer solution were effectively entrapped in the gel when the solution temperature was raised from 25°C to body temperature; and the gel showed no cytotoxicity. Moreover as opposed to a traditional cell-entrapping matrix of alginate [12], another significant advantage of the gel was its higher permeability (brought about by the gel's heterogeneous character), which then helped to facilitate insulin secretion from the entrapped islets. Chondrocytes immobilized in a thermo-reversible NiPAAM/acrylic acid copolymer gel demonstrated better phenotype expression with a round shape than that cultured in a two-dimensional matrix (culture dish) [13].

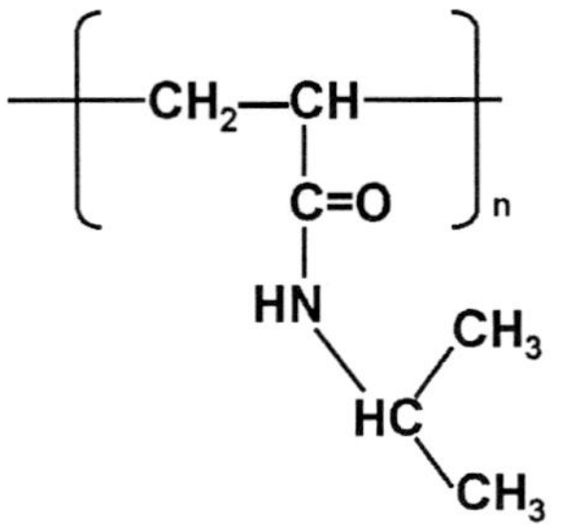

Figure 7–16   Chemical structure of poly(*N*–isopropyl acrylamide)   (Reprinted from reference [9] with permission)

7.4.3 Amphiphilic Triblock Copolymer Hydrogels

Recently, physical hydrogels formed by synthetic amphiphilic triblock copolymers and their potential applications in drug delivery have attracted special attention. As an illustration, the temperature-induced sol-gel transition behavior of block copolymers of poly(ethylene glycol)–poly(propylene glycol)–poly(ethylene glycol) (PEG–PPG–PEG as shown in Figure 7–17) have been extensively studied and utilized to deliver drugs such as polypeptides and proteins [14,15].

Another well-studied triblock copolymer that undergoes temperature-induced gelation is poly(ethylene glycol)–poly(L–lactide)–poly(ethylene glycol) (PEG–PLLA–PEG as shown in Figure 7–18) [16,17]. However PEG–PLLA–PEG differs from PEG–PPG–PEG in that it is biodegradable — due to the PLLA block. Further, the length of the middle PLLA block affects gelation concentration and temperature (as shown in Figure 7–19). In terms of drug release profile, a model drug — FITC-labeled dextran (MW 20,000) — was mixed with an aqueous solution of the 5000–2040–5000 triblock copolymer above the critical gelation temperature at a given polymer concentration. The mixture was then gelled by cooling to body temperature. Over the next 10 days, dextran was released at a constant rate with or without burst effect depending on the polymer concentration (Figure 7–20).

7.4.4 Other Novel Synthetic Copolymer Physical Hydrogels

More novel physical hydrogel systems formed with temperature- or pH-sensitive copolymers or based on complexation of enantiomeric polymer or polypeptide segments have also been reported recently. Graft copolymers of poly(*N*–isopropyl acrylamide)–poly(acrylic acid) were synthesized and found to undergo temperature-induced sol-gel phase transitions over a wide pH range [18].   Novel self-assembled hydrogels induced by stereocomplexation of aqueous solutions of enantiomeric lactic oligomers grafted to dextran [19,20], and by coiled-coil aggregation of artificial protein domains in polymer backbones [21] or side chains [22], were also reported.

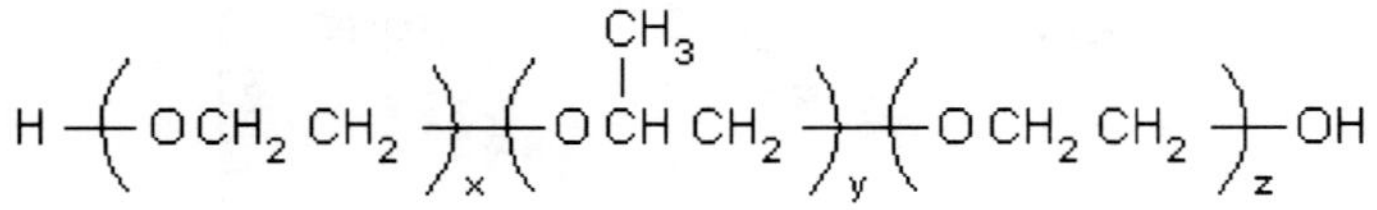

$$H\left(OCH_2\,CH_2\right)_x\left(O\overset{\displaystyle CH_3}{\underset{\displaystyle |}{CH}}\,CH_2\right)_y\left(OCH_2\,CH_2\right)_z OH$$

Figure 7–17 Chemical structure of PEG–PPG–PEG triblock copolymer

$$CH_3O\left(CH_2-CH_2-O\right)_x H$$

$$\Downarrow\quad LLA,\ (C_{16}H_{30}O_4)Sn$$

$$CH_3O\left(CH_2-CH_2-O\right)_x\left(\overset{O}{\overset{||}{C}}-\overset{CH_3}{\overset{|}{CH}}-O\right)_y H$$

$$\Downarrow\quad HMDI$$

$$CH_3O\left(CH_2-CH_2-O\right)_x\left(\overset{O}{\overset{||}{C}}-\overset{CH_3}{\overset{|}{CH}}-O\right)_y OCNH(CH_2)_6NHCO\left(O-\overset{CH_3}{\overset{|}{CH}}-\overset{O}{\overset{||}{C}}\right)_y\left(O-CH_2-CH_2\right)_x OCH_3$$

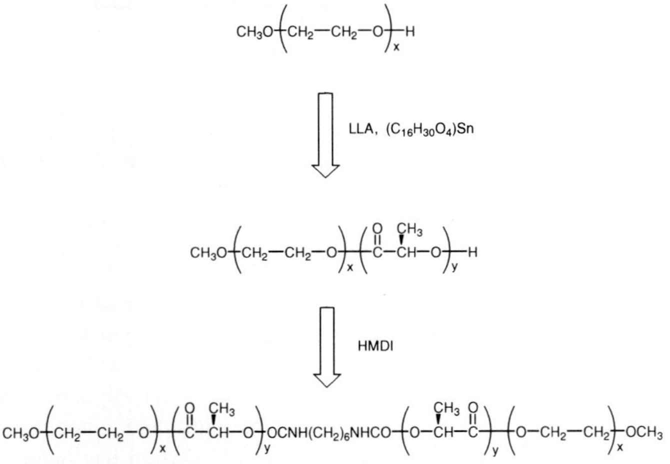

Figure 7–18 Preparation of PEG–PLLA–PEG triblock copolymer

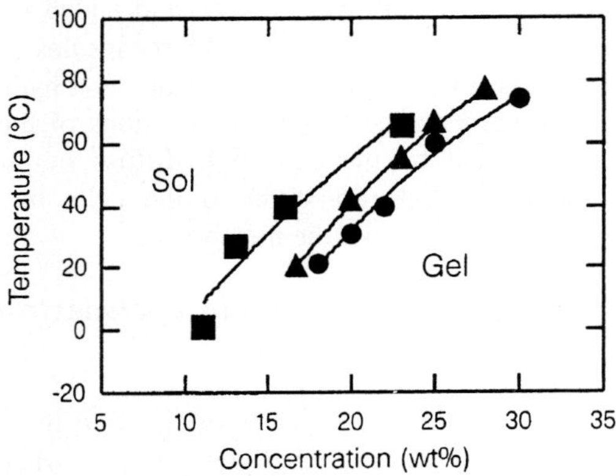

Figure 7–19 Gel-sol transition curves of PEG–PLLA–PEG triblock copolymers: (■) 5000–2040–5000; (▲) 5000–3000–5000; (●) 5000–5000–5000 (Reprinted from reference [16] with permission)

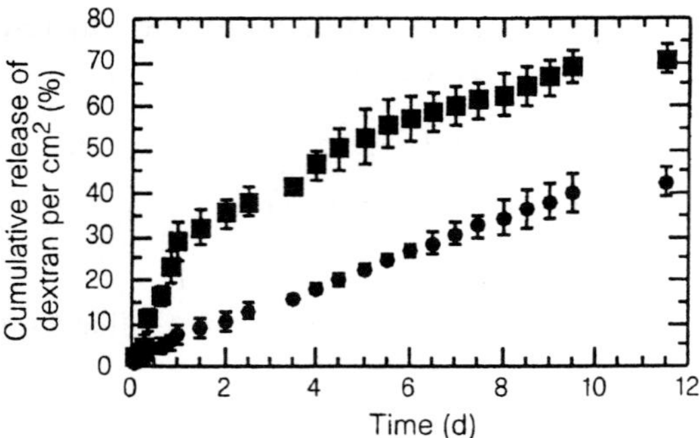

Figure 7–20 *In vitro* release of FITC-labeled dextran (MW 20,000) from PEG–PLLA–PEG (MW 5000–2040–5000) triblock copolymer; FITC-labeled dextran (5.4 mg) was mixed with 0.5 ml of aqueous polymer solution ((■) 23 wt%; (●) 35 wt% polymer) (Reprinted from reference [16] with permission)

7.4.5 Polyelectrolyte Complex Hydrogels

Some water-soluble polyelectrolyte copolymers can form hydrogels with metal ions or with another counter-charged polyelectrolyte polymer. Recently, we reported hydrogel formation between positively charged modified collagen and negatively charged synthetic polyelectrolyte terpolymer containing poly(methacrylic acid) under certain pH, ionic strength, and concentration of the polymers (Figure 7–21) [23]. The novel hydrogel system has been applied in tissue engineering for microencapsulation of hepatocytes that are used in bioartificial liver assist device. As shown in Figure 7–22, the cells are suspended in a solution of the modified collagen and added to the solution of HEMA–MMA–MAA terpolymers to form the microcapsules through complex coacervation reaction. The membrane of the capsules is a hydrogel permeable to nutrients required to maintain the metabolic functions of the cells. On the other hand, products secreted by the cells will diffuse out of the capsules, thereby providing immunological protection to the cells by restraining the migration of antibodies and cells across the membrane.

7.4.6 Supramolecular Hydrogels Formed by Cyclodextrins and Polymers

In the past decade, there have been extensive studies into the macromolecular self-assembly between polymers and cyclodextrins — when cyclodextrins thread onto the polymer chains [24,25,26]. Such supramolecular structures are called polyrotaxanes. A new class of polymer hydrogels with novel supramolecular systems, which is suitable for a wide range of biomedical applications, has been developed based on the formation of polyrotaxanes (Figure 7–23).

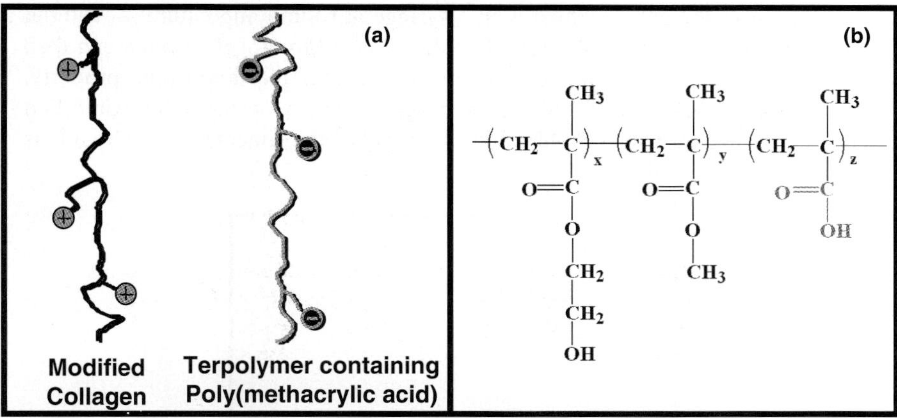

Figure 7–21 (a) Gel formation between modified collagen and terpolymer containing poly(methacrylic acid) by ionic complexation; (b) chemical structure of polyelectrolyte terpolymer

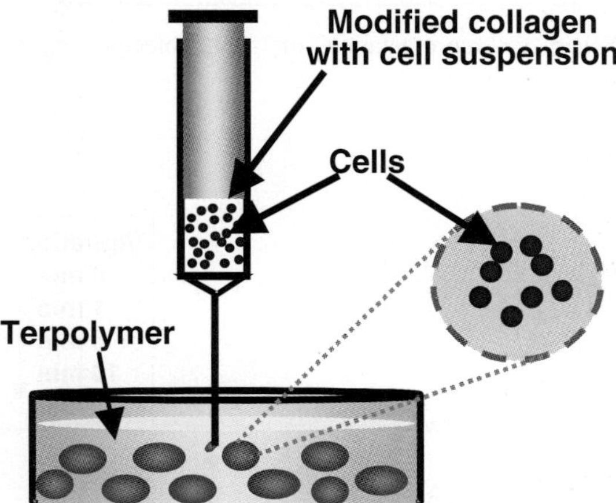

Figure 7–22 Schematic representation of the microencapsulation process of rat hepatocytes

The supramolecular hydrogels were found to be thixotropic and reversible [27]. The viscosity of the hydrogel greatly diminished as it was agitated (Figure 7–24(a)). This property renders the hydrogel formula injectable even through a fine needle. The diminished viscosity of the hydrogel eventually restored towards its original value, in most cases within hours, when there were no more agitations (Figure 7–24(b)). These thixotropic and reversible properties of the gel afford us with a unique injectable hydrogel drug delivery system. Now bioactive agents (such as drugs, proteins, vaccines, or plasmid DNAs) can be incorporated in the gel — which is in a syringe at room temperature — without any contact with organic solvents. The drug-loaded hydrogel formula can then be injected into the tissue under pressure because of the thixotropic property. After gelling is restored *in situ*, the hydrogel serves as a depot for controlled release.   Compared to implantable hydrogels, the injectable hydrogel is definitely more appealing.

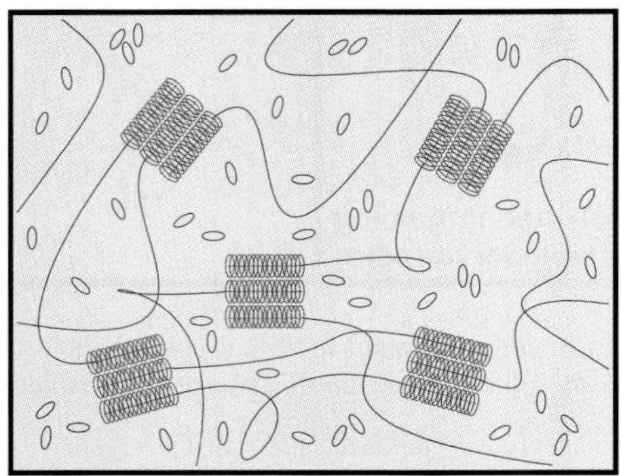

Figure 7–23   Schematic representation of supramolecular hydrogel formed by cyclodextrin and poly(ethylene glycol)

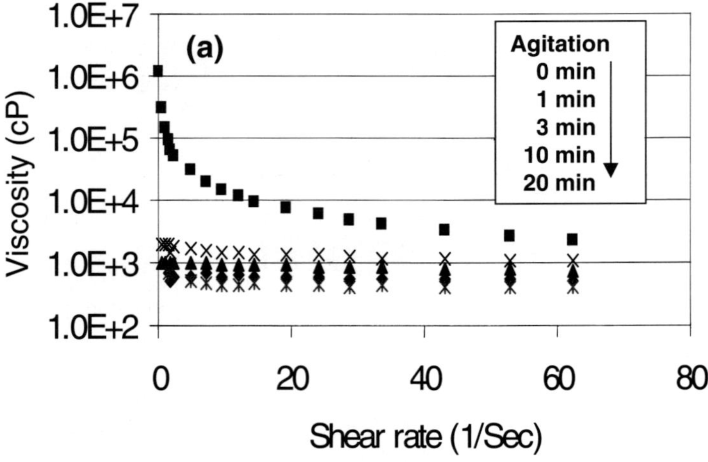

Figure 7–24(a)   Viscosity changes of Gel–20K–60 as function of agitation time at a shear rate of 120 s^{-1}

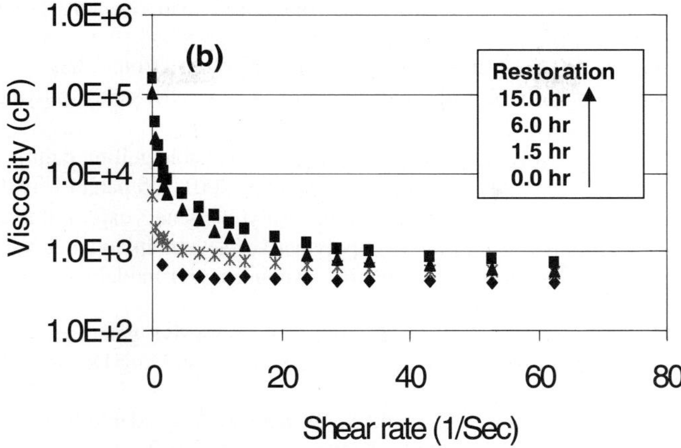

Figure 7–24(b) Restoration of gel viscosities after 20-min agitation at a shear rate of 120 s^{-1}

References

1. N. A. Peppas, Hydrogels in Medicine and Pharmacy, Vol. 1., (CRC Press, Florida, 1987).
2. K. Park, W. S. W. Shalaby, and H. Park, Biodegradable Hydrogels for Drug Delivery, (Technomic Publishing, Lancaster, 1993).
3. W. E. Hennink and C. F. van Nostrum, Novel cross-linking methods to design hydrogels, Adv. Drug Delivery Rev., 2002, 54:13.
4. A. S. Hoffman, Hydrogels for biomedical applications, Adv. Drug Delivery Rev., 2002, 43:3.
5. K. Ulbrich, V. Subr, L. W. Seymour, and R. Duncan, Novel biodegradable hydrogels prepared using the divinylic cross-linking agent N,O–dimethacryloylhydroxylamine. 1. Synthesis and characterization of rates of gel degradation, and rates of release of model drugs, *in vitro* and *in vivo*, J. Controlled Rel., 1993, 24:181.
6. W. E. Hennink, O. Franssen, W. N. E. van Dijk-Wolthuis, and H. Talsma, Dextran hydrogels for the controlled release of proteins, J. Controlled Rel., 1997, 48:107.
7. R. Tu, C. L. Lu, K. Thyagarajan, *et al.*, Kinetic study of collagen fixation with polyepoxy fixatives, J. Biomed. Mater. Res., 1993, 27:3.
8. J. M. Lee, C. A. Pereira, and K. W. K. Kan, Effect of molecular structure of poly(glycidyl ether) reagents on cross-linking and mechanical properties of bovine pericardial xenograft materials, J. Biomed. Mater. Res., 1994, 28:981.
9. B. Jeong, S. W. Kim, and Y. H. Bae, Thermosensitive sol-gel reversible hydrogels, Adv. Drug Delivery Rev., 2002, 54:37.
10. W. Friess, Collagen — biomaterials for drug delivery, Eur. J. Pharm. Biopharm., 1998, 45:113.

11. Y. Tabata and Y. Ikada, Protein release from gelatin matrices, Adv. Drug Delivery Rev., 1998, 31:287.

12. B. Vernon, S. W. Kim and Y. H. Bae, Insulin release from islets of langerhans entrapped in a poly(N–isopropylacrylamide–co–acrylic acid) polymer gel, J. Biomater. Sci. Polym. Ed., 1999, 10:183.

13. Y. H. Ahn, V. A. Mironov, and A. Gutowska, Reversible gelling culture media for *in vitro* cell culture in three-dimensional matrices, 2001, US patent US6103528.

14. P. Alexandridis and T. A. Hatton, Poly(ethylene oxide)–poly(propylene oxide)–poly(ethylene oxide) block copolymer surfactants in aqueous solutions and at interfaces: thermodynamics, structure, dynamics, and modeling, Coll. Surfaces, 1995, 96:1.

15. L. E. Bromberg and E. S. Ron, Temperature-responsive gels and thermogelling polymer matrices for protein and peptide delivery, Adv. Drug Delivery Rev., 1998, 31:197.

16. B. Jeong, Y. H. Bae, D. S. Lee, and S. W. Kim, Biodegradable block copolymers as injectable drug-delivery systems, Nature, 1997, 388:860.

17. B. Jeong, Y. H. Bae, and S. W. Kim, Drug release from biodegradable injectable thermosensitive hydrogel of PEG–PLGA–PEG triblock copolymers, J. Controlled Rel., 2000, 63:155.

18. G. H. Chen and A. S. Hoffman, Graft copolymer that exhibit temperature-induced phase transitions over a wide range of pH, Nature, 1995, 373:49.

19. S. J. de Jong, S. C. De Smedt, M. W. C. Wahls, J. Demeester, J. J. Kettenes-van den Bosch, and W. E. Hennink, Novel self-assembled hydrogels by stereocomplex formation in aqueous solution of enantiomeric lactic acid oligomers grafted to dextran, Macromolecules, 2000, 33:3680.

20. S. J. de Jong, S. C. de Smedt, J. Demeester, J. J. van Nostrum CF, Kettenes-van den Bosch, and W. E. Hennink, Biodegradable hydrogels based on stereocomplex formation between lactic acid oligomers grafted to dextran, J. Controlled Rel., 2001, 72:47.

21. W. A. Petka, J. L. Harden, K. P. McGrath, D. Wirtz, and D. A. Tirrell, Reversible hydrogels from self-assembling artificial proteins, Science, 1998, 281:389.

22. C. Wang, R. J. Stewart, and J. Kopecek, Hybrid hydrogels assembled from synthetic polymers and coiled-coil protein domains, Nature, 1999, 397:417.

23. S. M. Chia, K. M. Leong, J. Li, X. Xu, K. Y. Zeng, P. N. Er, S. J. Gao, and H. Yu, Hepatocyte encapsulation for enhanced cellular functions, Tissue Eng., 2000, 6:481.

24. A. Harada, J. Li, and M. Kamachi, The molecular necklace: a rotaxane containing many threaded α-cyclodextrins, Nature, 1992, 356:325.

25. J. Li, A. Harada, and M. Kamachi, Sol-gel transition during inclusion complex formation between α-cyclodextrin and high molecular weight poly(ethylene glycol)s in aqueous solution, Polym. J., 1994, 26:1019.

26. J. Li, X. Li, Z. Zhou, X. Ni, and K. W. Leong, Formation of supramolecular hydrogels induced by inclusion complexation between pluronics and cyclodextrin, Macromolecules, 2001, 34:7236.

27. J. Li, X. Ni, and K. W. Leong, Injectable drug-delivery systems based on supramolecular hydrogels formed by poly(ethylene oxide)s and cyclodextrin, J. Biomed. Mater. Res., 2003, 65(A):196.

CHAPTER 8

BIOACTIVE CERAMIC-POLYMER COMPOSITES FOR TISSUE REPLACEMENT

Min Wang

Medical Engineering and Mechanical Engineering
Faculty of Engineering, The University of Hong Kong
Pokfulam Road, Hong Kong
E-mail: memwang@hkucc.hku.hk

Bone, at the ultra-structural level, is a composite with mechanical properties that can be matched by man-made composites. It serves as the template for developing bone replacement materials. Research on biomaterials analogous to bone was started in the early 1980s by incorporating bioactive particles into biocompatible polymers in order to produce bone substitutes. Hydroxyapatite reinforced high-density polyethylene (HA/HDPE) is one of such materials and has been successfully used in human bodies. In this chapter, the structure and mechanical properties of bone are firstly reviewed. The production, structure, properties of HA/HDPE composites are then presented. Their biological performance is discussed subsequently, and examples of their clinical applications are given. Using the same or similar manufacturing processes, other bioactive composites have also been developed for tissue substitution or tissue regeneration.

8.1   Introduction

Numerous materials have been used for bone substitution ever since plaster of paris was tried for bone repair in the 19th century. In modern-day orthopedic surgery, metals (such as stainless steel and titanium alloy) and ceramics (such as alumina and toughened zirconia) are common in a variety of implants and devices. However, these materials, having been developed originally for other purposes rather than medical applications, are considerably stiffer than human bone. The modulus mismatch between an implant material and the host tissue can cause bone to resorb at the bone-implant interface, which leads to implant instability and hence its eventual failure [1]. A long-lasting bone replacement requires the establishment of a stable bone-implant interface, which necessitates the careful matching of the mechanical behavior as well as mechanical properties of synthetic implant materials with the natural tissue [2]. Furthermore, bone replacement materials must withstand any anticipated physical load imposed by body actions without substantial dimensional changes, catastrophic fracture, or failure due to impact, creep, or fatigue within their expected lifetime in the body.

It is now generally recognized that the best material for replacing a body tissue is the one that is similar, if not identical, to that tissue [3]. Advances in composite technology have led to the production of new composites that mimic the structure and match the properties of human tissues. These novel materials may overcome problems that have been encountered with the use of conventional implant materials [4].

8.2   Structure and Properties of Bone

Bone is the substantial unit of human skeletal system, which supports the body and its movements. Bone, as a natural tissue, has a complex structure in which several levels of organization, from macro- to micro-scale, can be identified [1]. Take a human long bone such as femur for an example (Figure 8–1). It consists of an outer load bearing shell of cortical bone with a medullary cavity containing cancellous bone towards the bone ends.

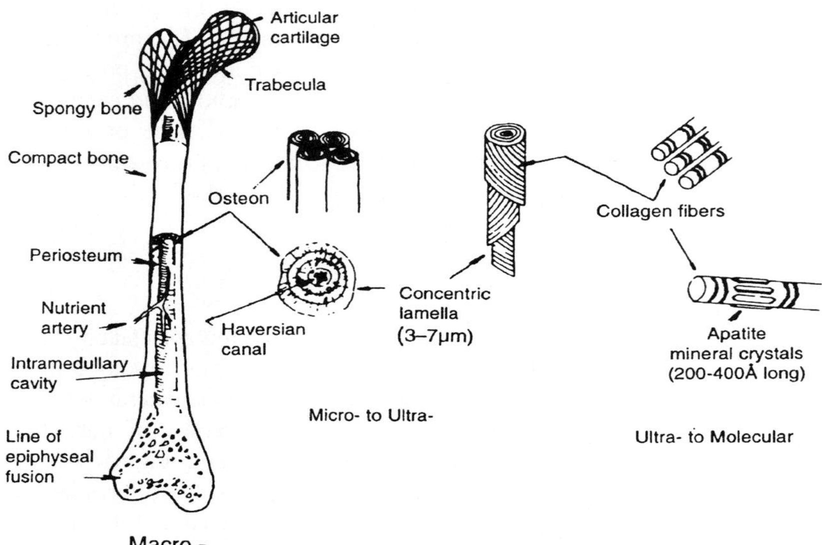

Figure 8–1 Structural organization in a human long bone (Reprinted from reference [1] with permission)

Cortical (or compact) bone as a material is anisotropic with osteons (also known as "Haversian systems") being oriented parallel to the long axis of the bone and interspersed in regions of non-oriented bone (Figure 8–2). Each osteon (about 100 to 300 μm in diameter) has a central Haversian canal (20 to 40 μm in diameter) containing a blood vessel, which supplies the elements required for bone remodeling. The Haversian canal is surrounded by 4 to 20 concentrically arranged lamellae with each lamella being 3 to 7 μm thick. Each adjacent lamellar layer has a different orientation of collagen fibers. Circumscribing the outermost concentric lamella of the osteon is a narrow zone known as cement line, which contains calcified mucopolysaccharides and is devoid of collagen. The cement line is 1 to 2 μm thick and is the weakest part of bone. The densely packed concentric lamellae in osteons are composed of two major components: fibrous collagen (which is a natural polymer) and bone mineral. The mineral crystallites that human bone contains are structurally calcium-deficient, carbonate-substituted hydroxyapatite. They are usually referred to as bone apatite, which normally has dimensions of 5 x 5 x 50 nm with a rod-like (or sometimes plate-like) habit and is embedded in collagen fibers. In mature bone, bone apatite occupies about 50 percent of the total volume. The precise microstructural organization of bone is a function of age and varies between different bones and between different locations of the same bone. Two levels of composite structure are considered when developing bone substitutes. First, the bone apatite reinforced collagen forming individual lamella (on the nanometer to micrometer scale) and, second, the osteon reinforced interstitial bone (on the micrometer to millimeter scale). It is the apatite-collagen composite at the microscopic level that provides the basis for producing bioceramic-polymer composites for bone replacement.

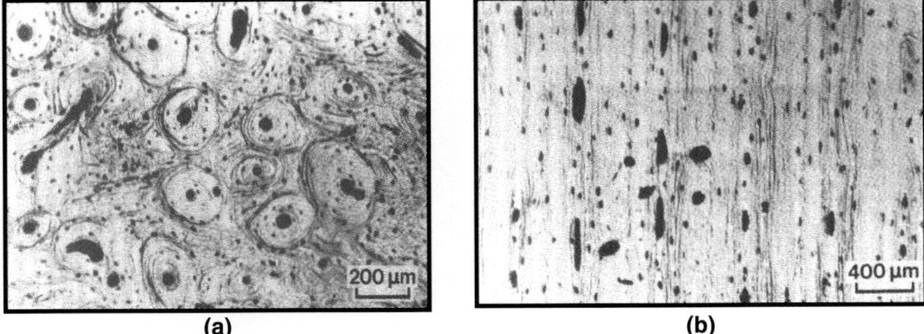

Figure 8–2 Reflected light optical micrographs of cortical bone showing the overall distribution of oriented osteons: (a) transverse section; (b) longitudinal section (Reprinted from reference [5] with permission)

The mechanical behavior of bone may be investigated by assessing whole bones *in vivo*. But the results obtained can be difficult to interpret due to irregular shapes of bones and the organizational hierarchy in bones. Normally, mechanical properties of bone (cortical or cancellous) are determined *in vitro* using standard or miniature specimens that conform to various standards originally designed for testing conventional materials such as metals and plastics. The conditions required to prepare and test dead bone specimens in order to gain meaningful results representative of living bone have been well established. It is very important to maintain water content of bone for mechanical assessment as the behavior of bone in the "wet" condition significantly differs from that of bone in a dry state [6]. Under the quasi-static testing condition, a tensile test of "wet" cortical bone at ambient temperature gives a stress-strain curve exhibiting a small viscoelastic component and culminating in brittle fracture at a total strain of 0.5–3.0 percent. As a result of orientation, location and age, cortical bone has a range of associated properties rather than a unique set of values (Table 8–1). Young's modulus of cortical bone therefore ranges between 7 and 30 GPa. It has been found that Young's modulus of cortical bone increases with an increase in the mineral content of bone [7]. Microhardness has been shown to be strongly related to Young's modulus for bone (Figure 8–3). Therefore, microhardness is a good predicator of Young's modulus of bone. It can also be seen from Table 8–1 that bone is significantly less stiff than the various alloys and ceramics currently utilized as prosthetic materials, but is stiffer than all biomedical polymers. Cortical bone fractures in a brittle fashion, with the ultimate tensile strength being 50 to 150 MPa. It is also known that fracture toughness — which is an important parameter for brittle solids — of bone is considerably lower than those of metallic implant materials. The structure and properties of cancellous (or spongy) bone are also well understood and documented [8].

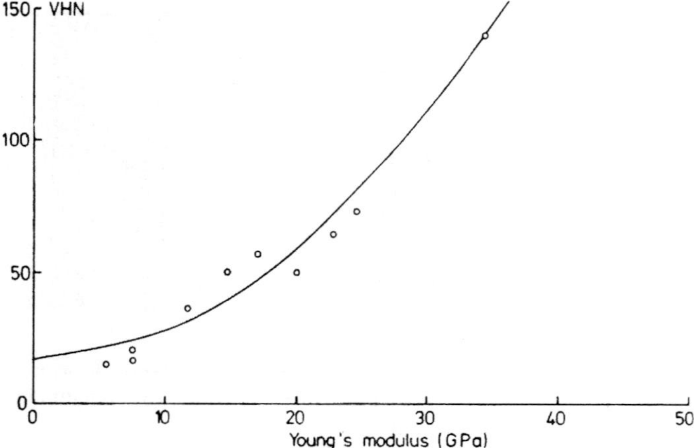

Figure 8–3 Correlation of microhardness (VHN) with Young's modulus for bone (Reprinted from reference [7] with permission)

Treating bone as a nanometer-scale composite, the mechanical behavior of bone may be explained using a simple composite model (Figure 8–4). Brittle apatite acts as a stiffening phase in bone, and ductile collagen provides a tough matrix. Consequently the tensile behavior of bone exhibits the combinational effect of these two major constituents of bone. A good understanding of the structure and properties of bone yields two-fold benefits. First, it gives good insight into the structural features of bone. Second, it provides the property range for approximating mechanical compatibility that is required of a bone analogue material for an exact structural replacement of bone with a stabilized bone-implant interface. It is important to bear in mind, however, that bone is unlike any engineering material in that it can alter its properties and configuration in response to changes in mechanical demand.

Table 8–1 Mechanical properties of bone and current implant materials

Material	E (GPa)	σ (MPa)	ε (%)	K_{IC} (MN m$^{-3/2}$)
Cortical bone	7–30	50–150	1–3	2–12
Cancellous bone	0.05–0.5	10–20	5–7	
Co–Cr alloys	230	900–1540	10–30	~100
Stainless steel	200	540–1000	6–70	~100
Ti–6Al–4V	106	900	12.5	~80
Alumina	400	450	~0.5	~3
Hydroxyapatite	30–100	60–190		~1
Polyethylene	1	30	>300	

E: Young's modulus σ: tensile strength (flexural strength for alumina)
ε: elongation at fracture K_{IC}: fracture toughness

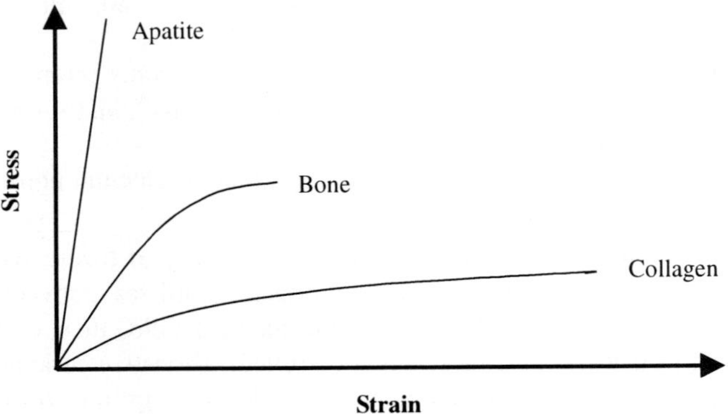

Figure 8–4 Schematic diagram showing the mechanical behavior of apatite, collagen, and compact bone

8.3   Bioceramics and Biopolymers

Some ceramics and polymers have been used as hard tissue replacement materials for several decades now. Quite a few of these materials have achieved clinical success due to their distinctive characteristics. Several materials in these two categories can be combined to form composites for various medical applications.

8.3.1 Bioactive Ceramics

Ceramics for medical uses have come into prominence over the last two decades. With the modern and now widely accepted definition, the group of materials that are termed "bioceramics" includes ceramics, glasses, and glass-ceramics which are used to repair and reconstruct diseased, damaged, or "worn out" parts of the body. Bioceramics have the advantage of being compatible with the human body environment. Their biocompatibility is a direct result of their chemical compositions which contain ions commonly found in the physiological environment (such as Ca^{2+}, K^+, Mg^{2+}, Na^+, *etc.*) and other ions which show very limited toxicity to body tissues (such as Al^{3+} and Ti^{2+}). For materials implanted in the body, there are four types of tissue response [9]:

(1) If the material is toxic, the surrounding tissue dies;
(2) If the material is non-toxic and biologically inactive, a fibrous tissue capsule of variable thickness forms around the material;
(3) If the material is non-toxic and biologically active, an interfacial bond forms between the material and tissue;
(4) If the material is non-toxic and dissolves, the surrounding tissue replaces the dissolved material.

In consideration of these tissue responses, there are three types of bioceramics that can fulfill their functions in the body:

(1) Bioinert ceramics, e.g., carbon, alumina, and zirconia ceramics;
(2) Bioactive ceramics, e.g., hydroxyapatite, Bioglass®, and A–W glass-ceramic;
(3) Bioresorbable ceramics, e.g., calcium sulfate, tricalcium phosphate, and calcium aluminate.

Bioceramics are manufactured and used in a variety of forms: particulates, fibers, monoliths, and coatings. Their production utilizes conventional and advanced technologies. For their use in the medical field, their composition, structure, and properties must be strictly controlled. Bioactive ceramics include calcium phosphates (with hydroxyapatite being the most prominent member of this group of compounds), bioactive glasses such as Bioglass®, and bioactive glass-ceramics such as A–W glass-ceramic. Calcium phosphate-based bioceramics have been in use in medicine and dentistry for over twenty years now. The interest in one particular group member, hydroxyapatite (HA), arises from its similarity to bone apatite (a biological apatite) — the major component of the inorganic phase of bone, which plays a key role in the calcification and resorption processes of bone.

Biological apatites constitute the mineral phase of calcified tissues such as bone, dentin, and enamel in the body and also some pathological calcifications. The general chemical formula for biological apatites is $(Ca, M)_{10}(PO_4, CO_3, Y)_6(OH, F, Cl)_2$, where M represents metallic elements such as Na, K and Mg, Y represents functional groups such as acid phosphate, sulfate, *etc.* As compared to synthetic HA with the chemical formula of $Ca_{10}(PO_4)_6(OH)_2$, substitution in biological apatites by the carbonate group for the phosphate group takes place in a coupled manner, *i.e.*, CO_3^{2-} for PO_4^{3-} while Na^+ for Ca^{2+}. Biological apatites are usually calcium-deficient as a result of various substitutions in regular HA lattice points.

HA is the most commonly used calcium phosphate in the medical field as it possesses excellent biocompatibility and is osteoconductive. Its production and properties have been well documented [10,11]. HA in the particulate form can be produced using a variety of methods. Characteristics of HA powders have significant effects on the subsequent products — where HA can be in the form of dense or porous structure, in coatings, or in composites. The production of HA powder generally falls into three categories: wet method, dry method, and hydrothermal method. The wet method can be used for the mass production of crystalline HA or non-crystalline calcium phosphate powder. One process with the wet method involves a neutral reaction of acid and alkaline solutions (Figure 8–5). The reaction temperature, reactant concentrations, and other production parameters should be carefully controlled in order to obtain high-purity, good-quality HA powder [12]. Particle size, particle size distribution, and particle morphology of HA powders must be optimized for their use as the secondary, bioactive phase in various composites.

HA has been used clinically on its own as a bioactive material in the form of powder, porous structure, or dense body. The successful utilization of HA as an implant material should be in the first place attributed to its good biocompatibility — which is a perceived advantage of being a material similar to the mineral phase in bone and teeth when replacing these tissues.

Another attractive member of the calcium phosphate family for medical applications is tricalcium phosphate (TCP). The chemical formula of TCP is $Ca_3(PO_4)_2$, and TCP has four polymorphs: α, β, γ, and super-α. The γ polymorph is a high-pressure phase and the super-α polymorph is observed at temperatures above approximately 1500°C. Therefore the most frequently encountered TCP polymorphs in the field of bioceramics are α- and β-TCP. TCP is a bioresorbable ceramic, and the dissolution rate increases in the following order:

$$HA < \beta\text{-TCP} < \alpha\text{-TCP} \tag{1}$$

TCP has been accepted and used as a biocompatible, bioresorbable material for bone repair in the form of ceramic blocks, granules, or calcium phosphate cements [13].

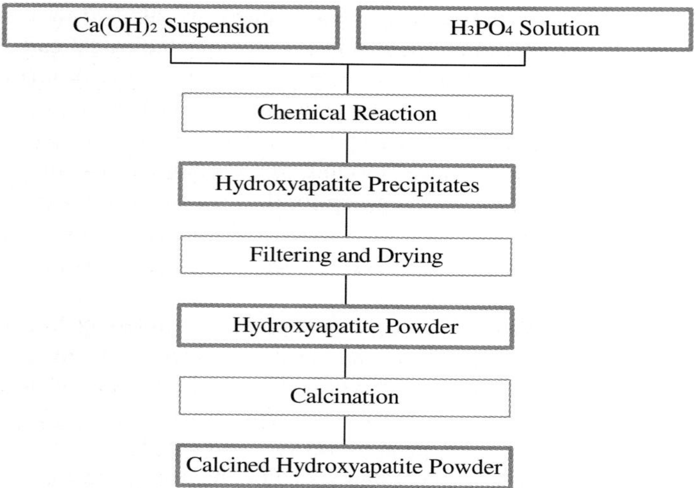

Figure 8–5 Synthesis of hydroxyapatite powder using the wet method

8.3.2 *Biocompatible Polymers*

Polymers are long-chain molecules that consist of small repeating units (*i.e.*, "mers"). There are a wide variety of polymers including natural materials (such as cellulose and collagen) and synthetic materials (such as polyethylene and poly(methyl methacrylate) (*i.e.*, PMMA)). Medical use of synthetic polymers has a long history. The success of polymers in medicine can be exemplified by the applications of PMMA and ultra high molecular weight polyethylene (UHMWPE) in total hip replacement. The great number of currently available synthetic polymers makes the selection of a suitable polymer for a particular biomedical application a difficult task. However, among all properties required for an application, biocompatibility of the polymer with tissues and biological fluids is always the foremost consideration for all candidate materials. On the basis of years of laboratory experimentation and clinical investigation, the following synthetic polymers are considered "biocompatible" [14,15]: polyethylene (PE), polypropylene (PP), polyurethane (PU), polytetrafluoroethylene (PTFE), poly(vinyl chloride) (PVC), polyamides (PA), poly(methyl methacrylate) (PMMA), polyacetal, polycarbonate (PC), poly(ethylene terephthalate) (PET), polyetheretherketone (PEEK), and polysulfone (PSU). These polymers are also considered "biostable" in the body and have found wide applications in the medical field, ranging from PTFE vascular grafts to UHMWPE acetabular cups.

Among all biostable polymers, polyethylene (PE) occupies a prominent position for medical devices. PE is a synthetic polymer and has the chemical formula of $(CH_2CH_2)_n$. It is produced from ethylene through various processes [16]. Depending on the manufacturing process used, different polyethylenes are made: low density polyethylene (LDPE), linear low density polyethylene (LLDPE), high density polyethylene (HDPE), cross-linked polyethylene (XLPE), and ultra high molecular weight polyethylene (UHMWPE). The properties of these polyethylenes depend on the length and degree of branching of the polyolefin chains. Generally the higher the degree of branching, the lower the density of the solid. The density of polyethylenes ranges from 0.92 to 0.97 g/cm^3 [16,17]. It is HDPE and UHMWPE that have found extensive applications in the medical field.

UHMWPE is a linear polyethylene that has an extremely high average molecular weight (M_w). Its M_w is approximately 4×10^6 g/mol, which is an order of magnitude greater than that of HDPE. It has outstanding resistance to wear and abrasion and low coefficient of friction. Due to its wear resistance and low friction characteristics when coupled with metals such as Co–Cr alloys and stainless steel, it has been used for acetabular cups in total hip prostheses for over thirty years now.

HDPE consists of molecules that are essentially linear, typically with fewer than one branch per 200 carbon atoms in the backbone. The linearity of polymer chains permits the development of high degrees of crystallinity which results in the highest modulus and the lowest permeability of all classes of polyethylenes. HDPE can thus have Young's modulus of up to 1 GPa, tensile strength above 20 MPa and elongation at break greater than 100 percent. HDPE has already been in use in tubing for drains and catheters due to its excellent toughness and its resistance to fats and oils. Furthermore, HDPE, having high content of particulate filler, can still be melt processed using current extrusion and molding technology, thereby providing the option of mass production of implants at reasonable manufacturing costs. The advantage that HDPE is a linear polymer with very few branches is very important. This is because when advanced polymer processing technology such as hydrostatic extrusion is used, polyethylene chains will be aligned in the extrusion direction and hence high modulus and high strength materials can be produced.

If biodegradation is desired of implants, biocompatible and biodegradable polymers can be used. These polymers include poly(lactic acid) (PLA), poly(glycolic acid) (PGA), poly(ε–caprolactone) (PCL), polyhydroxybutyrate (PHB), and a few other polymers [18]. It must be borne in mind that during the selection of a biodegradable polymer, apart from other required properties, the degradation rate of the material should be matched with the growth rate of the new tissue.

8.4 Hydroxyapatite Reinforced Polyethylene Composites for Bone Replacement

The success that metals, polymers, and ceramics have achieved in tissue substitution should not hinder the progress in pursuing better and smarter materials for implants and medical devices. And indeed the last twenty years have witnessed a rapid pace in the development of new biomaterials.

8.4.1 Combining Hydroxyapatite and Polyethylene for Bioactive Bone Analogues

As bone is an apatite-collagen composite material at the ultra-structural level, a polymer matrix composite containing a particulate, bioactive component appears a natural choice for substituting cortical bone. Bonfield *et al.* pioneered the use of hydroxyapatite (HA) particles as the bioactive and strengthening phase in polymers to produce bone analogues [19]. HA closely resembles bone apatite and exhibits excellent bioactivity. Polyethylene (PE) is a proven biocompatible polymer and widely used in orthopedics. It is therefore natural to combine these two materials to produce a composite that mimics the structure and matches the mechanical properties of cortical bone. The ductile polyethylene allows incorporation of relatively high volume percentages of HA particles in the polymer matrix, which is essential for obtaining bioactivity of the composite. With good bioactivity of the composite due to the presence of particulate HA, a strong bond should be formed between implants made of the composite and the surrounding tissue. As no other materials are used, all components of the composite are biocompatible and hence the composite should also be biocompatible.

8.4.2 Manufacture of Hydroxyapatite/polyethylene Composites

HA/HDPE composites containing up to 45 vol% (*i.e.*, 73 wt%) of HA can be routinely made through standardized procedures [20,21]. The process for manufacturing HA/HDPE composites is outlined in Figure 8–6.

Both commercially available HA powders and particulate HA produced in-house have been used to produce HA/HDPE composites. Either a twin screw extruder [20] or an internal mixer [21] was used for compounding the materials efficiently. Compounding using two-roll mills appeared to be unsuitable due to their inability to cope with composites of high HA volume fractions and also polymer degradation. Powdering of compounded materials usually took place in a centrifugal mill at below $-100°C$. Compression or injection molding could produce bulk materials for prostheses or even some small medical devices. Composite plates as thick as 20 mm could be made by compression molding using composite powders. These plates were void-free, as revealed by X-ray radiographs.

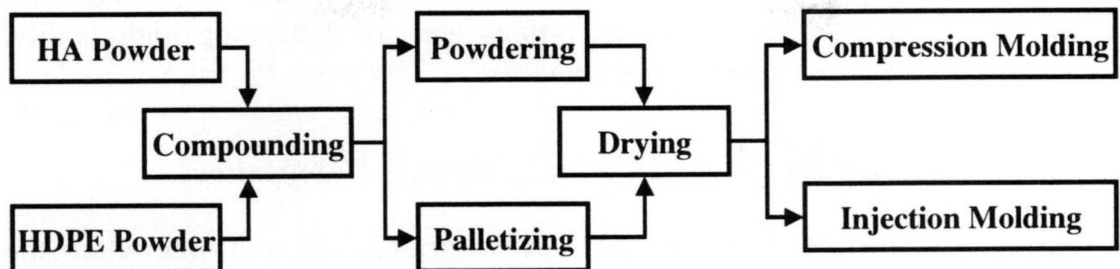

Figure 8–6 Manufacture of HA/HDPE composites

Rheological studies revealed that the incorporation of particulate HA into HDPE resulted in an increase in the viscosity of composites at their processing temperatures [22,23]. The presence of HA particles restricted molecular mobility of HDPE under shear and hence resulted in higher viscosity. This increase in viscosity was more pronounced at low shear rates (Figure 8–7).

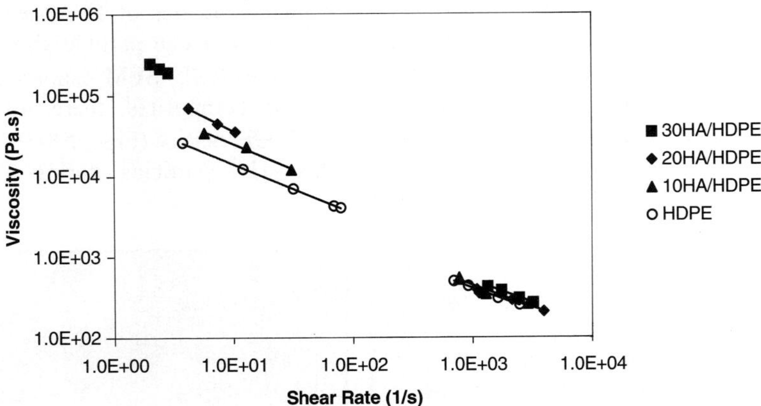

Figure 8–7 Apparent viscosity versus apparent shear rate for HA/HDPE composite at 190°C [23]

When the shear rate was increased, the viscosity of HA/HDPE composites approached that of the unfilled HDPE. Both HDPE and HA/HDPE composites showed pronounced shear thinning behavior. HA/HDPE composites at their processing temperatures exhibited discontinuity with a varying shear rate. As the HA content in the composite increased, the shear rates at which discontinuity occurred were reduced. The die swell ratio of HA/HDPE composite was reduced as the HA content was increased. It is possible that the presence of HA particles in the polymer matrix reduced the degree of recoiling of the HDPE molecular chains and hence led to the reduction in swelling of composite. Analysis of rheological behavior of HA/HDPE composites is important for optimizing composite processing conditions and for producing high-quality, net-shape (or near net-shape) medical devices.

8.4.3 *Structure of Hydroxyapatite/polyethylene Composites*

SEM examination of polished HA/HDPE surfaces showed that after the compounding process, HA particles were well dispersed, exhibiting a homogeneous distribution in the polymer matrix (Figure 8–8). Subsequent composite processing by compression molding preserved these characteristics. This uniform distribution of HA particles in composites is essential for mechanical as well as biological performance of implants. Using the image analysis technique and stereology, it was possible to calculate the average volume diameter of HA particles in composites from SEM micrographs (*i.e.*, from two-dimensional images to three-dimensional projections). The calculations indicated that the high shear forces generated during the compounding process broke up HA particle agglomerates into unit particles in the polymer matrix [24]. The average volume diameter of HA particles in compounded HA/HDPE was nearly the same as the mean particle size of HA powder used for producing the composites (Table 8–2). SEM examination of tensile fracture surfaces suggested that in the composites, there was only mechanical bond between HA particles and HDPE matrix (Figure 8–9) due to the shrinkage of HDPE around individual HA particles during thermal processing [20,25].

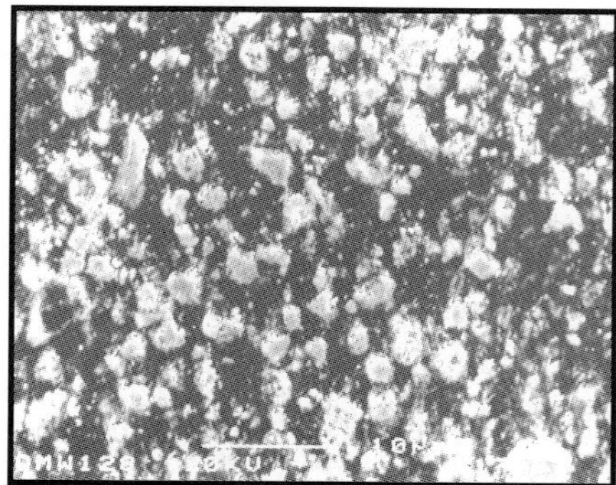

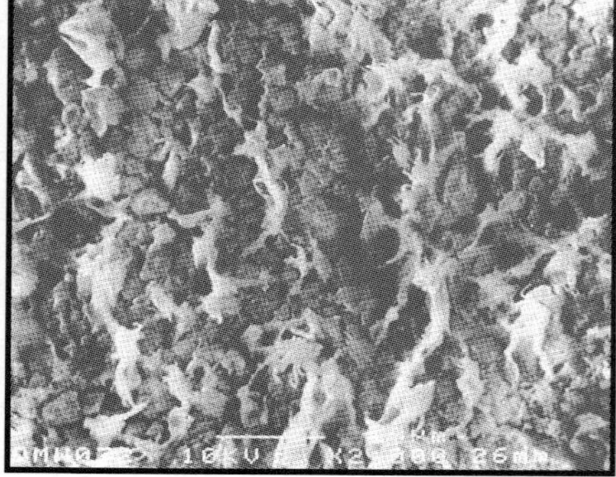

Figure 8–8 Uniform distribution of HA particles in HA/HDPE composite containing 40 vol% of HA [20]

Figure 8–9 Tensile fracture surface of HA/HDPE composite containing 45 vol% of HA [20]

Table 8–2 HA particle size at different stages of composite processing [24]

HA Volume (%)	Particle Size		
	$d_{0.5}$ (µm)	d_{2d} (µm)	d_{3d} (µm)
20	3.85	1.86	3.74
40	3.85	1.99	3.32

$d_{0.5}$: median volume diameter of particles from as-received powder
d_{2d}: average area diameter of particles on polished composite surface obtained by image analysis of SEM micrographs
d_{3d}: average volume diameter of particles calculated using stereology

It was found that compounding caused slight decreases in the weight average molecular mass (M_w) of HDPE, with the decrease being dependent on HA volume fraction [25]. Further thermal processing by compression or injection molding also reduced M_w. Differential scanning calorimetry (DSC) results indicated that the addition of HA particles caused decreases in the degree of crystallinity of HDPE, where composites of higher HA contents had lower degrees of crystallinity for the polymer matrix [21].

Thermogravimetric analysis (TGA) was used to determine the real HA content in HA/HDPE composites (Figure 8–10). Calculations made from the TGA curves showed that the difference between the actual mass percentages of HA in the composites produced and the "Rule of Mixtures (ROM)" values was negligible. Hence the intended compositions had been achieved (Table 8–3).

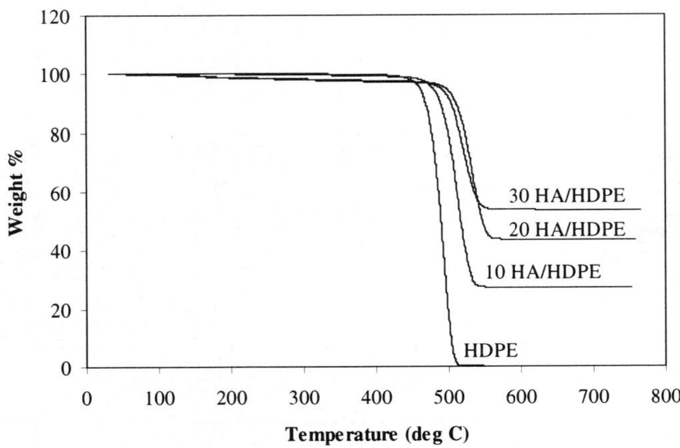

Figure 8–10 TGA curves obtained for the HA/HDPE composite [21]

Table 8–3 HA content in HA/HDPE composite

Nominal HA Volume (vol%)	Theoretical HA Mass[*] (wt%)	Real HA Mass[**] (wt%)
0	0.0	0.1
10	27.1	26.7
20	45.5	43.5
30	58.9	57.4
40	69.0	67.7

[*]: calculation based on "Rule of Mixtures", using $\rho_{HA} = 3.16$ g/cm^3 and $\rho_{HDPE} = 0.945$ g/cm^3
[**]: thermogravimetric analysis result

8.4.4 Mechanical Properties of Hydroxyapatite/polyethylene Composites

By varying the amount of HA in the composite, a range of mechanical properties of the material and biological responses to the material could be obtained. The incorporation of HA in HDPE evidently stiffened the composite (Figure 8–11). An increase in the HA volume percentage led to increases in the Young's modulus, shear modulus, and tensile strength of HA/HDPE, with a corresponding decrease in the strain to fracture [20,26].

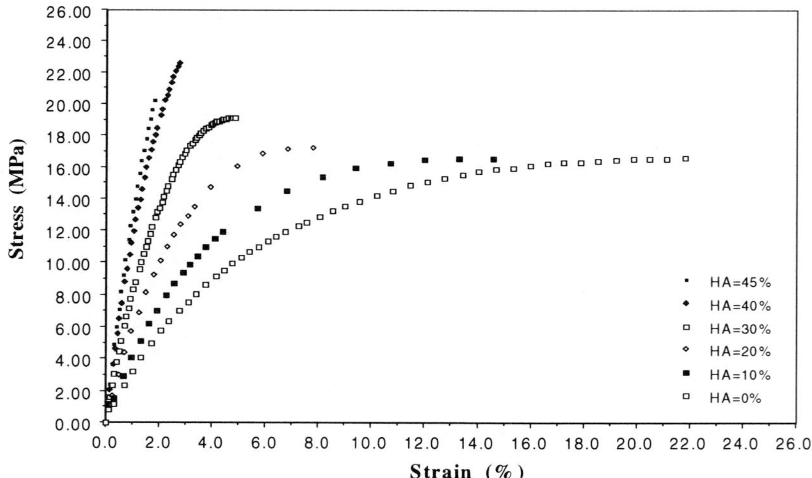

Figure 8–11 Tensile stress-strain curves of HA/HDPE composite (0 to 45 vol% of HA) up to respective peak stress

The particle morphology and average particle size of HA were found to affect mechanical properties of HA/HDPE composites [26]. HA/HDPE with 45 vol% of HA possessed a Young's modulus value of 5.54 GPa, approaching the lower bound for cortical bone (Table 8–4). HA/HDPE composites containing around 40 vol% appeared to be suitable for clinical use in bone substitution. But the actual composite to be used depends on the nature of bone being replaced and the anticipated physiological load.

Table 8–4 Mechanical properties of HA/HDPE composite [26]

HA Volume (%)	E (GPa)	G (GPa)	σ (MPa)	ε (%)
0	0.65±0.02	0.28±0.10	17.89±0.29	>360
10	0.98±0.02	0.39±0.16	17.30±0.27	>200
20	1.60±0.02	0.48±0.07	17.77±0.09	34.0±9.5
30	2.73±0.10	0.71±0.17	19.55±0.20	6.4±0.5
40	4.29±0.17	1.18±0.07	20.67±1.56	2.6±0.4
45	5.54±0.62	1.46±0.26	18.98±2.11	1.9±0.2

E: Young's modulus G: shear modulus σ: tensile strength ε: elongation at fracture

Using an instrumented falling weight impact tester, it was shown that for HA/HDPE composites an increase in HA content produced a decrease in impact energy for fracture [27]. However, the HA content seemed to have little effect on the maximum impact force for fracture as this force was at nearly the same level for composites of all compositions. Under this type of impact condition, the failure of composites containing various amounts of HA was classified as "brittle", since there were no evidences of gross plastic deformation when compared to the rupture of the matrix polymer itself.

Microhardness of HA/HDPE composites increased with an increase in HA content [7,21]. However for a given volume fraction of the ceramic phase (either HA or bone apatite), the hardness of HA/HDPE composites was considerably lower than that of the native tissue. This could be due to the different particle size, the distribution of ceramic phase, and the way in which ceramic particles are bonded to the matrix.

Dynamic properties and the damping capability of HA/HDPE composites were also studied in detail [21,25,28]. Dynamic mechanical analysis (DMA) results showed that the storage modulus of the composites increased with increase in HA content and decreased with increase in temperature (Figure 8–12). Unlike storage modulus which decreased monotonically with increase in temperature, the loss modulus of the composites decreased when the temperature rose from –100°C to –25°C. It then increased to peak at around 40°C, with a subsequent decrease towards higher temperatures. It was also shown that the addition of HA particles into HDPE reduced the damping capability (as indicated by tan δ values in the DMA analysis) of the polymer, with the degree of reduction depending upon the HA volume fraction (Figure 8–13).

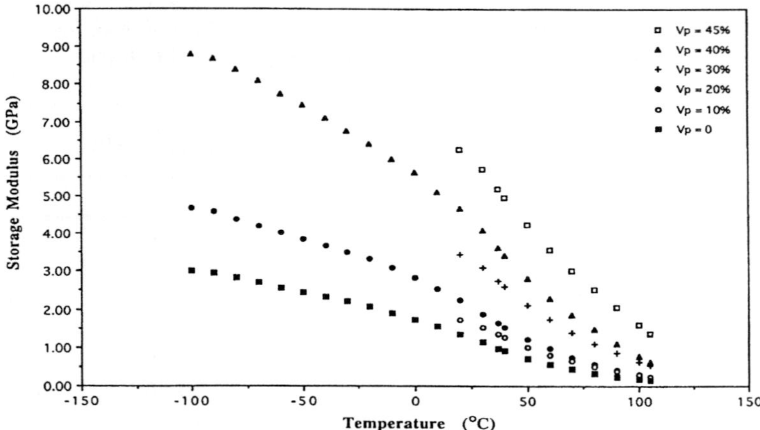

Figure 8–12   Variation of storage modulus with temperature for HA/HDPE composite [25]

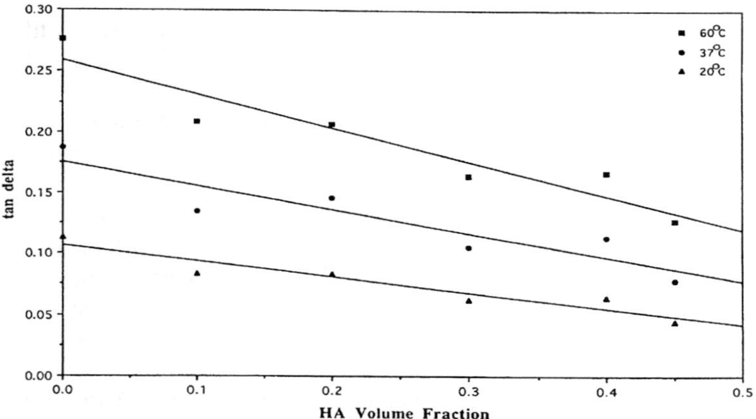

Figure 8–13 Variation of tan δ with HA volume fraction at different temperatures for HA/HDPE composite [25]

The creep behavior of HA/HDPE composites was investigated using a three-station tensile creep machine [29–31]. The inclusion of HA particles in HDPE improved the short-term creep resistance when specimens were subjected to similar stresses. Hence an increase in the HA volume fraction increased creep resistance (Figure 8–14). The increase of creep resistance is associated with the increase in moduli of the composites. However creep failure of composites could occur at prolonged times due to debonding at the HA-HDPE interface. Immersion in Ringer's solution reduced the creep resistance of HA/HDPE composites. This effect was due to the penetration of fluid into the composites. The decrease in creep resistance and hence the increase in the amount of fluid penetration were found to be a function of HA volume fraction [30].

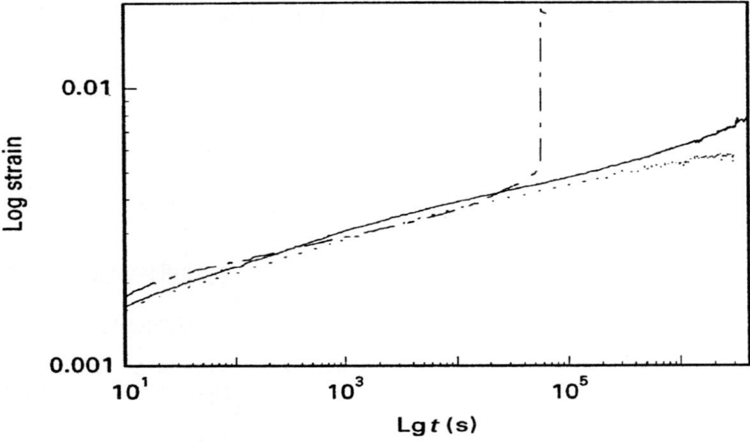

Figure 8–14 Creep strain versus time for HA/HDPE composite loaded at different stress levels in Ringer's solution (HDPE at 2 MPa, 20%HA/HDPE at 4 MPa, 40%HA/HDPE at 8 MPa) [29]

Biaxial (*i.e.*, axial and torsional) fatigue tests were conducted using standard fatigue specimens for HA/HDPE composites [32]. The ultimate shear strength of HDPE and HA/HDPE composite with 20 vol% of HA was determined to be 17.12 MPa and 17.46 MPa respectively. A fixed axial component of 50 percent of ultimate tensile strength (UTS) with the torsional component varying from zero percent to 50 percent of ultimate shear strength (USS) was used for fatigue tests. Generally the fatigue life of HDPE and that of the composite were reduced when shear stress increased in the biaxial stress condition (Figure 8–15). The addition of particulate HA in HDPE led to shorter fatigue life in low shear stress conditions. HDPE specimens did not fail after one million fatigue cycles with shear stress levels being zero percent and 12.5 percent of USS, whereas composite specimens failed at finite numbers of cycles under the same stress conditions. In high shear stress conditions, the effects of shear stress became dominant and the fatigue lives of both HDPE and HA/HDPE were about the same.

Tribological properties (*i.e.*, coefficient of friction, wear rate, and lubrication in the presence of proteins) of HDPE and HA/HDPE composite were evaluated against duplex stainless steel under dry and lubricated conditions [33].

Lubricants included distilled water and aqueous solutions of proteins (egg albumen or glucose). It was found that HA/HDPE composite had lower coefficients of friction than HDPE under certain conditions. However the addition of HA beyond 10 vol% deteriorated the tribological properties of HA/HDPE composite by forming an abrasive slurry of HA in the lubricants. Both egg albumen and glucose were shown to be corrosive to steel and adversely reactive for HDPE and HA/HDPE composite. HA/HDPE composite appeared unsuitable for implants with articulating surfaces.

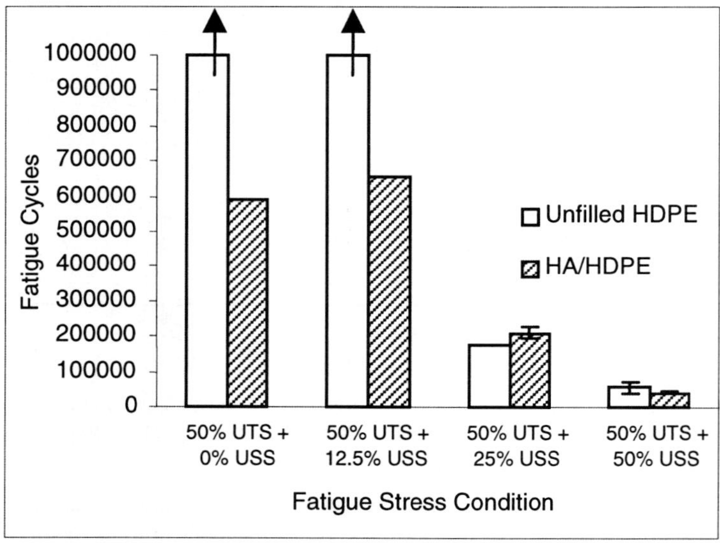

Figure 8–15 Fatigue lives of HDPE and HA/HDPE under various biaxial fatigue stress conditions [32]

8.4.5 In Vitro and In Vivo Assessments

For implant materials, it is essential to demonstrate that they are biocompatible with host tissues. It is well established now that the response of the body to an implant is to produce a fibrous capsule which may be remodeled with time. If the material is toxic, the fibrous capsule will increase in thickness; if the material is inert, the fibrous capsule will be of constant thickness [1]. However with a bioactive implant material such as hydroxyapatite, which releases calcium and phosphate ions from its surfaces and encourages the deposition of an apatite layer on the implant surface, the fibrous capsule will thin and disappear. When a bone analogue material is implanted into the body, the response to the material depends on a combination of responses to the constituents of the composite.

The biological performance of implant materials can be evaluated by *in vitro* tests using simulated body fluid or cell cultures, or by *in vivo* assessments. In *in vitro* experiments using human osteoblast cell primary cultures, it was observed that the osteoblast cells attached to "islands" of HA in the composite and subsequently proliferated (Figure 8–16), thus showing clearly the biocompatibility and bioactivity of HA/HDPE composite [34].

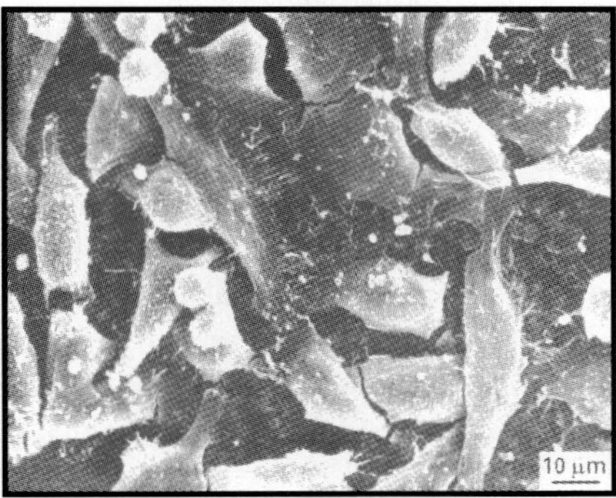

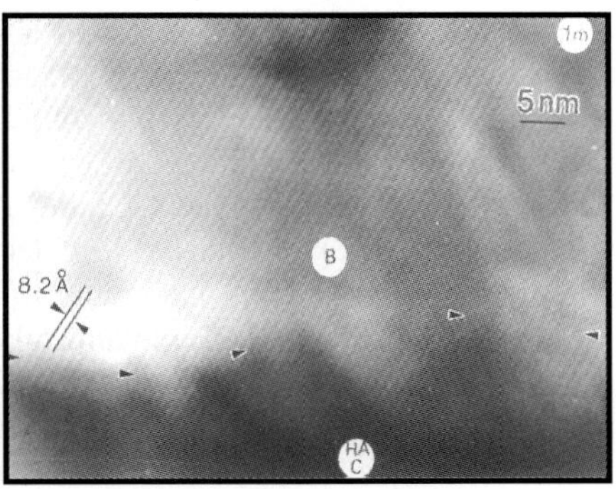

Figure 8–16 Human osteoblast cells attached to the surface of a HA/HDPE composite [34]

Figure 8–17 High-resolution TEM image of the bone-implant interface for a HA/HDPE implant [36]

For *in vivo* experiments, following sterilization by γ irradiation, machined pins (φ 2.4mmx5mm) of HA/HDPE composite were implanted in the lateral femoral condyle of adult New Zealand white rabbits [35]. It was demonstrated that cortical and cancellous bones responded positively to the presence of HA/HDPE implant by localized apposition adjacent to the implant surface. The implant was initially surrounded by a fibrous layer, which was in turn surrounded by a layer of new bone. With time the fibrous layer was locally replaced by newly formed bone, which created a strong bond between the natural bone and the implant. After six months' implantation, the areas of direct bone apposition — as measured from histological sections — had reached 40 percent of the implant surface. As the limb of rabbits was not immobilized during the *in vivo* tests, this favorable bone response to the HA/HDPE implant occurred during physiological loading. Such an observation indicated that the mechanical compatibility of the HA/HDPE composite with natural bone had resulted in the absence of significant relative movement at the bone-implant interface, thus encouraging bone growth around the implant. Ultra-microtomed specimens were also prepared for TEM examinations of the bone-implant interface [36]. At one month, the new bone was mainly seen adjacent to the interface where HA particles were present. At six months, the bone tissue was seen growing along the whole length of composite implant including exposed HA particles and polyethylene matrix. High-resolution TEM imaging revealed lattice fringes of bone apatite in bone and HA in HA/HDPE implant. The image of lattice planes at the bone-implant interface after three months' implantation is shown in Figure 8–17. It exhibited continuity across the interface, thus indicating epitaxial growth of apatite crystals from the implant into new bone.

8.4.6 Clinical Applications

Since the late 1980s, subperiosteal orbital floor implants made from HA/HDPE composites have been used in the correction of volume deficient sockets and in orbital floor reconstruction following trauma [37,38]. All the implants remained in position, and no infections or extrusions occurred. Clinical examination found the implants to feel stable. After six months' implantation computer tomography (CT) was unable to detect any gap between the implant and bone, implying at least partial integration of the implant with the orbital floor, which accounted for the marked implant stability (Figure 8–18). More recently middle ear implants were made from HA/HDPE composites, and satisfactory clinical results have been obtained [39]. Figure 8–19 shows a middle ear implant that is commercially available since mid-1990s.

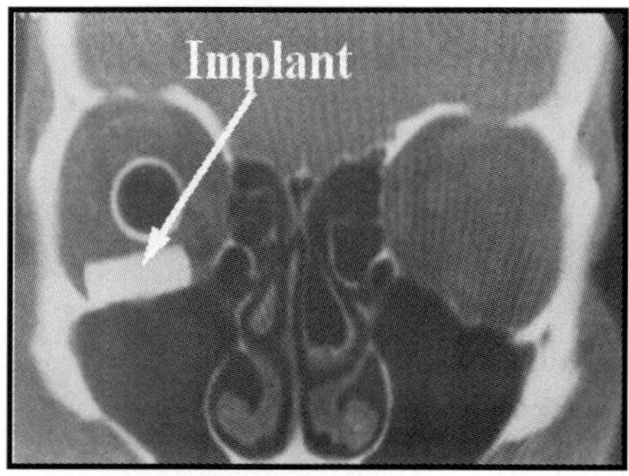

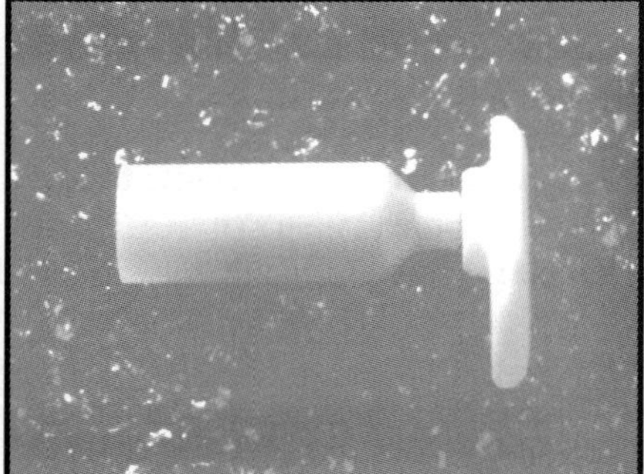

Figure 8–18 CT scan of orbits of a patient 24 months after operation [37]

Figure 8–19 A middle ear implant made from HA/HDPE composite (the diameter of the implant shaft is 1.68 mm) [39]

8.4.7 Enhanced Hydroxyapatite/polyethylene Composites

HA/HDPE composites exhibit required bioactivity which promotes the formation of biological bond between bone and implants made of the composites. To improve mechanical properties of HA/HDPE composites for load bearing implant applications, hydrostatic extrusion of the composites was investigated [40]. It was found that higher extrusion ratios led to higher Young's modulus and tensile strength of HA/HDPE composites which are within the bounds for mechanical properties of cortical bone (Figure 8–20). The fracture strain of HA/HDPE was also substantially increased by hydrostatic extrusion. Extruded HA/HDPE containing 40 vol% of HA possessed a strain to fracture which was far greater than that of human cortical bone (9.4% versus 1–3%). Furthermore the bioactivity of the composites was retained after extrusion. Therefore HA/HDPE which has been further processed via hydrostatic extrusion exhibits great potential for major load bearing applications.

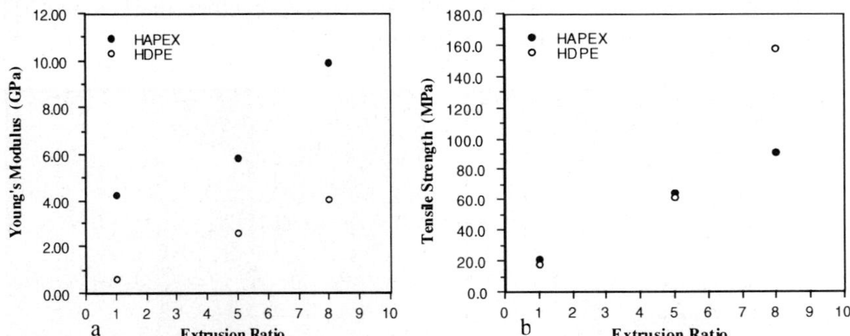

Figure 8–20 Effects of hydrostatic extrusion on mechanical properties of HA/HDPE composite (HAPEX: HA/HDPE containing 40 vol% of HA): (a) effect on Young's modulus; (b) effect on tensile strength [40]

An alternative method to enhance mechanical properties of the composites, *i.e.*, using chemical coupling for HA with HDPE, was also studied [41]. However only limited improvements in tensile strength and ductility were achieved, and Young's modulus was slightly decreased. It was observed that the chemical bond established between HA and HDPE delayed the dewetting and cavitation processes, but could not prevent interfacial debonding which caused eventual failure of the composites.

Using chopped high-modulus PE fibers as the matrix material for HA reinforced PE composites was also investigated [42]. Chopped PE fibers could provide a matrix with much higher modulus and strength values. It was found that the fiber morphology of the matrix had a positive contribution to the mechanical properties of the composites. However the uneven distribution of particulate HA in the composites of PE fiber matrix remains a major problem.

8.5   Other Bioceramic-Polymer Composites for Medical Applications

To establish a stronger bone-implant interface within a shorter period of time, glasses or ceramics that are more bioactive than HA can be used as the bioactive phase in the composites. Therefore using the same or similar manufacturing processes, bioactive composites such as Bioglass®/high-density polyethylene

[43] and A–W glass-ceramic/high-density polyethylene [44] have been developed for tissue substitution. These composites exhibited enhanced bioactivity (Figure 8–21).

Apart from polyethylene, there are a few other biomedical polymers that could be used for producing bone analogue materials. With the same rationale, bioactive and biostable composites such as Bioglass®/polysulfone [47], bioactive glass/UHMWPE [48], bioactive glass fiber/polysulfone [49], hydroxyapatite/polysulfone [50], and hydroxyapatite/polyetheretherketone [51] were produced for potential medical applications.

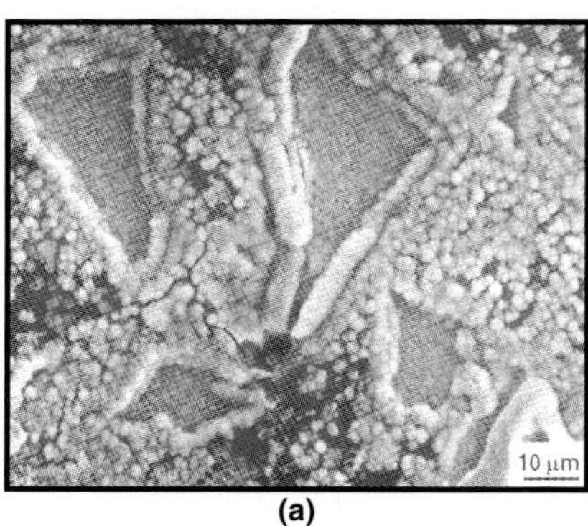
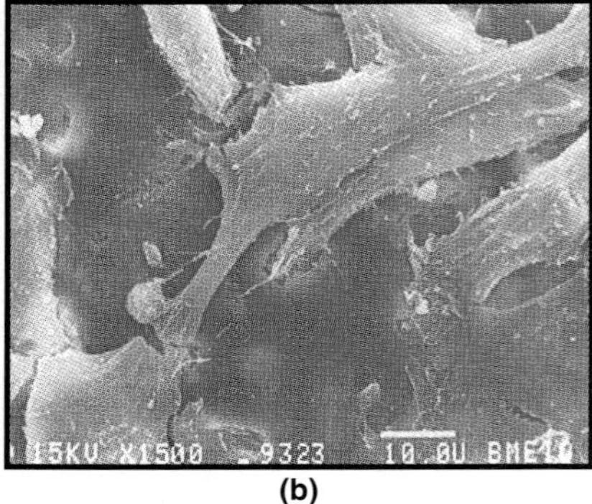

(a)   (b)

Figure 8–21 *In vitro* bioactivity of Bioglass®/HDPE composite: (a) formation of bone-like apatite on the composite after immersion in a simulated body fluid [45]; (b) human osteoblast-like cells cultured on the composite, showing cell attachment to Bioglass® particles in the composite [46]

When a biodegradable polymer is used as matrix of the composite, a bioactive and biodegradable composite is developed. After implantation in the body, a biodegradable bone-substituting material will have gradual decreases in strength and stiffness over a clinically determined optimal period. As bone repairs itself, the external load will be transferred from the biodegrading implant to bone. This approach provides the best biomaterials solution to tissue replacement and regeneration, if requirements for the initial stiffness and strength and other short-term performance criteria can be met. To date, the bioactive and biodegradable composites developed include hydroxyapatite/poly(L–lactide) [52], hydroxyapatite/PEG/PBT [53], hydroxyapatite/poly(DL–lactide) [54], tricalcium phosphate/poly-hydroxybutyrate [55,56], hydroxyapatite/polyhydroxybutyrate [57], hydroxyapatite/SEVA [58], and a few other systems.

In recent years, tissue engineering as a multidisciplinary endeavor has shown promises in combating medical problems of tissue loss and organ failure. One of the key issues in tissue engineering is the development of suitable materials and scaffolds for seeding cells and for subsequent growth of tissues.

Efforts have been made to produce bioactive and biodegradable scaffolds for such purposes. There have been reports on scaffolds based on composites such as hydroxyapatite/poly(DL–lactic–co–glycolic acid) [59,60], hydroxyapatite/poly(caprolactone) [61], hydroxyapatite/chitin and calcium phosphate/poly(L–lactic acid) [62]. Both bioactivity and biodegradability of these composite scaffolds are clearly shown in Figure 8–22.

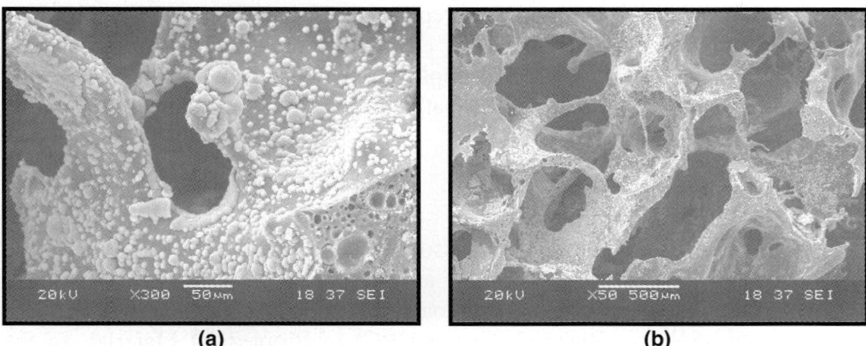

Figure 8–22 Ca–P/PLLA composite scaffold after immersion in a simulated body fluid: (a) formation of bone-like apatite on scaffold surface; (b) degradation of some struts [62]

The use of bioactive particles or short fibers in composites is not confined to the area of tissue replacement and tissue regeneration. The concept of bioactive composites has also been extended to other areas such as bone cement and dental materials. Investigations into bioactive bone cement started nearly twenty years ago, and work on hydroxyapatite/poly(methylmethacrylate) [63], hydroxyapatite/poly(ethylmethacrylate) [64], and tricalcium phosphate/poly (propylene fumarate) [65] has been reported. Research on bioactive dental composites has also been conducted [66,67].

8.6   Concluding Remarks

Most tissues in the human body are natural composite materials, and they serve as templates in the development of replacement materials. Over the last few decades, composites science and technology has matured and established itself as a new discipline. Great advances have been made in developing various composite materials to meet requirements firstly in the aerospace industry, then in the automotive industry and civil engineering sector, and more recently in the healthcare industry. Man-made composites have distinctive properties that their constituents do not possess. Very often, these properties are required to meet specific needs. Bioactive polymeric matrix composites have shown their efficacy and can find wide applications. However, to date, no one material can exactly match the structure and properties of any particular human tissue. Perhaps no material will do, bearing in mind that biological materials such as bone have the exceptional ability of self-repair. Nevertheless, materials scientists and engineers will certainly use their knowledge and expertise to invent new materials and devise viable systems to help improve the quality of life of people who unfortunately have diseased or damaged tissues. Man learns from nature, man may imitate nature, but man cannot beat nature.

The future development in tissue repair may also depend on research in the emerging field of tissue engineering. However the traditional approach in designing new materials for specific applications will still remain as an essential and viable means in the course of combating problems in the medical field.

Acknowledgements

The author would like to thank Professor William Bonfield (formerly with the University of London and presently at University of Cambridge, UK) for involving him in various projects on bioactive composites when he was working in the Interdisciplinary Research Center (IRC) in Biomedical Materials of the University of London. He also thanks his colleagues and students in the University of London, UK, and Nanyang Technological University, Singapore, for their assistance and discussions. Funding for the research in bioactive composites from various sources is gratefully acknowledged. Permissions granted by various publishers for reproducing figures and tables, which appeared in previous publications, in this chapter are acknowledged.

References

1. J. B. Park, Biomaterials: An Introduction, (Plenum Press, New York, 1979).
2. W. Bonfield, Materials for the replacement of osteoarthritic hip joints, Metals and Materials, 1987, 3:712–716.
3. W. Bonfield, M. Wang, and K. E. Tanner, Interfaces in analogue biomaterials, Acta Materialia, 1998, 46:2509–2518.
4. W. Bonfield, Present problems, future solutions, in Bioceramics, Vol. 8, eds. J. Wilson, L. L. Hench, and D. Greenspan, (Pergamon, Oxford, 1995) pp:375–380.
5. W. Bonfield, Can materials stimulate advances in orthopedics?, in The science of new materials, ed. A. Briggs, (Blackwell Publishers, Oxford, 1992) pp:168–176.
6. Y. C. Fung, Biomechanics: Mechanical properties of living tissues, 2nd Edition, (Springer–Verlag, New York, 1993).
7. G. P. Evans, J. C. Behiri, J. D. Currey, and W. Bonfield, Microhardness and Young's modulus in cortical bone exhibiting a wide range of mineral volume fractions, and in a bone analogue, J. Matls. Sci. Matls. Med., 1990, 1:38–43.
8. L. J. Gibson and M. F. Ashby, Cellular solids: structure and properties, 2nd Edition, (Cambridge University Press, Cambridge, 1997).

9.　L. L. Hench, Bioceramics: from concept to clinic, Journal of the American Ceramic Society, 1991, 74:1487–1510.

10.　H. Aoki, Medical Applications of Hydroxyapatite, (Ishiyaku EuroAmerica, Tokyo and St. Louis, 1994).

11.　J. C. Elliott, Structure and chemistry of the apatites and other calcium orthophosphates, (Elsevier Science, Amsterdam, 1994).

12.　H. Y. Yang and M. Wang, Effects of reaction parameters on the thermostability of spray-dried hydroxyapatite powders, in Processing and fabrication of advanced materials VIII, eds. K. A. Khor, T. S. Srivatsan, M. Wang, W. Zhou, and F. Boey, (World Scientific, Singapore, 2000) pp:307–316.

13.　M. Bohner, J. Lemaître, A. P. Legrand, J. B. d'Espinose de la Caillerie, and P. Belgrand, Synthesis, X-ray diffraction and solid-state ^{31}P magic angle spinning NMR study of α-tricalcium orthophosphate, J. Matls. Sci. Matls. Med., 1996, 7:457–463.

14.　S. H. Teoh, Z. G. Tang, and G. W. Hastings, Thermoplastic polymers in biomedical applications: structures, properties and processing, in Handbook of biomaterial properties, eds. J. Black and G. Hastings, (Chapman & Hall, London, 1998) pp:270–301.

15.　D. Hill, Design engineering of biomaterials for medical devices, (John Wiley & Sons, Chichester, 1998).

16.　A. J. Peacock, Handbook of polyethylene: structures, properties, and applications, (Marcel Dekker, New York, 2000).

17.　W. D. Callister, Jr., Materials science and engineering: an introduction, 4th Edition, (John Wiley & Sons, New York, 1997).

18.　B. D. Ratner, A. S. Hoffman, F. J. Schoen, and J. E. Lemons, Biomaterials science: an introduction to materials in medicine, (Academic Press, San Diego, 1996).

19.　W. Bonfield, M. D. Grynpas, A. E. Tully, J. Bowman, and J. Abram, Hydroxyapatite reinforced polyethylene — a mechanically compatible implant material for bone replacement, Biomaterials, 1981, 2:185–186.

20.　M. Wang, D. Porter, and W. Bonfield, Processing, characterization, and evaluation of hydroxyapatite reinforced polyethylene composites, British Ceramic Transactions, 1994, 93:91–95.

21.　F. Tang, Production and evaluation of hydroxyapatite–polyethylene composites for tissue replacement, (MEng Thesis, Nanyang Technological University, Singapore, 2000).

22.　F. Tang, B. Chua, and M. Wang, Production and rheological behavior of hydroxyapatite reinforced polymers, in Transactions of the 6th World Biomaterials Congress, (Hawaii, USA, 2000) p539.

23.　F. Tang and M. Wang, Production and rheological behavior of hydroxyapatite reinforced polyethylene, in Processing and fabrication of advanced materials VIII, eds. K. A. Khor, T. S. Srivatsan, M. Wang, W. Zhou, and F. Boey, (World Scientific, Singapore, 2000) pp:299–306.

24.　M. Wang and W. Bonfield, Processing of highly filled polyethylene for medical applications, in Polymer processing towards AD2000, (Singapore, 1996) pp:203–204.

25. M. Wang, R. Joseph, and W. Bonfield, Hydroxyapatite–polyethylene composites for bone substitution: effects of ceramic particle size and morphology, Biomaterials, 1998, 19:2357–2366.

26. M. Wang, C. Berry, M. Braden, and W. Bonfield, Young's and shear moduli of ceramic particle filled polyethylene, J. Matls. Sci. Matls. Med., 1998, 9:621–624.

27. P. J. Hogg, J. Behiri, A. Brandwood, J. Bowman, and W. Bonfield, Impacting testing of hydroxyapatite-high density polyethylene composites, in Proceedings of the 1st International Conference of Composites in Bio-Medical Engineering, (London, UK, 1985) pp29.1–29.9.

28. F. Tang, C. H. Ng, and M. Wang, Manufacture and thermophysical properties of hydroxyapatite reinforced high density polyethylene, in Proceedings of the International Conference on Thermophysical Properties of Materials, (Singapore, 1999) pp:502–508.

29. J. Suwanprateeb, K. E. Tanner, S. Turner, and W. Bonfield, Creep in polyethylene and hydroxyapatite reinforced polyethylene composites, J. Matls. Sci. Matls. Med., 1995, 6:804–807.

30. J. Suwanprateeb, K. E. Tanner, S. Turner, and W. Bonfield, Influence of Ringer's solution on creep resistance of hydroxyapatite reinforced polyethylene composites, J. Matls. Sci. Matls. Med., 1997, 8:469–472.

31. J. Suwanprateeb, K. E. Tanner, S. Turner, and W. Bonfield, Influence of sterilization by gamma irradiation and of thermal annealing on creep of hydroxyapatite reinforced polyethylene composites, J. Biomed. Matls. Res., 1998, 39:16–22.

32. M. Wang, B. Chua, and F. Tang, Biaxial fatigue behavior of bioceramic-polymer composites developed for bone replacement, in Proceedings of the 10th International Conference on Biomedical Engineering, (Singapore, 2000) pp:219–220.

33. M. C. Neo, M. Chandrasekaran, M. Wang, N. L. Loh, and W. Bonfield, Tribology of HA/HDPE composites against stainless steel in the presence of proteins, in Bioceramic, Vol. 12, eds. H. Ogushi, G. W. Hastings, and T. Yoshikawa, (World Scientific, Singapore, 1999) pp:449–452.

34. J. Huang, L. Di Silvio, M. Wang, K. E. Tanner, and W. Bonfield, *In vitro* mechanical and biological assessment of hydroxyapatite-reinforced polyethylene composite, J. Matls. Sci. Matls. Med., 1997, 8:775–779.

35. W. Bonfield, J. C. Behiri, C. Doyle, J. Bowman, and J. Abram, Hydroxyapatite reinforced polyethylene composites for bone replacement, in Biomaterials and Biomechanics, eds. P. Ducheyne, G. Van der Perre, and A. E. Aubert, (Elsevier Science, Amsterdam, 1984) pp:421–426.

36. W. Bonfield and Z. B. Luklinska, High-resolution electron microscopy of a bone implant interface, in The bone-biomaterial interface, ed. J. E. Davies, (University of Toronto Press, Toronto, 1991) pp:89–93.

37. R. N. Downs, S. Vardy, K. E. Tanner, and W. Bonfield, Hydroxyapatite–polyethylene composite in orbital surgery, in Bioceramics, Vol. 4, eds. W. Bonfield, G. W. Hastings, and K. E. Tanner, (Butterworth–Heinemann, Oxford, 1991) pp:239–246.

38. K. E. Tanner, R. N. Downes, and W. Bonfield, Clinical applications of hydroxyapatite reinforced materials, British Ceramic Transactions, 1994, 93:104–107.
39. R. E. Swain, M. Wang, B. Beale, and W. Bonfield, HAPEX™ for otologic applications, Biomedical Engineering: Applications, Basis & Communications, 1999, 11:315–320.
40. M. Wang, I. M. Ward, and W. Bonfield, Hydroxyapatite–polyethylene composites for bone substitution: effects of hydrostatic extrusion, in Proceedings of the 11th International Conference on Composite Materials, (Gold Coast, Australia, 1997), Vol. 1, pp:488–495.
41. M. Wang, S. Deb, K. E. Tanner, and W. Bonfield, Hydroxyapatite–polyethylene composites for bone substitution: effects of silanation and polymer grafting, in Proceedings of the 7th European Conference on Composite Materials, Vol. 2, (London, UK, 1996) pp:455–460.
42. N. H. Ladizesky, E. M. Pirhonen, D. B. Appleyard, I. M. Ward, and W. Bonfield, Fiber reinforcement of ceramic/polymer composites for a major load-bearing bone substitute material, Composites Science and Technology, 1998, 58:419–434.
43. M. Wang, W. Bonfield, and L. L. Hench, Bioglass®/high density polyethylene composite as a new soft tissue bonding material, in Bioceramics, Vol. 8, eds. J. Wilson, L. L. Hench, and D. Greenspan, (Pergamon, Oxford, 1995) pp:383–388.
44. M. Wang, T. Kokubo, and W. Bonfield, A–W glass-ceramic reinforced polyethylene composite for medical applications, in Bioceramics, Vol. 9, eds. T. Kokubo, T. Nakamura, and F. Miyaji, (Pergamon, Oxford, 1996) pp:387–390.
45. J. Huang, L. Di Silvio, M. Wang, I. Rehman, C. Ohtsuki, and W. Bonfield, Evaluation of *in vitro* bioactivity and biocompatibility of Bioglass® reinforced polyethylene composite, J. Matls. Sci. Matls. Med., 1997, 8:809–813.
46. J. Huang, L. Di Silvio, M. Wang, K. E. Tanner, and W. Bonfield, *In vitro* assessment of hydroxyapatite and Bioglass® reinforced polyethylene composites, in Bioceramics, Vol. 10, eds. L. Sedel and C. Rey, (Pergamon, Oxford, 1997) pp:519–522.
47. R. L. Orefice, G. P. LaTorre, J. K. West, and L. L. Hench, Processing and characterization of bioactive polysulfone–Bioglass® composites, in Bioceramics, Vol. 8, eds. J. Wilson, L. L. Hench, and D. Greenspan, (Pergamon, Oxford, 1995) pp:409–414.
48. R. L. Reis, A. M. Cunha, M. H. Ferdandez, and R. N. Correia, Bionert and biodegradable polymeric matrix composites filled with bioactive SiO_2–3CaO. P_2O_5–MgO glasses and glass-ceramics, in Bioceramics, Vol. 10, eds. L. Sedel and C. Rey, (Pergamon, Oxford, 1997) pp:415–418.
49. M. Marcolongo, P. Ducheyne, J. Garino, and E. Schepers, Bioactive glass fiber/polymeric composites bond to bone tissue, J. Biomed. Matls. Res., 1998, 39:161–170.
50. M. Wang, C. Y. Yue, B. Chua, and L. C. Kan, Hydroxyapatite reinforced polysulfone as a new biomaterial for tissue replacement, in Bioceramics, Vol. 12, eds. H. Ogushi, G. W. Hastings, and T. Yoshikawa, (World Scientific, Singapore, 1999) pp:401–404.

51. M. M. Abu Bakar, P. Cheang, and K. A. Khor, Thermal processing of hydroxyapatite reinforced polyetheretherketone composites, Journal of Materials Processing Technology, 1999, 89–90:462–466.
52. C. C. P. M. Verheyen, J. R. de Wijn, C. A. van Blitterswijk, and K. de Groot, Evaluation of hydroxylapatite/poly(L–lactide) composites: mechanical behavior, J. Biomed. Matls. Res., 1992, 26:1277–1296.
53. Q. Liu, J. R. de Wijn, and C. A. van Blitterswijk, Composite biomaterials with chemical bonding between hydroxyapatite filler particles and PEG/PBT copolymer matrix, J. Biomed. Matls. Res., 1998, 40:490–497.
54. X. Guo, Q. Zheng, J. Du, D. Duan, Y. Yan, and S. Li, Biodegradation and mechanical properties of hydroxyapatite/poly-DL-lactide composites for fracture fixation, Journal of Wuhan University of Technology, 1998, 13:9–15.
55. M. Wang, C. X. Wang, J. Weng, and J. Ni, Developing biodegradable composites using polyhydroxybutyrate and its co-polymer, in Transactions of the 6th World Biomaterials Congress, (Hawaii, USA, 2000) p81.
56. M. Wang, J. Weng, C. H. Goh, J. Ni, and C. X. Wang, Developing tricalcium phosphate/polyhydroxybutyrate composite as a new biodegradable material for clinical applications, in Bioceramics, Vol. 13, eds. S. Giannini and A. Moroni, (Trans Tech Publications, Zurich, 2000) pp:741–744.
57. M. Wang, C. X. Wang, J. Weng, J. Ni, and P. Y. Quek, Production and evaluation of biodegradable hydroxyapatite/polyhydroxybutyrate composite, in Proceedings of the 10th International Conference on Biomedical Engineering, (Singapore, 2000) pp:545–546.
58. R. A. Sousa, R. L. Reis, A. M. Cunha, and M. J. Bevis, Structure and properties of hydroxyapatite reinforced starch bone analogue composites, in Bioceramics, Vol. 13, eds. S. Giannini and A. Moroni, (Trans Tech Publications, Zurich, 2000) pp:669–672.
59. R. C. Thomson, M. J. Yaszemski, J. M. Powers, and A. G. Mikos, Hydroxyapatite fiber reinforced poly(alpha-hydroxy ester) foams for bone regeneration, Biomaterials, 1998, 19:1935–1943.
60. R. Zhang and P. X. Ma, Poly(alpha-hydroxyl acids)/hydroxyapatite porous composites for bone-tissue engineering, I: Preparation and morphology, J. Biomed. Matls. Res., 1999, 44:446–455.
61. D. W. Hutmacher, I. Zein, and S. H. Teoh, Processing of bioresorbable scaffolds for tissue engineering of bone by applying rapid prototyping technologies, in Processing and fabrication of advanced materials VIII, eds. K. A. Khor, T. S. Srivatsan, M. Wang, W. Zhou, and F. Boey, (World Scientific, Singapore, 2000) pp:201–206.
62. M. Wang, L. J. Chen, J. Ni, J. Weng, and C. Y. Yue, Manufacture and evaluation of bioactive and biodegradable materials and scaffolds for tissue engineering, J. Matls. Sci. Matls. Med., 2001, 12:855–860.
63. R. Olmi, A. Moroni, A. Castaldini, A. Cavallini, and R. Romagnoli, Hydroxyapatites alloyed with bone cement: physical and biological characterization, in Ceramics in surgery, ed. P. Vincenzini, (Elsevier Science, Amsterdam, 1983) pp:91–96.

64. E. J. Harper, J. C. Behiri, and W. Bonfield, Flexural and fatigue properties of a bone cement based upon polyethylmethacrylate and hydroxyapatite, J. Matls. Sci. Matls. Med., 1995, 6:799–803.
65. S. J. Peter, P. Kim, A. W. Yasko, M. J. Yaszemski, and A. G. Mikos, Cross-linking characteristics of an injectable poly(propylene fumarate)/beta-tricalcium phosphate paste and mechanical properties of the cross-linked composite for use as a biodegradable bone cement, Biomed. Matls. Res., 1999, 44:314–321.
66. R. Labella, M. Braden, and S. Deb, Novel hydroxyapatite-based dental composites, Biomaterials, 1994, 15:1197–1200.
67. C. Domingo, R. W. Arcis, A. Lopez-Macipe, R. Osorio, R. Rodriguez-Clemente, J. Murtra, M. A. Fanovich, and M. Toledano, Dental composites reinforced with hydroxyapatite: Mechanical behavior and absorption/elution characteristics, J Biomed. Matls. Res., 2001, 56:297–305.

CHAPTER 9

COMPOSITES IN BIOMEDICAL APPLICATIONS

Zheng-Ming Huang[1] and S. Ramakrishna[2]

[1]*Department of Engineering Mechanics, Tongji University,*
1239 Siping Road, Shanghai 200092, P. R. China,
E-mail: huangzm@mail.tongji.edu.cn

[2]*Biomaterials Laboratory, Division of Bioengineering,*
Department of Mechanical Engineering, National University of Singapore,
10 Kent Ridge Crescent, Singapore 119260

Composites are materials that contain two or more distinct constituent phases on a scale larger than that of atomic. Compared with traditional homogeneous materials such as metals, ceramics, and polymers, the main advantage of the composites is that their mechanical, biological, and other physical properties can be tailored to the requirements of specific applications. This chapter focuses on composites that are suitable for biomedical applications. Various application practices documented in literature have been summarized in the chapter. Some of the commonly used methods for composite fabrications are introduced. Attention has been given to the mechanics of composites: a study which aims at estimating the mechanical properties of different composites using only the material parameters and geometric information of their constituents. Some future trends are also given at the end of the chapter.

9.1 Introduction

A composite material is a physical mixture of two or more distinct constituents. It has radically different properties from those of each constituent. Except for some interfacial reactions to ensure good bonding, no chemical reactions or any alloying exist between the constituents in a composite. Though a composite can be made of two or more constituents, in most cases the composite comprises only two constituents: the matrix phase and the reinforcing phase. The matrix phase is continuous and provides the overall form. A reinforcing phase — such as fibers or particulates — is generally stronger than the matrix. Biocomposites are a special form of composites which can be used in biomedical applications, either inside or in contact with the human body. A key advantage of composites over monolithic materials is that the material properties of the composites can be tailored according to different requirements in the mechanical, chemical, biological, and other physical aspects. This is achieved by altering the composition, interfacial bonding, and physical arrangement of the constituent phases in the composites.

The composites in common use can be classified based on either the reinforcing phase or the matrix phase. For classification based on the reinforcing phase, there are mainly three kinds of reinforcements: continuous fibers, short or chopped fibers, and particulates.

- A continuous fiber has an aspect ratio (the ratio of its length over its diameter) generally greater than 10^5 — the resulting composites are called continuous fiber reinforced composites.
- The short or chopped fibers have an aspect ratio between 5 to 200 (included in this category are whiskers and blades also) — the resulting composites are called short (chopped) fiber reinforced composites.
- The particulates or powders have an aspect ratio from less than 1 to about 2 — the resulting composites are called particulate reinforced composites.

These three kinds of composites together with their biomedical application examples are summarized in Figure 9–1. Note that among various kinds of continuous fiber composites, a unidirectional (UD) fiber reinforced composite is fundamental. This composite, which is abbreviated as UD composite, is fabricated by arranging all the fibers in the same direction.

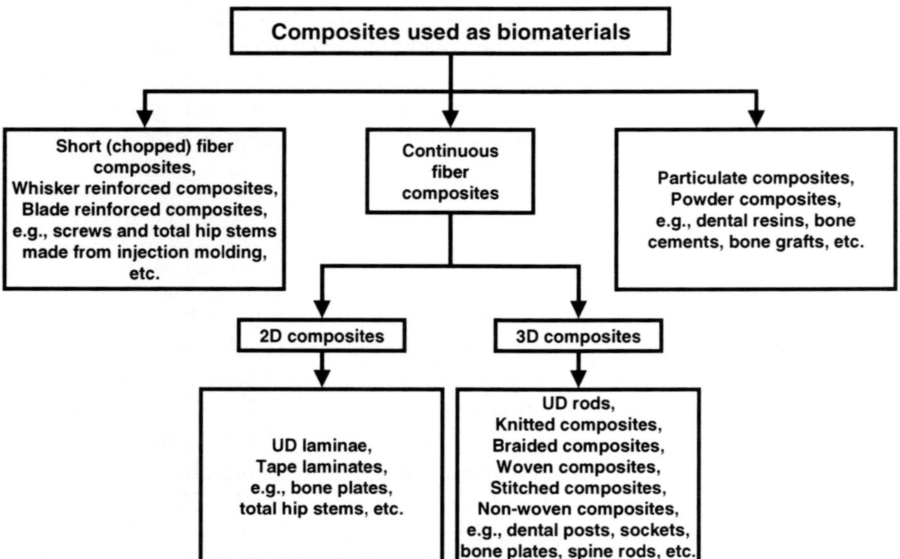

Figure 9–1 Classification of composites based on reinforcing phase

Besides classification by the reinforcing phase, composites can also be classified according to the matrix materials used. For example, monolithic metals, ceramics, and polymer materials can be used as matrix materials. The resulting composites are then classified as metal matrix composites, ceramic matrix composites, and polymer matrix composites. As most composites in biomedical applications are polymer matrix composites, this chapter will thus focus on this type of composites.

Polymers can be either thermoset or thermoplastic, according to their thermal behaviors. A thermoplastic polymer can be molten at high temperature and solidified at low temperature many times. Hence a thermoplastic composite can be re-shaped to some extent after its fabrication. On the other hand, a thermoset polymer cannot be molten at high temperature. Hence a thermoset composite, once it is made, cannot be re-shaped without destroying its structure.

Apart from categorization by thermal behaviors, polymer matrix composites can also be grouped by their biodegradable property. A biodegradable material is one that can be absorbed by human body once it is implanted within the body. If both the polymer matrix phase and the reinforcing phase (such as fiber) are biodegradable, the resulting composite is called a fully resorbable composite. If only the polymer matrix is biodegradable but the reinforcing phase is not, the resulting composite is partially resorbable. A non-resorbable composite is one where all of its constituent substances are not biodegradable.

To date, the majority of biomedical devices used either as implants in the human body or as external prostheses are made of biocompatible homogeneous materials such as metals, ceramics, or polymers. However, there are recognized limitations in these monolithic material devices. For example, though most implants in orthopedic surgery are made of metals, their drawbacks include:
1) Too stiff such that a stress protection of the fractured bone can occur during healing [1];
2) Considerable artifacts are produced under X-ray, which make the interpretation of radiographs difficult [2];
3) Metal sensitization can occur and the implants may cause mutagenicity.

In contrast, these drawbacks can be overcome if implants were made of polymer matrix composites. Moreover, biodegradable implants can be developed based on composite technology, which no longer needs a second operation to remove the implants once they are fixed into host tissues [3]. This unique feature is not present in any metal implant.

Composite materials can offer numerous advantages over the traditional homogeneous materials in biomedical applications. As such, a fundamental knowledge of composite materials is necessary for the development of biomaterials as well as for the design of medical devices. The purpose of this chapter is to provide an introductory description on composite theory, fabrication, characterization, the potential in biomedical applications as well as the outlook in future advances.

9.2   Biomedical Applications

As aforementioned, a biomedical device can be an external prosthesis or an implant used within the human body. An implant then needs to be in contact with host tissues. The human tissues can be categorized as hard and soft tissues. Only bones, teeth, and cartilages are hard tissues [4]. All other tissues are of the soft category. In this respect, the biomedical applications of composites can be grouped into those for hard tissues and some others for soft tissues. A schematic show of various possible composite biomaterials in the human body is given in Figure 9–2. Following which, some medical devices (such as bone plates, dental materials, and vascular grafts) are discussed in more detail.

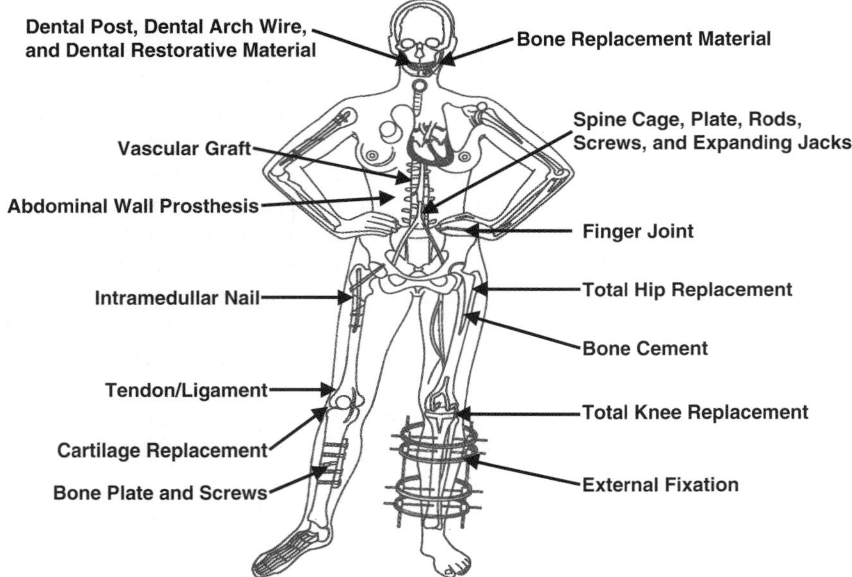

Figure 9–2 Medical devices which can be fabricated using composites

9.2.1 Bone Plates

The majority of composites used in biomedical applications are targeted for bone repairing purpose. Bone constitutes the skeleton of a human being and sustains all kinds of loads including gravity applied to the human body. Therefore bone can be easily injured under an external load. There are many types of bone fractures depending on the crack size, orientation, morphology, and location — which have to be treated in different ways. In general, medical devices are necessary to fix the fractured bone for proper healing. The most commonly used of such devices are the bone plates.

Bone plates, also known as osteosynthesis plates, are conventionally made of stainless steel, Cr–Co, and Ti alloys. The rigid fixation is designed to provide high axial pressures (also known as dynamic compression) in the fragments of the bone, in order to facilitate primary bone healing without the formation of external callus. A secondary operation is generally required to remove the plate once the bone healing is completed — which may take one to two years. However, the high rigidity of the metal plate fixation can result in bone atrophy. The bone underneath the plate adapts to the low stress and becomes less dense and weak. Due to bone atrophy, there is a possibility of bone refracture after the plate is removed. This is recognized as the "stress shielding" effect. It may be noted that the modulus of stainless steel (210–230 GPa) is much higher than the 10–18 GPa modulus of the bone. In the plate and the fractured bone system, the amount of stress carried by each of them is directly related to its stiffness. Thus bone is insufficiently loaded compared to the implanted plate, resulting in "stress-shielding" or stress protection. Many investigators [5,6,7] have shown that the degree of stress protection is proportional to the degree of stiffness mismatch. This suggests that 'less rigid fixation plates' diminish the stress-shielding problem, and that it is desirable to use plates whose stiffness is close to that of the bone. However, low stiffness should not be accompanied with low fatigue strength, since the plate/bone system will have to sustain severe cyclic loading while the bone is healing. Polymer composite materials offer the desired high strength and bone-like elastic properties, and hence have been proposed for bone plate applications (Figure 9–3). They may be grouped into non-resorbable, partially resorbable, and fully resorbable bone plates.

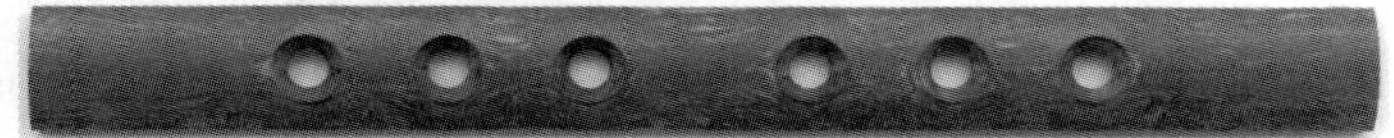

Figure 9–3 A composite bone plate

Non-resorbable bone plates are made of either thermoset or thermoplastic polymer composite materials. CF/epoxy, GF/epoxy are a few examples of non-resorbable thermoset composites [8,9,10]. However, there is a concern over the toxic effects of monomers in partially cured epoxy composite materials [11,12]. Thermoplastic composite bone plates using carbon fibers (CF) and various polymer matrix materials have been made available, including CF/PMMA, CF/PP, CF/PS, CF/PE, CF/nylon, CF/PBT, and CF/PEEK [13]. Amongst which, the CF/PEEK material system has shown promising characteristics [14]. Unlike the thermoset composites, thermoplastic composites are considered free from the complications associated with unused monomers. Moreover, like a metal alloy plate, a thermoplastic composite plate can be bent or contoured to the shape of the bone at the time of surgery.

As the bone healing progresses, it is desirable that the bone be subjected to gradual increase of stress, thus reducing the stress-shielding effect. In other words, the stress on the plate should decrease with time whereas the stress on the bone should increase. This is possible only if the plate looses rigidity in the body environment. The non-resorbable polymer composites do not display this desired characteristic. To meet this need, resorbable polymer composites have been introduced for bone plate applications. Polymers such as poly(lactic acid) (PLA) and poly(glycolic acid) (PGA) resorb or degrade upon implantation into the human body. Many bioresorbable polymers are found to loose most of their mechanical properties in a few weeks. Tormala *et al.* (1991) [3] and Choueka *et al.* (1995) [15] proposed fully resorbable composites by reinforcing resorbable matrices with resorbable fibers such as poly(L–lactic acid) (PLLA) fibers. One of the advantages often cited for resorbable composite prostheses is that they need not be removed with a second operative procedure, as is recommended with metallic or non-resorbable composite implants. However, the low mechanical property of resorbable materials remains a drawback, and hence they are only limited to applications where the loads are moderate.

To improve the mechanical properties, resorbable polymers are reinforced with a variety of non-resorbable materials including carbon fibers [16,17,18] and polyamide fibers. Due to the non-resorbable nature of reinforcements used, these composites are called partially resorbable composites. According to Zimmerman *et al.* (1987) [16], CF/PLA composites possessed superior mechanical properties before implantation. However, they lost mechanical properties too rapidly in the human body because of delamination.

9.2.2 Intramedullary Nails

Intramedullary nails or rods are mainly used to fix long bone fractures. It is inserted into the intramedullary cavity of the bone and fixed in position using screws or friction fit method (Figure 9–2). The insertion often requires reaming of the medullary canal, and can affect intramedullary blood vessels and nutrient arteries. The nail must have a sufficient strength to carry the weight of the patient without bending in either flexure or torsion, and should not completely disrupt the blood supply. Stainless steel is one of the widely used materials in intramedullary nails. Recently, Lin *et al.* (1997) [19] developed short GF/PEEK composite material for intramedullary applications, whereas Kettunen *et al.* (1999) [20] made an intramedullary rod from a unidirectional carbon fiber reinforced liquid crystalline (Vectra A950) polymer composite. It was reported that the non-resorbable composite nails were biologically inert with good flexural strength and elastic modulus close to the bone.

To date, the most successful applications of fully bioresorbable implants are in the forms of pins, rods, and screws [21]. Most implants are manufactured from hydroxy fatty acids — such as PGA (polyglycolic acid), PLA (polylactic acid), and copolymers — with a self-reinforcing technique in which oriented filaments are used as a scaffold for the matrix of the same chemical structure to produce strong implants [22,23]. Due to their modest mechanical properties, these implants were restricted to low-stress applications in cancellous bone, mainly in the small fracture regions of ankle and foot, knee, elbow, wrist and hand [24]. These biodegradable devices have a key advantage in that they dissolve during implantation. Hence this advantage obviates the need for a second operation to remove the biodegradable implants. However a new type of infectious complication, the sterile sinus formation, has been observed. Santavirta *et al.* (1990) [25] reported an incidence of this aseptic inflammatory response that varies from 3 percent in Chevron osteotomies to 22 percent in distal radius fractures. Bostman *et al.* (1992) [26] made another survey and found that out of 216 patients with malleolar fractures, 24 developed a transient local inflammatory reaction with a painful erythematous fluctuant swelling. Average postoperative period in these studies was three months.

9.2.3 Spine Instrumentation

Spine is a linked structure consisting of 33 vertebrae superimposed one on another. The vertebrae are separated by fibrocartilaginous intervertebral discs (IVD) and are united by articular capsules and ligaments. Spine disorders commonly include metastasis of vertebral body and disc, disc herniation, facet degeneration, stenosis, and structural abnormalities such as kyphosis, scoliosis, and spondylolistheses. These disorders are caused by various reasons such as birth deformities, aging, tumorous lesions (metastasis), and mechanical loads induced by work and sports.

When the spine defect is limited to some vertebrae, alternative treatments such as spinal fusion and disc replacement are used. Ignatius *et al.* (1997) [27] and Claes *et al.* (1999) [28] developed Bioglass/PU composite material for vetebral body replacement, whereas Marcolongo *et al.* (1998) [29] proposed Bioglass/PS composite material for bone grafting purposes. Preliminary experiments indicated that these materials are bioactive, and that they facilitate direct bone bonding (osseous integration). Brantigan *et al.* (1991) [30] and Ciappetta *et al.* (1997) [31] developed CF/PEEK and CF/PS composite cages for lumbar interbody fusion. The composite cage has an elastic modulus close to that of the bone, thus eliciting maximum bone growth into the cage. The composite cages are radiolucent and hence do not hinder radiographic evaluation of bone fusion. Moreover they produce fewer artifacts on CT images than other implants constructed of metal alloys. Researchers also developed CF/PEEK and CF/PS [7] composite plates and screws for stabilizing the replacement body and spine. Flexural and fatigue properties of CF/PEEK composites are comparable to those of stainless steel, which is normally used for spine plates and screws.

Problems related to intervertebral disc are treated by replacing affected nucleus with a substitute material or by replacing the total disc (nucleus and annulus) with an artificial disc [32]. A variety of materials such as stainless steel, Co–Cr alloy, PE, SR, PU, PET/SR [33,34], and PET/hydrogel [35] composites have been proposed for disc prostheses — either being utilized alone or in combinations. However, their performance has not yet been acceptable for long-term applications. To date, no artificial disc is able to reproduce the unique mechanical and transport behaviors of natural disc satisfactorily.

Structural abnormalities or curvatures (lordosis, kyphosis, and spondylolistheses) of spine are corrected using either external or internal fixations. Splints and casts form the external fixation devices. The internal fixations require surgery, and many types of instrumentation (screws, plates, rods, and expanding jacks) are available [36]. In some cases, adjustable stainless steel rod — also known as Harrington spinal distraction rod — is used to stabilize or straighten the curvature. Schmitt-Thomas *et al.* (1997) [37] made initial attempts to develop a polymer composite rod using unidirectional and braided carbon fibers and biocompatible epoxy resin. The main motivation for this work is to overcome the problems of metal alloys such as corrosion and interference with the diagnostic techniques. To date, specific mechanical and physical properties required for ideal spine instrumentation have not yet been attained.

9.2.4 *Total Hip Replacement (THR)*

Joints enable the movement of body and its parts. THR is the most common artificial joint in human beings. For example, over 150,000 THRs are conducted each year in USA alone. A typical THR consists of a cup-type acetabular component and a femoral component (also called the femoral stem). The latter's head is designed to fit into the acetabular cup and enables joint articulations. Conventional THRs use stainless steel, Co–Cr and Ti alloys for the femoral stem. Acetabular cups are often made of UHMWPE. Although the short-term function of UHMWPE acetabular cups is satisfactory, their long-term performance has been a concern for many years. To improve creep resistance, stiffness, and strength, researchers proposed reinforcing UHMWPE with carbon fibers [38] or UHMWPE fibers [39]. Deng and Shalaby (1997) [39] found no appreciable difference in wear properties of reinforced and unreinforced UHMWPE. However, the effect of carbon fibers on the wear characteristics of UHMWPE is a controversial subject because of the negatively opposite results reported in the literature.

Although metal THRs are used widely, one of the major unresolved problems is the mismatch between the stiffness of femur bone and that of the prosthesis. It has been acknowledged that metallic stems, due to stiffness mismatch, induce unphysiological stresses in the bone and hence lead to bone resorption and eventual aseptic loosening of the prosthesis. This may cause severe pain and clinical failure, thus necessitating a repeat surgery. Gese *et al.* (1992) [40] demonstrated that Ti alloy stems result in a 50 percent reduction in the femur peak stress compared to the Co–Cr alloy stem. This suggests that implant loosening and eventual failure could be reduced through improvement in the prosthesis design and the use of a less stiff material with mechanical properties close to those of bone. Researchers introduced CF/PS [41] and CF/C [42] composite stems. They reported faster bone bonding in the case of composite implants as compared to high-stiffness conventional implants. The composite stems were found to be stable with no release of soluble compounds, and also favorably possessing high static and fatigue strengths. Chang *et al.* (1990) [43] proposed CF/epoxy stems by laminating 120 layers of unidirectional plies in a predetermined orientation and stacking sequence. Simoes *et al.* (1999) [44] made composite stems using braided hybrid carbon–glass fiber preforms and epoxy resin. Some researchers [45,46,47] also designed CF/PEEK composite stems (Figure 9–4) through injection molding, which exhibit a mechanical behavior similar to that of the femur. Animal studies indicated that CF/PEEK composite elicits minimal response from muscular tissue.

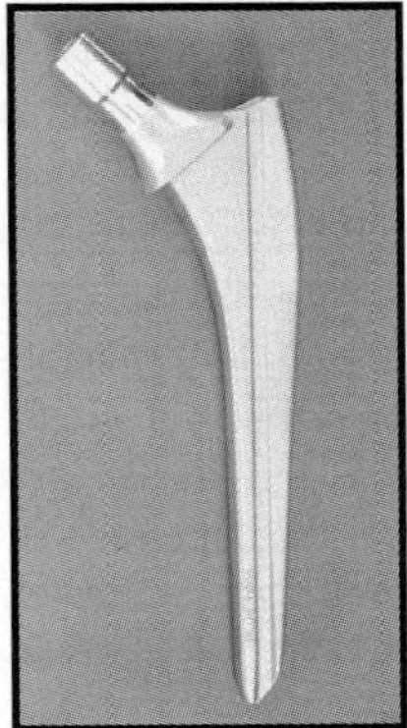

Figure 9–4 A total hip replacement stem made of CF/PEEK composite

9.2.5 Bone Grafts

Synthetic bone grafts are necessary to fill bone defects or replace fractured bones. The bone graft material must be sufficiently strong and stiff, and also capable of bonding to the residual bones. PE is considered biocompatible from its satisfactory utilization in hip and knee joint replacements for many years. However, its stiffness and strength are much lower than those of the bone. To improve the mechanical properties, bioactive HA particulates have been used to reinforce PE. The resulting composite has an elastic modulus of 1–8 GPa, and a strain-to-failure value from over 90 percent to 3 percent as the volume fraction of HA increases from 0 percent to 50 percent. It was reported that when HA particulate volume fraction is above 40 percent, the composite becomes brittle. Moreover the bioactivity of the composite is less than optimal because the surface area of HA available is low and the bonding rate between bone and HA is slow. To increase the interface between HA particles and the bone tissues, some researchers developed partially resorbable composites. They reinforced resorbable polymers such as PEG, PBT [57], PLLA [58], PHB [59], alginate, and gelatin [60] with bioactive particles. Upon implantation, as the matrix polymer resorbs, more and more bioactive particles come in contact with the growing tissues — thus resulting in good integration of the biomaterial into the bone. The wide range of material combinations offers the possibility of making composites with various desired properties such as stiffness, strength, biodegradation, and bioactivity.

9.2.6 Dental Materials

Dental treatment is one of the most frequent medical treatments for human beings, which ranges from filling cavities to replacing fractured or decayed teeth. Dental restorative materials — as the name suggests — are used to fill tooth cavities (caries), and sometimes to mask discoloration (veneering) or correct contour and alignment deficiencies. Amalgam, gold, alumina, zirconia, acrylic resins, and silicate cements have been traditionally used for restoring decayed teeth. Dental composite resins — which are translucent with refractive index matching that of the enamel — have virtually replaced some of these traditional materials; presently, they are very commonly used to restore posterior teeth as well as anterior teeth. The dental composite resin comprises BIS–GMA as the matrix polymer and quartz, barium glass, and colloidal silica as fillers. Polymerization can be started by a thermochemical initiator, or by a photochemical initiator that generates free radicals when subjected to ultraviolet light from a lamp used by the dentist. In other types of composites, a urethane dimethacryate resin is used rather than BIS–GMA. The filler particle concentration varies from 33 percent to 78 percent by weight, and size varies from 0.05 μm to 50 μm. The glass fillers reduce the shrinkage during resin polymerization as well as the coefficient of thermal expansion mismatch between the resin and the teeth. Strong bonding between the fillers and resin is achieved using silane-coupling agents [61]. Active research is still being carried out to develop dental composite resins with improved performance.

When a severely damaged tooth lacks the structure to adequately retain a filling or restoration, a dental post or cast dowel is used to reinforce the remaining tooth structure. The post is normally inserted in the root canal and fixed in position using dental cement. Traditional posts made of stainless steel, Ni–Cr, Au–Pt or Ti alloys are attributed to the hypothesis that the post should be rigid. In recent years this old basic tenet has been strongly challenged. As a result, it has been suggested to reduce the modulus mismatch between the post and the dentine so as to minimize the occurrence of root fractures (where root fracture frequency is between 2 to 4 percent) and restoration failures. Newer posts made of zirconia, short glass fiber reinforced polyester, and unidirectional carbon fiber reinforced epoxy composite [62] are introduced. These new posts are adequately rigid, and resistant to corrosion and fatigue. In addition to providing support to the core, the dental post also helps to direct occlusal and excursive forces more apically along the length of the root. Recent findings have suggested that an ideal post should have varying stiffness along its length. Specifically, the coronal end of the post should have higher stiffness for better retention and rigidity of the core, while the apical end of the post should have lower stiffness matching that of the dentine to overcome root fractures (that arise due to stress concentration). A post with varying stiffness but no change in the cross-sectional geometry along its length is only possible by using functionally graded composite materials. Ramakrishna *et al.* (1998) [63] proposed a functionally graded dental post using braided CF/epoxy composite technology. It has a high stiffness in the coronal region, and this stiffness gradually reduces to a value comparable to the stiffness of dentine at the apical end.

Orthodontic arch wires (approximately 0.5 mm in diameter) are used to correct teeth alignment. An arch wire is placed through orthodontic brackets and retained in position using ligature — a small plastic piece. By changing the tension in the arch wire, the alignment of the teeth is adjusted. Traditionally, arch wires are made of stainless steel and Ni–Ti (beta titanium) alloys. To date, composite arch wires based on glass fiber reinforcement have been developed [64,65]. The advantages of using composite arch wires include improved aesthetics, easy forming in the clinic, and the possibility of varying stiffness without changing component dimensions [66].

9.2.7 Prosthetic Sockets

Artificial legs are designed primarily to restore walking of the amputees, and were previously made of wood or metallic materials. These materials are limited by their weight, and poor durability due to corrosion and moisture induced swelling. A typical artificial leg system consists of three parts: socket, shaft, and foot (Figure 9–5). The most highly customized and important part of the prosthesis is the socket, which has to be fabricated individually to the satisfaction of each amputee. Sockets can be divided into two categories: direct and indirect sockets. A widely used indirect socket is fabricated by wrapping several layers of knitted or woven fabrics [67] on a customized plastic mold, vacuuming the fabrics enclosed in a plastic bag, and impregnating the vacuumed fabrics with a polyester resin. The socket is formed after the resin is cured under vacuum pressuring condition. It is reported that the performance of an indirect socket depends on the quality of the mold, and especially on the prosthesist skills. A direct socket — as the name suggests — is fabricated directly on the stump of a patient, without using any mold. Compared with indirect sockets, the benefit of direct socket fabrication is that it helps to reduce reliance on socket molding/creation skills, hence leading to reduction of fitting errors between the stump and the socket. In addition, direct socket fabrication also reduces the number of patient visits, hence improving the quality of service to the physically disabled people. The direct sockets appeared in the market only in recent years. They are made using a combination of knitted or braided carbon or glass fiber fabrics and water-curable (water-activated) resins. As expected braided fabric reinforced sockets are stiff and strong, whereas knitted fabric reinforced sockets are flexible and more conformable to the patient's stump [68].

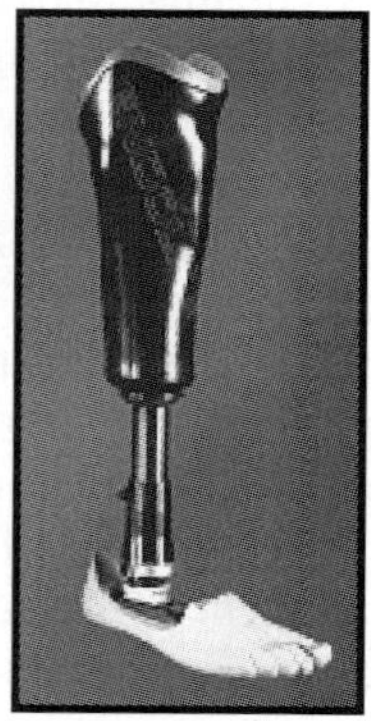

Figure 9–5 An artificial leg consisting of a socket, shank, and foot [68]

9.2.8 Tendons and Ligaments

Tendons and ligaments hold the bones of a joint, thus facilitating their stability and movement. They are essentially composite materials comprising undulated collagen fiber bundles aligned along the length and immersed in a ground substance — which is a complex made of elastine and mucopolysaccharide hydrogel [69]. Synthetic biomaterials used thus far in repairing tendons/ligaments include UHMWPE, PP, PET, PTFE, PU, Kevlar 49, carbon, and reconstituted collagen fibers in a multi-filament or braided form. Clinical experience with synthetic prostheses has been disappointing thus far. Problems with synthetic prostheses include difficulty to anchor to the bone, and abrasion and wear of prostheses — whose strength deteriorates in the long term and leads to mechanical failure (such as fatigue). Furthermore, particulate matter generated by abrasion against rough bony surfaces may cause synovitis, as well as inflammation of the lymph nodes should the size of the particulate matter produced allow its migration to the nodes [70]. To reduce particle migration and improve handling properties, prostheses are coated with polymers such as SR, poly(2–hydroxyethyl methacrylate) (PHEMA), and PLA. Pradas and Calleja (1991) [69] reported that by combining flexible polymer such as PMA or PEA with crimped Kevlar–49 fibers, the stress-strain behavior of natural ligaments can be reproduced to a certain extent. Iannace *et al.* (1995) [71] and Ambrosio *et al.* (1998) [72] developed a ligament prosthesis by reinforcing a hydrogel matrix (PHEMA) with helically wound rigid PET fibers, and demonstrated that both static and dynamic mechanical behavior of natural ligaments can be reproduced. Note that PET maybe sensitive to hydrolytic, stress-induced degradation. Surgeons are still looking for suitable synthetic materials to adequately reproduce the mechanical behavior of natural tissue for long-term applications. To many researchers, a combination of autegenous tissue and synthetic materials maybe an ideal choice for tendon/ligament prostheses.

9.2.9 Vascular Grafts

Arterial blood vessels are complex, multi-layered structures comprising collagen and elastin fibers, smooth muscle, ground substance, and endothelium. The blood vessel is anisotropic because of the orientation of inherent fibrous components. Vascular grafts are used to replace displaced or blocked segments of the natural cardiovascular system, such as in atherosclerosis — where deposits on the inner surface of blood vessels restrict the flow of blood and increase blood pressure. However, the use of vascular grafts is mainly successful in the case of blood vessels with lumen diameter exceeding 5 mm. Most widely used vascular grafts are woven or knitted fabric tubes of PET material or extruded porous wall tubes of PTFE and PU materials. The most important property of a graft is its porosity. Appropriate degree of porosity is desirable as it promotes tissue growth and acceptance of the graft by the host tissues. However, excessive porosity leads to blood leakage. In addition to porosity, other key requirements of vascular graft include good handling and suturing characteristics, satisfactory healing (*i.e.*, rapid tissue growth), and mechanical and chemical stability (*i.e.*, good tensile strength and resistance to deterioration). Since vascular grafts are subjected to static pressure and repeated stress of pulsation in application, they should have good dilation and creep resistance. Therefore fabric tubes are crimped to make them bulky, resilient, and soft. This is because crimping facilitates extensibility and enables bending of fabric tubes without kinks and stress concentrations — which are very important considerations in blood transporting vascular grafts.

Conventional vascular prostheses are predominantly rigid structures that lack anisotropy and non-linear compliance. Gershon *et al.* (1990, 1992) [73,74] and Klein *et al.* (1993) [75] developed composite grafts which comprised Lycra-type polyurethane fibers and Pellathane-type polyurethane matrix with PELA (block copolymer of lactic acid and polyethylene glycol) mixture. The non-linear stress-strain behavior of the composite graft was obtained by controlling the fiber orientation. The composite graft is anisotropic, and isocompliant with the natural artery. The matrix material is designed to resorb in animal testing conditions. At the time of implantation the impervious graft prevents any blood loss. The resorption of matrix material during healing process will result in pores. The ingrowth of granulation tissue into the pores provides a stable anchorage for the development of a viable cellular lining. The optimum pore size of the outer and inner layers of the graft can be designed to meet the exact needs of ingrowth and anchorage. Presently, the composite grafts are still in the clinical research phase and yet to be used clinically.

9.3   Composite Fabrication

A number of methods on how to fabricate polymer matrix composites have been proposed in numerous literature works. Most methods are applicable to specific kinds of composites: some may be suitable for thermoplastic composites, others for thermoset composites, but only a few for both composite types. In terms of fabrication techniques, some are limited to particulate and short fiber reinforcements, whereas others are best suited for handling continuous fiber reinforcements. In terms of fabrication processes, some make use of dry reinforcement, whereas others use prepregs — in which fibers are already combined with the polymer matrix — as raw materials. Brief descriptions of some of the most widely used fabrication methods are given in the following sections. Before making his own composites, the reader may refer to other references such as Agarwal and Broutman (1990) [76], Astrom (1997) [77], and Chawla (1998) [78] for more detailed information.

9.3.1 Filament Winding

Filament winding (Figure 9–6) is a process in which continuous fiber yarns are passed through a low viscosity resin bath for impregnation, and then precisely wound over a rotating or stationary mandrel. Successive layers are laid on at a constant or varying angle until the desired thickness is obtained. After the wound part is cured, the mandrel will be removed if necessary. Sometimes (such as for thermoplastic polymers), a hot-melt or solvent-dip process is used to impregnate the fibers. In another approach (called tow winding), thermoplastic prepreg tape is heated to the melting point of the polymer just before it is wound onto the mandrel. To avoid uneven cooling across the laminate's thickness — which may generate residual stresses, mandrel is normally heated to a temperature which is above the glass transition temperature of the polymer.

Filament winding is best suited for making parts with rotational symmetry (e.g., tubes and cylinders). Due to good control of fiber orientation, this process can generate higher fiber contents by up to 65 percent by volume. Care should be taken to avoid void formation at yarn crossover and at regions between layers of different fiber orientations. As the process uses only one-sided tooling, some cases may lead to poor surface finishing (depending on the process control).

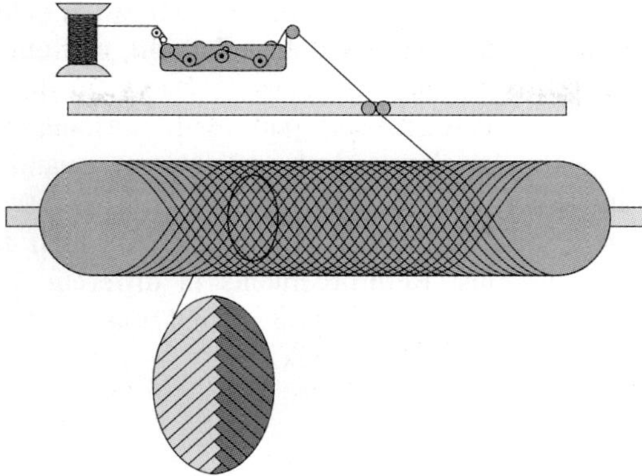

Figure 9–6 Illustration of filament winding for composite fabrication

9.3.2 Pultrusion

Many composite biomedical devices can be made through pultrusion (Figure 9–7). It is a process that involves pulling the reinforcement through a bath of liquid thermosetting resin, and then directly and continuously through a heated die to produce a continuous section. While passing through the bath, the reinforcement is properly impregnated with the resin. The die has a constant cross-sectional cavity almost along its entire length, except at the tapered entrance — which is designed to squeeze out any excess resin from the reinforcement. The heated die permits curing of the thermosetting resin and determines the cross-sectional shape. Subsequently, the hot solid is cooled and cut to the required lengths. In some special cases, prepregs are also pultruded to make good quality components.

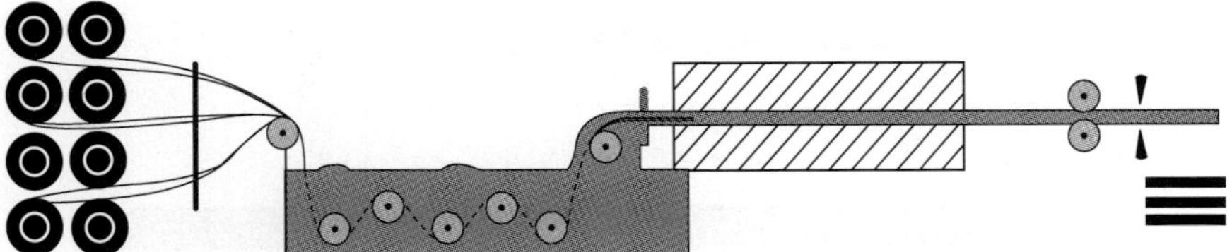

Figure 9–7 Schematic diagram of pultrusion in composite fabrication

This process can also be applied to produce thermoplastic composites. In such a case, the feedstock (prepreg) possesses both the reinforcement fibers and matrix polymer either in pre-consolidated or in non-preconsolidated form (e.g., a commingled yarn containing both reinforcement and thermoplastic polymer matrix fibers). A preheating system is used to heat the feedstock to a temperature near to or in excess of the softening point of the matrix. The feedstock then enters a heated die, which melts the matrix polymer and determines the cross-sectional shape of the composite. Subsequently the composite is consolidated in a cooling die, pulled out, and cut according to the desired lengths.

Pultrusion is best suited for making parts with constant cross-section (e.g., rods, tubes, pipes, beams, angles, and sheets) in large quantities. Very good fiber alignment and fiber volume fractions (as high as 60 percent) can be obtained. However, there are some limitations to which this process can achieve on fiber orientations. Reinforcements in different forms — such as unidirectional fibers (rovings), continuous strand mat, braided, woven, and stitched fabrics — can be used as feedstock.

9.3.3 Extrusion

An extrusion machine (Figure 9–8) consists mainly of rotating screws in a heated barrel. At one end of the barrel, a die is attached — design of the die cavity is based on the desired cross-sectional geometry of the component. The feedstock is a combined form of polymer matrix and reinforcement fibers. It is fed in the form of pellets from a hopper at the other end of the barrel. The feedstock is mixed and heated to plasticity and then passed through the die. The extruded product is cooled and cut according to the desired dimensions.

This process is limited to particulate and short fiber reinforcements with sections of uniform cross-section. The capital cost is high. Typical reinforcement contents are in the range of 10 to 30 percent by volume.

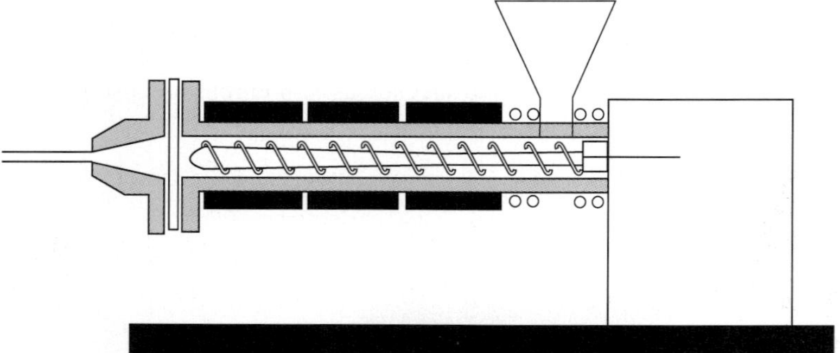

Figure 9–8 Schematic diagram of an extrusion process

9.3.4 Injection Molding

In injection molding (IM) (Figure 9–9), the feedstock containing polymer matrix and reinforcement in a combined form is heated to plasticity in a cylindrical barrel at controlled temperature. By means of a rotating screw inside the barrel, the material is forced through a nozzle into spruces, runners, gates, and cavities of the mold. Upon solidification or cross-linking of the polymer, the mold is opened and the part ejected. This process is widely used for making thermoplastic composites and to a lesser extent, thermoset composites.

The fierce rotating action of the screw inside the barrel aids in reducing the reinforcement's length. As such, this process is limited to particulate or short fiber reinforcement, where typical reinforcement contents are in the range of 10 to 30 percent by volume. Moreover this process is capable of mass producing complicated parts with very accurately controlled dimensions, which is another contributing factor to the high capital cost of the injection molding equipment.

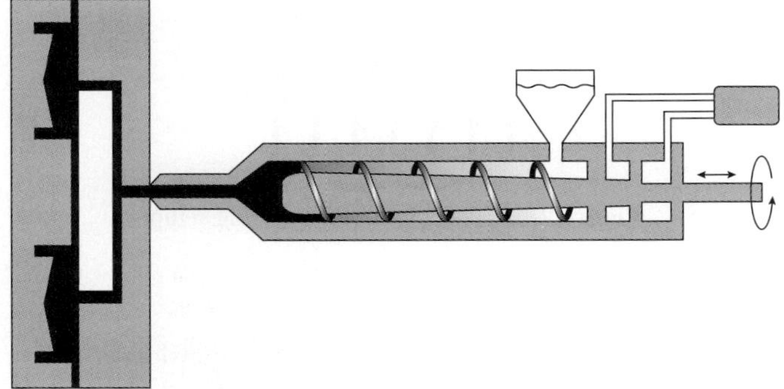

Figure 9–9 Schematic show of injection molding

9.3.5 Compression Molding

Compression molding, as shown in Figure 9–10, is widely used for making composites from prepregs such as sheet molding compound (SMC), bulk molding compound (BMC), or glass mat reinforced thermoplastic (GMT). This process uses matching male and female mold halves. A pre-weighed charge cut to the size is placed inside the mold, which is then closed, and suitable pressure and temperature are applied using a hot press. The applied temperature and pressure force the material to fill the mold cavity, hence facilitating the polymerization (or cross-linking) and consolidation of the composite material. The aforementioned prepregs contain short and randomly distributed fibers, and they readily flow to fill the mold. In the case of prepregs with aligned and continuous fibers — such as fabric prepregs, the mold filling ability is limited. Nevertheless, this technique is used widely to make flat laminates or simple shapes from fabric prepregs.

Compression molding is suitable for making both thermoset and thermoplastic composites. Extremely intricate parts — such as undercuts, side draws, small holes, and delicate inserts — with close tolerances and of good quality are difficult to produce. This is because the quality of a composite is determined by mold design, molding temperature cycle, and the application of pressure in the correct sequence. Ideally, the pressure should be applied slowly as the charge softens and before it starts to gel. It is also essential that the mold be adequately vented to allow water vapor and other volatiles to escape during the curing/consolidation process.

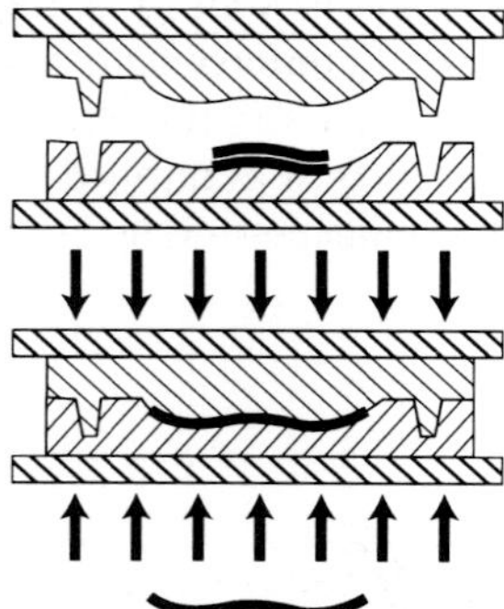

Figure 9–10 A compression molding setup

9.3.6 Thermoforming

Thermoforming (Figure 9–11) is a technique that transforms a flat sheet of composite into a three-dimensional shape. 'Press forming' or 'sheet forming' is the simplest of such method. The composite sheet, heated to a temperature above the softening point of the polymer, is squeezed into shape between two tools. Both tools may be made of metal (as in the case of compression molding), or one tool made of metal and the other made of rubber (the latter is called rubber-block molding). The rubber tool generates an even pressure and reduces the risk of wrinkles on the part. A related method called 'hydroforming' uses hydraulic fluid pressure and membrane to force the composite sheet into shape.

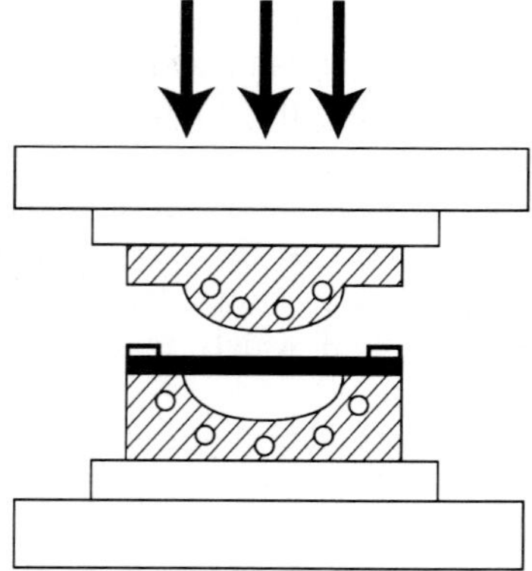

Figure 9–11 A thermoforming process

A variant is the 'diaphragm forming' method, in which stacked composite sheets are sandwiched between two diaphragms (super-plastic aluminium sheets or polyamide films). The edges of the diaphragms (not the composite sheets) are clamped to a frame and heated to a temperature above the melting point of the polymer. Pressure is applied to one side, which conforms the diaphragms to the shape of a one-sided tool. To aid the forming process, air is evacuated from between the assembly and the tool. The component is formed after the assembly is cooled and the diaphragms removed. This process is also carried out in purpose-built autoclaves.

9.3.7 A Fabrication Example

Besides the aforesaid fabrication techniques, many composites in laboratory-development level are fabricated through some simple methods by hand. Such an example is given here. The composite was developed for bone plate application (Figure 9–3) using carbon fiber and PEEK matrix material system. The PEEK matrix, also in a fiber form, was combined with the reinforcing carbon fibers through a micro-braiding technique [14] to form a commingled yarn (Figure 9–12(a)). In the next step, the micro-braiding yarns were made into braided fabrics using a flat braiding machine, as seen in Figure 9–12(b). Then, the fabrics were placed in a stainless steel mold to make the composite bone plate. As screws are necessary to fix the plate to human bone, the bone plate must be fabricated with the screw holes. It is recognized that drilling a hole on a fabricated composite can drastically reduce its load carrying capacity due to breakage of fiber continuity. Conversely, if the hole is done before matrix impregnation and without causing significant fibers damage, good fracture resistance around the hole can be expected [79]. In this regard, a fabrication mold with six inserted pins was prepared. The diameter of each pin was equal to that of the screws (Figure 9–13). The female mold consisted of three parts — all connected through screw bolts. The central part had a convex curvature, giving a curve form for the bone plate. Flat braided fabrics — of nine layers — were placed in between the mold. The pins were carefully penetrated through the fabrics, without breaking the continuity of yarns. The mold was then put into a vacuumed hot press machine for a further melt-and-press treatment, with an average holding pressure of 5.6 MPa and a heating temperature of 400°C for 60 minutes. The bone plate (Figure 9–3) was achieved when the mold was cooled down to room temperature and removed, with an average fiber volume fraction of 48.1 percent (measured through a burning method). Good impregnation of PEEK matrix into carbon fiber braided fabrics was recognized.

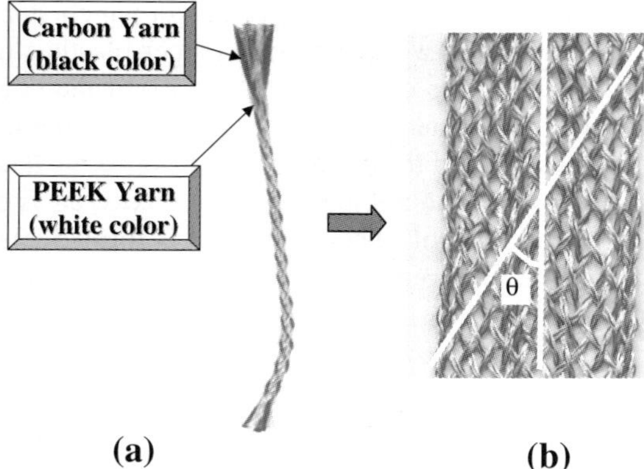

Figure 9–12 (a) A micro-braiding CF/PEEK yarn; (b) a flat braided fabric using such yarns

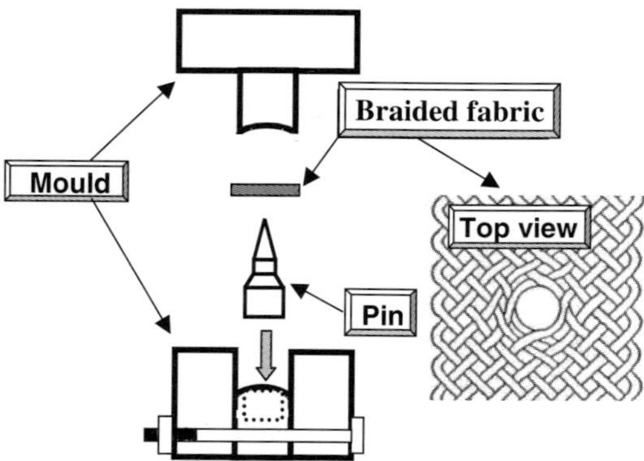

Figure 9–13 Schematic show for braided composite bone plate

9.4   Mechanics of Composites

A key advantage for composites to be used in biomedical applications is that their mechanical properties can be customized to meet the specific requirements of each application.   To achieve this, the composite's structure-property relationship must be clearly understood.   The study of the mechanics of composites aims to explore this relationship based upon the knowledge of the behaviors and geometries of the composites' constituents.

9.4.1 RVE and Effective Property

In composites, mechanical properties such as stress, strain, modulus, strength, *etc.* are not quantified point-wise.   Instead, they are expressed on an averaged sense with respect to a finite volume element called Representative Volume

Element or RVE. The resulting quantities are called effective quantities. Figure 9–14 depicts a UD composite of which its RVE geometry is shown in Figure 9–15.

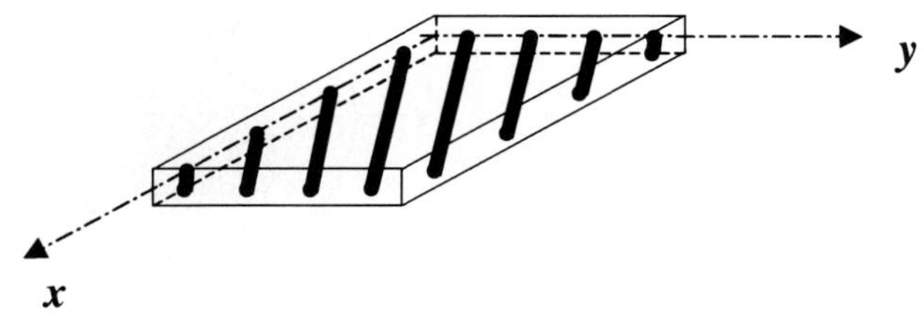

Figure 9–14 A UD composite with an off-axial direction

Let V' denote the RVE volume. The RVE volumes of fiber and matrix are V'_f and V'_m respectively. Suppose the ith point-wise stress and strain in RVE are σ_i and ε_i, which may be different at a different point. The volume-averaged stress $\overline{\sigma}_i$ of the composite is defined as:

$$\overline{\sigma}_i = \frac{1}{V'}\int_{V'}\sigma_i dV = \frac{1}{V'}\left[\int_{V'_f}\sigma_i dV + \int_{V'_m}\sigma_i dV\right]$$

$$= \left(\frac{V'_f}{V'}\right)\left(\frac{1}{V'_f}\int_{V'_f}\sigma_i dV\right) + \left(\frac{V'_m}{V'}\right)\left(\frac{1}{V'_m}\int_{V'_m}\sigma_i dV\right)$$

$$= V_f\overline{\sigma_i^f} + V_m\overline{\sigma_i^m} \tag{1}$$

where $V_f = V'_f /V'$ and $V_m = V'_m /V'$ are volume fractions of the fiber and matrix, and $\overline{\sigma_i^f}$ and $\overline{\sigma_i^m}$ are volume-averaged internal stresses in the fiber and matrix respectively. Similarly, the volume-averaged strain of the composite is given by:

$$\overline{\varepsilon}_i = V_f\overline{\varepsilon_i^f} + V_m\overline{\varepsilon_i^m} \tag{2}$$

In all of the above and following equations, the suffixes (either superscripts or subscripts) "f" and "m" stand for fiber and matrix phases respectively. A quantity without any suffix denotes a composite, or sometimes, a special kind of material. Equations (1) and (2) are valid for every i=1, 2, …, 6. As this chapter focuses on volume-averaged quantities only, the over-bars in equations (1) and (2) can be omitted. Thus, we obtain the following two relationships for unidirectional composites.

$$\{\sigma_i\} = V_f\{\sigma_i^f\} + V_m\{\sigma_i^m\} \tag{3}$$

$$\{\varepsilon_i\} = V_f\{\varepsilon_i^f\} + V_m\{\varepsilon_i^m\} \tag{4}$$

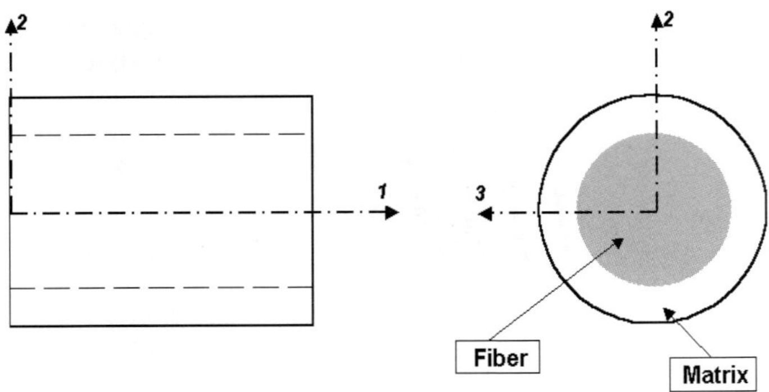

Figure 9–15 A RVE geometry for UD composite

Further, suppose that $[S_{ij}^{f}]$ and $[S_{ij}^{m}]$ are the compliance matrices of the fiber and matrix materials respectively. These two matrices are invariant with respect to a volume average. Thus,

$$\left\{\varepsilon_{i}^{f}\right\}=[S_{ij}^{f}]\{\sigma_{j}^{f}\} \tag{5a}$$

$$\left\{\varepsilon_{i}^{m}\right\}=[S_{ij}^{m}]\{\sigma_{j}^{m}\} \tag{5b}$$

$$\{\varepsilon_{i}\}=[S_{ij}]\{\sigma_{j}\} \tag{6}$$

where $[S_{ij}]$ denotes the compliance matrix of the composite. Note that any fiber reinforced composite can be subdivided into a series of UD composites. Thus, the study of UD composites plays a key role in the development of composite theories.

9.4.2 *Moduli of UD Composite — Rule of Mixture Approach*

A micromechanices theory is defined as an approach where the effective quantities of a composite are obtained based on only the quantities of its constituent materials. Amongst the micromechanics models to calculate a composite's elastic properties, one of the simplest is the Rule of Mixture approach. Consider a UD composite with its fiber axis along the x direction (Figure 9–16). The basic assumption used in the rule of mixture approach is that the volume-averaged longitudinal (*i.e.*, the fiber axis directional) strains in the fiber, matrix, and composite are the same when a uniaxial load is applied longitudinally. On the other hand, the volume-averaged transverse and shear stresses in the fiber, matrix, and composite are, respectively, equal to each other when any other kind of uniaxial load is applied.

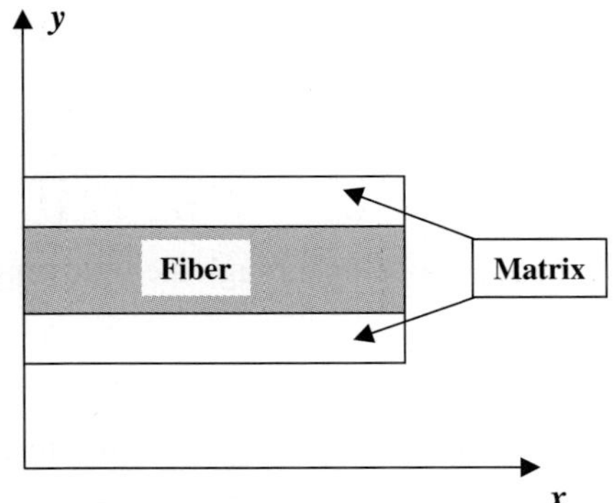

Figure 9–16 A UD composite model in rule of mixture approach

Different uniaxial loads are then applied to the composite. First, only a longitudinal stress is applied. Under such a load condition, the above basic assumption gives the following:

$$\varepsilon_{xx} = \varepsilon_{xx}^{f} = \varepsilon_{xx}^{m}, \ \sigma_{yy} = \sigma_{yy}^{f} = \sigma_{yy}^{m} = 0, \text{ and } \sigma_{xy} = \sigma_{xy}^{f} = \sigma_{xy}^{m} = 0$$

Due to uniaxial stress state, we obtain the following:

$$\sigma_{xx} = E_{xx}\varepsilon_{xx} = V_f \sigma_{xx}^{f} + V_m \sigma_{xx}^{m} = V_f E_{xx}^{f}\varepsilon_{xx}^{f} + V_m E_{xx}^{m}\varepsilon_{xx}^{m} = (V_f E_{xx}^{f} + V_m E_{xx}^{m})\varepsilon_{xx}$$

Therefore, the overall longitudinal Young's modulus of the composite is given as follows:

$$E_{xx} = V_f E_{xx}^{f} + V_m E_{xx}^{m}$$

Similarly, from:

$$\varepsilon_{yy} = -v_{xy}\varepsilon_{xx} = V_f \varepsilon_{yy}^{f} + V_m \varepsilon_{yy}^{m} = V_f (-v_{xy}^{f}\varepsilon_{xx}^{f}) + V_m (-v_{xy}^{m}\varepsilon_{xx}^{m}) = -(V_f v_{xy}^{f} + V_m v_{xy}^{m})\varepsilon_{xx}$$

it follows that:

$$v_{xy} = V_f v_{xy}^{f} + V_m v_{xy}^{m}$$

Next, a transverse stress is applied alone. According to the basic assumption, the stress states generated in the fiber, matrix, and composite are:

$$\sigma_{xx} = \sigma_{xx}^{f} = \sigma_{xx}^{m} = 0, \ \sigma_{yy} = \sigma_{yy}^{f} = \sigma_{yy}^{m} \neq 0, \text{ and } \sigma_{xy} = \sigma_{xy}^{f} = \sigma_{xy}^{m} = 0$$

The overall strain in the y direction is derived as:

$$\varepsilon_{yy} = \frac{\sigma_{yy}}{E_{yy}} = V_f \varepsilon_{yy}^{f} + V_m \varepsilon_{yy}^{m} = V_f (\frac{\sigma_{yy}^{f}}{E_f}) + V_m (\frac{\sigma_{yy}^{m}}{E_m}) = \left(\frac{V_f}{E_f} + \frac{V_m}{E_m}\right)\sigma_{yy}$$

Hence, the resulting transverse Young's modulus is obtained from the following:

$$\frac{1}{E_{yy}} = \frac{V_f}{E_f} + \frac{V_m}{E_m}$$

Finally, applying a pure shear stress, σ_{xy}, to the composite yields:

$$\sigma_{xx} = \sigma_{xx}^{f} = \sigma_{xx}^{m} = 0, \ \sigma_{yy} = \sigma_{yy}^{f} = \sigma_{yy}^{m} = 0, \ \text{and} \ \sigma_{xy} = \sigma_{xy}^{f} = \sigma_{xy}^{m} \neq 0$$

From the overall shear strain,

$$\varepsilon_{xy} = \frac{\sigma_{xy}}{G_{xy}} = V_f \varepsilon_{xy}^{f} + V_m \varepsilon_{xy}^{m} = V_f \left(\frac{\sigma_{xy}^{f}}{G_f}\right) + V_m \left(\frac{\sigma_{xy}^{m}}{G_m}\right) = \left(\frac{V_f}{G_f} + \frac{V_m}{G_m}\right)\sigma_{xy}$$

we obtain the longitudinal shear modulus through the following:

$$\frac{1}{G_{xy}} = \frac{V_f}{G_f} + \frac{V_m}{G_m}$$

In summary, the rule of mixture approach gives the formulae for effective moduli as follows (using *1*, *2*, and *3* instead of *x*, *y*, and *z*):

$$E_{11} = V_f E_{11}^{f} + V_m E^{m} \tag{7a}$$

$$V_{12} = V_f V_{12}^{f} + V_m V^{m} \tag{7b}$$

$$E_{22} = \frac{E^{m}}{1 - V_f (1 - E^{m} / E_{22}^{f})} \tag{7c}$$

$$G_{12} = \frac{G^{m}}{1 - V_f (1 - G^{m} / G_{12}^{f})} \tag{7d}$$

$$G_{23} = \frac{G^{m}}{1 - V_f (1 - G^{m} / G_{23}^{f})} \tag{7e}$$

where E_{11}^{f}, V_{12}^{f}, and G_{12}^{f} are longitudinal Young's modulus, Poisson's ratio, and shear modulus of the fiber material, whereas E_{22}^{f} and G_{23}^{f} are transverse Young's and shear moduli of the fiber. E^{m}, V^{m}, and G^{m} are the elastic modulus, Poisson's ratio, and shear modulus of the matrix, with $G^{m} = 0.5 E^{m} / (1 + V^{m})$.

Note that the longitudinal Young's modulus and Poisson's ratio formulae, *i.e.*, equations (7a) and (7b), have been shown to be sufficiently accurate. On the other hand, the transverse Young's modulus and shear modulus are much underestimated when equations (7c) and (7d) are used.

9.4.3 *Strengths of UD Composite — Bridging Model Formulae*

It is difficult to calculate the strength of a composite by using only the properties of its constituent materials. Limited number of micromechanics strength formulae exists in the literature. This is because composite strength depends significantly on the load direction, and that a superposition is no longer applicable due to the inelastic deformation of the constituent materials. Given below is a set of micromechanics strength formulae, which are applicable only when the composite is subjected to uniaxial loads [80].

9.4.3.1 *Longitudinal tensile strength*

If the UD composite is subjected only to a longitudinal tensile load (σ_{11}), its strength is given as follows:

$$\sigma_{11}^{u} = \min\left\{ \frac{\sigma_u^f - (\alpha_{e1}^f - \alpha_{p1}^f)\sigma_{11}^0}{\alpha_{p1}^f}, \frac{\sigma_u^m - (\alpha_{e1}^m - \alpha_{p1}^m)\sigma_{11}^0}{\alpha_{p1}^m} \right\} \tag{8a}$$

$$\sigma_{11}^0 = \min\left\{ \frac{\sigma_Y^m}{\alpha_{e1}^m}, \frac{\sigma_u^f}{\alpha_{e1}^f} \right\} \tag{8b}$$

$$\alpha_{e1}^f = \frac{E_{11}^f}{V_f E_{11}^f + (1 - V_f)E^m} \tag{8c}$$

$$\alpha_{e1}^m = \frac{E^m}{V_f E_{11}^f + (1 - V_f)E^m} \tag{8d}$$

$$\alpha_{p1}^f = \frac{E_{11}^f}{V_f E_{11}^f + (1 - V_f)E_T^m} \tag{8e}$$

$$\alpha_{p1}^m = \frac{E_T^m}{V_f E_{11}^f + (1 - V_f)E_T^m} \tag{8f}$$

In the above, σ_u^f is the fiber tensile strength (in axial direction) and σ_u^m the matrix tensile strength. σ_Y^m and E_T^m are the yield strength and hardening modulus of the matrix (Figure 9–17). Note that a bilinear elastic-plastic behavior has been assumed for the matrix, and that the fiber material has been assumed to be linearly elastic until rupture.

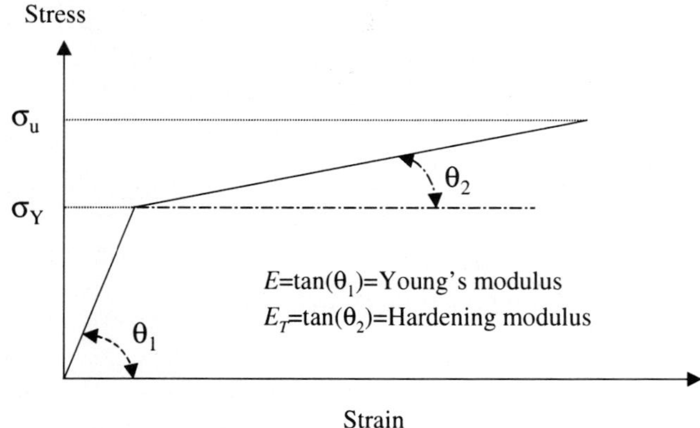

Figure 9–17 Schematic bilinear stress-strain curve of a matrix material

9.4.3.2 *Transverse tensile strength*

If the composite is subjected only to a transverse tensile load (σ_{22}), its strength is determined from:

$$\sigma_{22}^u = \min\left\{\frac{\sigma_u^f - (\alpha_{e2}^f - \alpha_{p2}^f)\sigma_{22}^0}{\alpha_{p2}^f}, \frac{\sigma_u^m - (\alpha_{e2}^m - \alpha_{p2}^m)\sigma_{22}^0}{\alpha_{p2}^m}\right\} \tag{9a}$$

where $$\sigma_{22}^0 = \min\left\{\frac{\sigma_Y^m}{\alpha_{e2}^m}, \frac{\sigma_u^f}{\alpha_{e2}^f}\right\} \tag{9b}$$

$$\alpha_{e2}^f = \frac{E_{22}^f}{V_f E_{22}^f + 0.5(1-V_f)(E^m + E_{22}^f)} \tag{9c}$$

$$\alpha_{e2}^m = \frac{0.5(E_{22}^f + E^m)}{V_f E_{22}^f + 0.5(1-V_f)(E^m + E_{22}^f)} \tag{9d}$$

$$\alpha_{p2}^f = \frac{E_{22}^f}{V_f E_{22}^f + 0.5(1-V_f)(E_T^m + E_{22}^f)} \tag{9e}$$

$$\alpha_{p2}^m = \frac{0.5(E_{22}^f + E_T^m)}{V_f E_{22}^f + 0.5(1-V_f)(E_T^m + E_{22}^f)} \tag{9f}$$

9.4.3.3 *In-plane shear strength*

The ultimate strength of the composite due to an in-plane shear load (σ_{12}) alone is calculated through:

$$\sigma_{12}^u = \min\left\{\frac{\sigma_u^f - (\alpha_{e3}^f - \alpha_{p3}^f)\sigma_{12}^0}{\alpha_{p3}^f}, \frac{\sigma_u^m - (\alpha_{e3}^m - \alpha_{p3}^m)\sigma_{12}^0}{\alpha_{p3}^m}\right\} \tag{10a}$$

where $$\sigma_{12}^0 = \min\left\{\frac{\sigma_Y^m}{\sqrt{3}\alpha_{e3}^m}, \frac{\sigma_u^f}{\alpha_{e3}^f}\right\} \tag{10b}$$

$$\alpha_{e3}^f = \frac{G_{12}^f}{V_f G_{12}^f + 0.5(1-V_f)(G^m + G_{12}^f)} \tag{10c}$$

$$\alpha_{e3}^m = \frac{0.5(G_{12}^f + G^m)}{V_f G_{12}^f + 0.5(1-V_f)(G^m + G_{12}^f)} \tag{10d}$$

$$\alpha_{p3}^f = \frac{3G_{12}^f}{3V_f G_{12}^f + 0.5(1-V_f)(E_T^m + 3G_{12}^f)} \tag{10e}$$

$$\alpha_{p3}^m = \frac{0.5(3G_{12}^f + E_T^m)}{3V_f G_{12}^f + 0.5(1-V_f)(E_T^m + 3G_{12}^f)} \tag{10f}$$

9.4.4 Example

A SiC-fiber reinforced titanium (Ti) matrix UD composite has properties of E^f=400 GPa, v^f=0.25, σ_u^f =3480 MPa, E^m=110 GPa, v^m=0.33, E_T^m =2.16 GPa, σ_Y^m =850 MPa, and σ_u^m =1000 MPa [81]. The fiber volume fraction is 0.15. Calculate uniaxial strengths of this composite and identify its corresponding failure modes.

SOLUTION

A) *Longitudinal Strength*

Substituting the relevant parameters into equations (8a) – (8f), we have:

α_{e1}^f =(400)/[(0.15)(400)+(0.85)(110)]=2.606,

α_{e1}^m =(110)/[(0.15)(400)+(0.85)(110)]=0.717,

α_{p1}^f =(400)/[(0.15)(400)+(0.85)(2.16)]=6.550,

α_{p1}^m =(2.16)/[(0.15)(400)+(0.85)(2.16)]=0.0349,

σ_{11}^0 =min{(850)/(0.717),(3480)/(2.606)}=min{1185.5,1335.4}=1185.5,

σ_{11}^u =min{[3480-(2.606-6.55)(1185.5)]/6.55,

        [1000-(0.717-0.0349)(1185.5)]/(0.0349)}

    =min{1245.1,5483.4} =1245.1 (MPa)

The last expression indicated that it was fiber fracture that caused the composite failure (since under the longitudinal load the fiber failure corresponded stress is 1245.1 MPa, whereas the matrix failure corresponded stress is 5483.4 MPa).

B) *Transverse Strength*

According to equations (9a) – (9f), we obtain:

α_{e2}^f =(400)/[(0.15)(400)+(0.5)(0.85)(110+400)]=1.445,

α_{e2}^m =(0.5)(110+400)/[(0.15)(400)+(0.5)(0.85)(110+400)]=0.921,

α_{p2}^f =(400)/[(0.15)(400)+(0.5)(0.85)(2.16+400)]=1.732,

α_{p2}^m =(0.5)(400+2.16)/[(0.15)(400)+(0.5)(0.85)(402.16)]=0.871,

σ_{22}^0 =min{(850)/(0.921),(3480)/(1.445)}=min{922.9,2408.3}=922.9,

σ_{22}^u =min{[(3480)-(1.445-1.732)(922.9)]/(1.732),

        [1000-(0.921-0.871)(922.9)]/(0.871)}

    =min{2162.2, 1095.1} =1095.1 (MPa)

The last expression indicated that it was matrix fracture that caused the composite failure (since under the transverse load the fiber failure corresponded stress is 2162.2MPa, whereas the matrix failure corresponded stress is 1095.1MPa).

C) In-plane Shear Strength

First, we have G^f=(400)/[(2)(1+0.25)]=160GPa and G^m=(110)/[(2)(1+0.33)]= 41.4GPa, as both the fiber and matrix are isotropic. Then, equations (10a) – (10f) give:

$$\alpha_{e3}^{f} = (160)/[(0.15)+(0.5)(0.85)(160+41.4)]=1.460,$$

$$\alpha_{e3}^{m} = (0.5)(201.4)/[(0.15)(160)+(0.5)(0.85)(201.4)]=0.919,$$

$$\alpha_{p3}^{f} = (3)(160)/[(3)(0.15)(160)+(0.5)(0.85)(2.16+480)]=1.733,$$

$$\alpha_{p3}^{m} = (0.5)(480+2.16)/[(3)(0.15)(160)+(0.5)(0.85)(2.16+480)]=0.871,$$

$$\sigma_{12}^{0} = \min\{(850)/[(1.732)(0.919)],(3480)/(1.46)\}$$
$$= \min\{563.4,2383.6\}=563.4$$

$$\sigma_{12}^{u} = \min\{[3480-(1.46-1.733)(563.4)]/(1.733),$$
$$[1000-(0.919-0.871)(563.4)]/(0.871)\}$$
$$= \min\{2096.8, 1118.4\} = 1118.4 \ (MPa)$$

The last expression indicated that it was matrix fracture that caused the composite failure (since under the in-plane shear load the fiber failure corresponded stress is 2096.8 MPa, whereas the matrix failure corresponded stress is 1118.4 MPa).

9.4.5 Structure-Property Relationship

The stiffness and strength formulae given in the preceding subsections are applicable only to the simplest cases, *i.e.*, UD composites subjected to uniaxial loads. In most cases, UD composites are used as laminae to construct multidirectional tape laminates in which the UD composites are subjected to a planar load condition. Even for such conditions, the previous micromechanics strength formulae are not applicable and sufficient. In reality, we often have to deal with problems such as a textile composite laminate (*i.e.*, a laminate consisting of multi-layer textile fabric reinforced composites) which can be much more complicated. In order to tackle these real problems, we need a more powerful micromechanics theory — thus leading to more complicated mathematical formulae.

9.4.5.1 *Mechanical properties of UD composite*

Suppose the UD composite is subjected to an arbitrary planar stress state, $\{\sigma\}=\{\sigma_{11}, \sigma_{22}, \sigma_{12}\}^{\mathrm{T}}$ (Figure 9–18(a)). What will be the composite's response up to failure? In other words, what will be the composite's instantaneous compliance matrix if an incremental description is adopted for the composite's stresses and strains (similar to equation (6))? To understand such a response, we need to identify internal stress states in the constituent fiber and matrix materials. This can be accomplished using the Bridging Model [82], in which an incremental solution strategy (Figure 9–18(b)) is generally applied when the analysis is out of an inelastic deformation range. The benefit for applying the incremental solution is that the composite stiffness (compliance) at the current load level can be regarded as unchanged when incremental loads are applied subsequently.

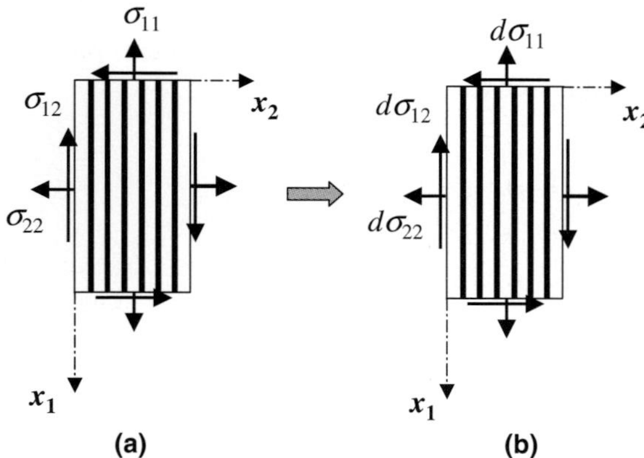

Figure 9–18 (a) UD composite subjected to any planar load; (b) an incremental approach

Internal Stresses

The stress increments in the fiber and matrix are given as follows:

$$\begin{Bmatrix} d\sigma_{11}^{f} \\ d\sigma_{22}^{f} \\ d\sigma_{12}^{f} \end{Bmatrix} = \begin{bmatrix} b_{11} & b_{12} & b_{13} \\ 0 & b_{22} & b_{23} \\ 0 & 0 & b_{33} \end{bmatrix} \begin{Bmatrix} d\sigma_{11} \\ d\sigma_{22} \\ d\sigma_{12} \end{Bmatrix} = [B] \begin{Bmatrix} d\sigma_{11} \\ d\sigma_{22} \\ d\sigma_{12} \end{Bmatrix} \qquad (11\mathrm{a})$$

$$\begin{Bmatrix} d\sigma_{11}^{m} \\ d\sigma_{22}^{m} \\ d\sigma_{12}^{m} \end{Bmatrix} = \begin{bmatrix} a_{11} & a_{12} & a_{13} \\ 0 & a_{22} & a_{23} \\ 0 & 0 & a_{33} \end{bmatrix} \begin{bmatrix} b_{11} & b_{12} & b_{13} \\ 0 & b_{22} & b_{23} \\ 0 & 0 & b_{33} \end{bmatrix} \begin{Bmatrix} d\sigma_{11} \\ d\sigma_{22} \\ d\sigma_{12} \end{Bmatrix} = [A][B] \begin{Bmatrix} d\sigma_{11} \\ d\sigma_{22} \\ d\sigma_{12} \end{Bmatrix} \qquad (11\mathrm{b})$$

where $[A]$ is a bridging matrix and $[B]$ is closely related to $[A]$. The total stresses in the fiber, matrix, and composite are updated *via*

$$[\sigma_{ij}^f]^{(k+1)} = [\sigma_{ij}^f]^{(k)} + [d\sigma_{ij}^f] \text{ and } [\sigma_{ij}^m]^{(k+1)} = [\sigma_{ij}^m]^{(k)} + [d\sigma_{ij}^m], \; k=0, 1, \ldots \quad (12)$$

where $[\sigma_{ij}]^{(0)} = [\sigma_{ij}^f]^{(0)} = [\sigma_{ij}^m]^{(0)} = [0]$, if no thermal residual stresses are involved. For an otherwise case, refer to Huang (2001b) [83].

Instantaneous Compliance Matrix

Under an incremental load condition, $\{d\sigma\} = \{d\sigma_{11}, \; d\sigma_{22}, \; d\sigma_{12}\}^{\mathrm{T}}$, the composite generates an incremental strain response, $\{d\varepsilon\} = \{d\varepsilon_{11}, \; d\varepsilon_{22}, \; 2d\varepsilon_{12}\}^{\mathrm{T}}$, following the expression below:

$$\{d\varepsilon_i\} = [S_{ij}]\{d\sigma_j\} \quad (13)$$

where the instantaneous compliance matrix is determined through:

$$[S] = [S_{ij}] = (V_f[S_{ij}^f] + V_m[S_{ij}^m][A])[B] \quad (14)$$

where $[S_{ij}^f]$ and $[S_{ij}^m]$ are the instantaneous compliance matrices of the fiber and matrix materials respectively.

Bridging Matrix Elements

The bridging elements — which are dependent on the constituents' properties — are expressed as:

$$a_{11} = E_m / E_{11}^f \quad (15a)$$

$$a_{22} = 0.5(1 + E_m / E_{22}^f) \quad (15b)$$

$$a_{33} = 0.5(1 + G_m / G_{12}^f) \quad (15c)$$

$$a_{12} = (S_{12}^f - S_{12}^m)(a_{11} - a_{22})/(S_{11}^f - S_{11}^m) \quad (15d)$$

$$a_{13} = \frac{d_2\beta_{11} - d_1\beta_{21}}{\beta_{11}\beta_{22} - \beta_{12}\beta_{21}} \quad (15e)$$

$$a_{23} = \frac{d_1\beta_{22} - d_2\beta_{12}}{\beta_{11}\beta_{22} - \beta_{12}\beta_{21}} \quad (15f)$$

$$d_1 = S_{13}^m(a_{11} - a_{33})$$

$$d_2 = S_{23}^m(V_f + V_m a_{11})(a_{22} - a_{33}) + S_{13}^m(V_f + V_m a_{33})a_{12}$$

$$\beta_{11} = S_{12}^m - S_{12}^f, \; \beta_{12} = S_{11}^m - S_{11}^f, \; \beta_{22} = (V_f + V_m a_{22})(S_{12}^m - S_{12}^f)$$

$$\beta_{21} = V_m(S_{12}^f - S_{12}^m)a_{12} - (V_f + V_m a_{11})(S_{22}^f - S_{22}^m)$$

$$E_m = \begin{cases} E^m, when \;\; \sigma_e^m \le \sigma_Y^m \\ E_T^m, when \;\; \sigma_e^m > \sigma_Y^m \end{cases}$$

$$G_m = \begin{cases} 0.5E^m/(1 + v^m), when \;\; \sigma_e^m \le \sigma_Y^m \\ E_T^m/3, when \;\; \sigma_e^m > \sigma_Y^m \end{cases}$$

$$\sigma_e^m = \sqrt{(\sigma_{11}^m)^2 + (\sigma_{22}^m)^2 - (\sigma_{11}^m)(\sigma_{22}^m) + 3(\sigma_{12}^m)^2}$$

The elements of $[B]$ are then found to be:

$$b_{11}=(V_f+V_m a_{22})(V_f+V_m a_{33})/c, \quad b_{12}=-(V_m a_{12})(V_f+V_m a_{33})/c \tag{16a}$$

$$b_{13}=[(V_m a_{12})(V_m a_{23})-(V_f+V_m a_{22})(V_m a_{13})]/c, \quad b_{22}=(V_f+V_m a_{11})(V_f+V_m a_{33})/c \tag{16b}$$

$$b_{23}=-(V_m a_{23})(V_f+V_m a_{11})/c, \quad b_{33}=(V_f+V_m a_{22})(V_f+V_m a_{11})/c \tag{16c}$$

$$c=(V_f+V_m a_{11})(V_f+V_m a_{22})(V_f+V_m a_{33})$$

Constituent Compliances

The instantaneous compliance matrices of the constituents are assumed to be known. For example, Hooke's law can be used to define the fiber compliance matrix if it is linearly elastic until rupture and Prandtl–Reuss theory can be used to define the matrix compliance matrix if it is an elasto-plastic material [82].

Ultimate Strength

When a composite fails, the corresponding applied load is defined as an ultimate stress state for the composite and the ultimate strength follows. How to identify composite failure? As there are only two constituents, composite failure occurs as soon as one of the constituents attains a failure stress state. Constituent failure can be detected using the maximum normal stress criterion — that is, composite failure is attained if any of the following conditions is fulfilled:

$$\frac{\sigma_{11}^f + \sigma_{22}^f}{2} + \frac{1}{2}\sqrt{(\sigma_{11}^f - \sigma_{22}^f)^2 + 4(\sigma_{12}^f)^2} \geq \sigma_u^f \tag{17a}$$

$$\frac{\sigma_{11}^f + \sigma_{22}^f}{2} - \frac{1}{2}\sqrt{(\sigma_{11}^f - \sigma_{22}^f)^2 + 4(\sigma_{12}^f)^2} \leq -\sigma_{u,c}^f \tag{17b}$$

$$\frac{\sigma_{11}^m + \sigma_{22}^m}{2} + \frac{1}{2}\sqrt{(\sigma_{11}^m - \sigma_{22}^m)^2 + 4(\sigma_{12}^m)^2} \geq \sigma_u^m \tag{17c}$$

$$\frac{\sigma_{11}^m + \sigma_{22}^m}{2} - \frac{1}{2}\sqrt{(\sigma_{11}^m - \sigma_{22}^m)^2 + 4(\sigma_{12}^m)^2} \leq -\sigma_{u,c}^m \tag{17d}$$

In the above equations, $\sigma_{u,c}^f$ and $\sigma_{u,c}^m$ denote the fiber (in axis direction) and matrix compressive strengths.

9.4.5.2 *Mechanical properties of laminated composite*

Suppose a laminated composite consists of N layers of UD laminae stacked in different ply-angles (Figure 9–19). A global coordinate system, (x, y, z), is assumed to have its origin on the middle surface of the laminate, with x and y in the laminate plane and z along the thickness direction. Let the fiber direction of the kth lamina have an inclined ply-angle θ_k with the global x direction, where θ is measured in anti-clockwise direction from x ($0°$) to the fiber axis direction of the ply.

                     Z.-M. Huang & S. Ramakrishna

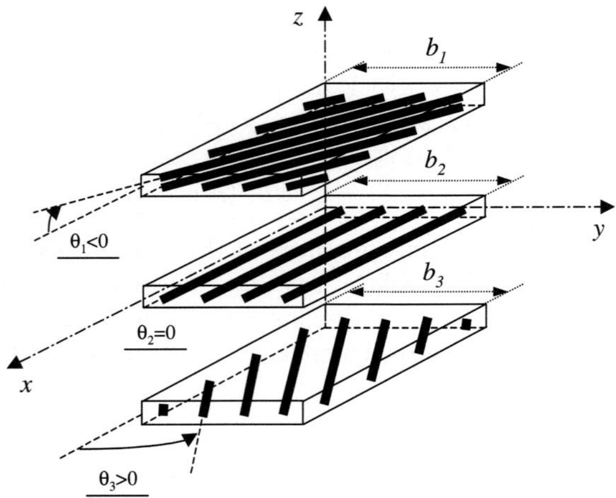

Figure 9–19 Schematic show of multi-layer laminae to constitute a laminate

The analysis of the laminate is based on the classical lamination theory [84]. A schematic procedure of the analysis is shown in Figure 9–20. For each lamina in the laminate, only in-plane stress and strain increments, *i.e.*, $\{d\sigma\}^G = \{d\sigma_{xx}, d\sigma_{yy}, d\sigma_{xy}\}^T$ and $\{d\varepsilon\}^G = \{d\varepsilon_{xx}, d\varepsilon_{yy}, 2d\varepsilon_{xy}\}^T$ are retained, where "G" refers to the global coordinate system (Figure 9–20(b)). They are correlated by equation (13), but in the global system — as shown in Figure 9–20(b) below.

$$\{d\sigma\}^G = [C_{ij}^G]\{d\varepsilon\}^G = [T]_c[S]^{-1}[T]_c^T\{d\varepsilon\}^G \tag{18}$$

where $[S]$ is the lamina's instantaneous compliance matrix and is determined using equation (14), and $[T]_c$ is a coordinate transformation matrix dependent on the ply-angle and is given by:

$$[T]_c = \begin{bmatrix} l_1^2 & l_2^2 & 2l_1l_2 \\ m_1^2 & m_2^2 & 2m_1m_2 \\ l_1m_1 & l_2m_2 & l_1m_2+l_2m_1 \end{bmatrix}, \; l_1=m_2=\cos\theta, \; l_2=-m_1=\sin\theta \tag{19}$$

According to the classical laminate theory, the global strain increments of the kth lamina in the laminate can be expressed as:

$$\{d\varepsilon\}_k^G = \{d\varepsilon_{xx}^0 + \frac{z_k+z_{k-1}}{2}d\kappa_{xx}^0, d\varepsilon_{yy}^0 + \frac{z_k+z_{k-1}}{2}d\kappa_{yy}^0, 2d\varepsilon_{xy}^0 + (z_k+z_{k-1})d\kappa_{xy}^0\}^T \tag{20}$$

where z_{k-1} and z_k are the z-coordinates of the bottom and top surfaces of the kth ply, and $d\varepsilon_{xx}^0$ etc. and $d\kappa_{xx}^0$ etc. are the strain and curvature increments of the middle surface respectively. They can be determined from the following formulae:

$$
\begin{Bmatrix} dN_{xx} \\ dN_{yy} \\ dN_{xy} \\ dM_{xx} \\ dM_{yy} \\ dM_{xy} \end{Bmatrix} = \begin{bmatrix} Q_{11}^{I} & Q_{12}^{I} & Q_{16}^{I} & Q_{11}^{II} & Q_{12}^{II} & Q_{16}^{II} \\ Q_{12}^{I} & Q_{22}^{I} & Q_{26}^{I} & Q_{12}^{II} & Q_{22}^{II} & Q_{26}^{II} \\ Q_{16}^{I} & Q_{26}^{I} & Q_{66}^{I} & Q_{16}^{II} & Q_{26}^{II} & Q_{66}^{II} \\ Q_{11}^{II} & Q_{12}^{II} & Q_{16}^{II} & Q_{11}^{III} & Q_{12}^{III} & Q_{16}^{III} \\ Q_{12}^{II} & Q_{22}^{II} & Q_{26}^{II} & Q_{12}^{III} & Q_{22}^{III} & Q_{26}^{III} \\ Q_{16}^{II} & Q_{26}^{II} & Q_{66}^{II} & Q_{16}^{III} & Q_{26}^{III} & Q_{66}^{III} \end{bmatrix} \begin{Bmatrix} d\varepsilon_{xx}^{0} \\ d\varepsilon_{yy}^{0} \\ 2d\varepsilon_{xy}^{0} \\ d\kappa_{xx}^{0} \\ d\kappa_{yy}^{0} \\ 2d\kappa_{xy}^{0} \end{Bmatrix}
\tag{21a}
$$

$$
Q_{ij}^{I} = \sum_{k=1}^{N} (C_{ij}^{G})_{k} (z_{k} - z_{k-1}) , \quad Q_{ij}^{II} = \frac{1}{2} \sum_{k=1}^{N} (C_{ij}^{G})_{k} (z_{k}^{2} - z_{k-1}^{2}) ,
$$

$$
Q_{ij}^{III} = \frac{1}{3} \sum_{k=1}^{N} (C_{ij}^{G})_{k} (z_{k}^{3} - z_{k-1}^{3})
\tag{21b}
$$

In equation (21a), the quantities dN_{xx}, dN_{yy}, dN_{xy}, dM_{xx}, dM_{yy}, and dM_{xy} are the overall incremental in-plane forces and moments per unit length exerted on the laminate respectively. Once the overall stress increments of the kth lamina are calculated through equation (18), they should be transformed into the local system (Figure 9–20(c)) before being substituted into the right hand side of equations (11a) and (11b) to determine the internal stress increments. The transformation formula from the global to the local systems is:

$$
\{d\sigma\} = [T]_{s}^{T} \{d\sigma\}^{G}
\tag{22}
$$

$$
\text{where} \quad [T]_{s} = \begin{bmatrix} l_{1}^{2} & l_{2}^{2} & l_{1}l_{2} \\ m_{1}^{2} & m_{2}^{2} & m_{1}m_{2} \\ 2l_{1}m_{1} & 2l_{2}m_{2} & l_{1}m_{2} + l_{2}m_{1} \end{bmatrix}
\tag{23}
$$

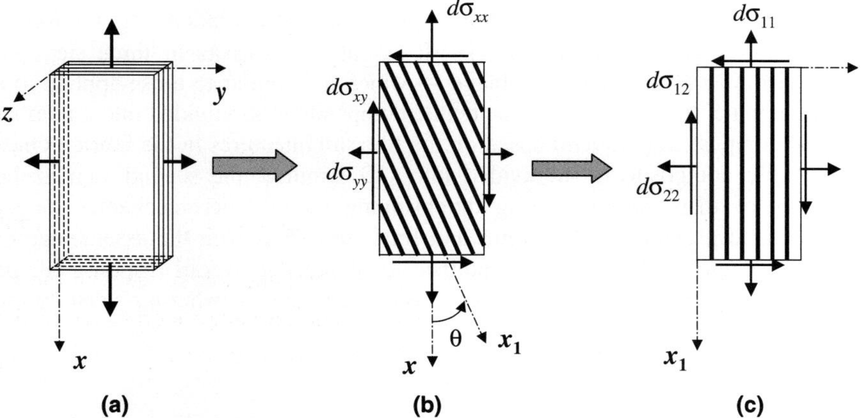

Figure 9–20 Analysis procedure for a tape laminate

As with the application of external loads, some laminae must fail before the others. Once a lamina fails, it no longer contributes to the remaining analysis of the laminate [85]. The overall instantaneous stiffness matrix of the laminate must be discounted from the failed lamina. Supposing the k_0^{th} lamina ply has failed, the remaining laminate stiffness elements are defined as follows [82]:

$$Q_{ij}^{I} = \sum_{\substack{k=1 \\ k \neq k_0}}^{N} (C_{ij}^{G})_k (z_k - z_{k-1}) , \quad Q_{ij}^{II} = \frac{1}{2} \sum_{\substack{k=1 \\ k \neq k_0}}^{N} (C_{ij}^{G})_k (z_k^2 - z_{k-1}^2) ,$$

$$Q_{ij}^{III} = \frac{1}{3} \sum_{\substack{k=1 \\ k \neq k_0}}^{N} (C_{ij}^{G})_k (z_k^3 - z_{k-1}^3) \tag{24}$$

In this way, a progressive failure process of the laminate can be identified and accordingly, its ultimate strength can be determined.

9.4.5.3 *Modeling procedure for a textile composite*

As shown in Figure 9–1, composites reinforced with textile fabrics are widely used in biomedical applications. A textile fabric refers to a fibrous structure made of continuous fiber yarns (bundles) by means of a textile technique. Three basic textile techniques can be employed to develop fibrous preforms (fabric structures) for bio-composite reinforcement. They are namely, weaving, braiding, and knitting. Correspondingly, the resulting composites are called woven fabric composites, braided fabric composites, and knitted fabric composites.

Although the fibrous structure of a textile composite is much more complicated than that of a tape laminate, the structure-property relationship of the former is analyzed in a manner somewhat similar to that of the latter. A schematic diagram to show the analysis procedure for a textile fabric reinforced composite is given in Figure 9–21. It essentially consists of three steps — subdivision, analysis, and assemblage — which are similar to those applied to a tape laminate. In the first step, the textile composite is subdivided into a number of UD composites (laminae) based on the fiber architectures in the fabric. Once the textile composite is subdivided into UD laminae, the second step is the analysis of these laminae using the bridging model micromechanics theory summarized previously. The third and final step deals with the assemblage of the contributions of all the UD laminae to obtain the overall response of the textile composite. Roughly speaking, the last step is somewhat a reverse to the first step.

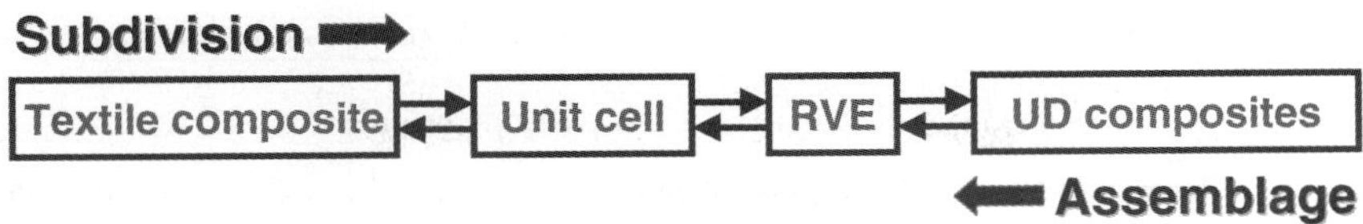

Figure 9–21 Analysis procedure for a textile fabric reinforced composite

9.4.5.4 *Analysis outline for a braided fabric composite*

As can be understood from the aforementioned procedure, the difference in the analyses of different fabric reinforced composites lies in the first (discretization) and last (assemblage) steps, which are more related to a geometrical rather than mechanical analysis.   A schematic diagram to show the discretization of a diamond braided composite into UD laminae is graphed in Figure 9–22. The whole fabric structure (Figure 9–22(a)) can be constructed by repeating some unit cell (Figure 9–22(b)), which can be further divided into four identical or symmetrical sub-cells. One such sub-cell together with the surrounding matrix is taken as a representative volume element (RVE) for the composite (Figure 9–22(a)). Thus, the analysis for the braided fabric composite can be achieved by the analysis of the RVE.

The RVE is subdivided in the fabric plane into sub-elements, as shown in Figure 9–22(c). Each sub-element (Figure 9–22(d)) has at most four material layers: braider yarn 1 (e.g., warp yarn), braider yarn 2 (e.g., fill yarn), and the top and bottom pure matrix layers. Note that the warp and fill yarns have already been impregnated with the polymer matrix. These material layers are considered as UD laminae in their respective local coordinate systems, while both the pure matrix layers are regarded as a UD composite with zero fiber volume fraction — as indicated in Figures 9–22(e) to 9–22(g). The mechanical responses of these UD laminae are determined by using the bridging model summarized previously. An assemblage of the three UD laminae gives the responses of a sub-element. An assemblage of the contributions of all the sub-elements then gives rise to the overall properties of the composite (RVE). For more details, refer to Huang (2000) [86].

To successfully accomplish the subdivision followed by assemblage, the fiber yarn orientation in the RVE must be specified. For a plain weave or a diamond braid, Huang (2000) [86] proposed a geometric model in which only limited geometric parameters such as the yarn thickness and width and the inter-yarn gap are required. Huang and Ramakrishna (2002) [87] also gave a general description of the geometric model for a 2D biaxial woven or braided fabric structure.

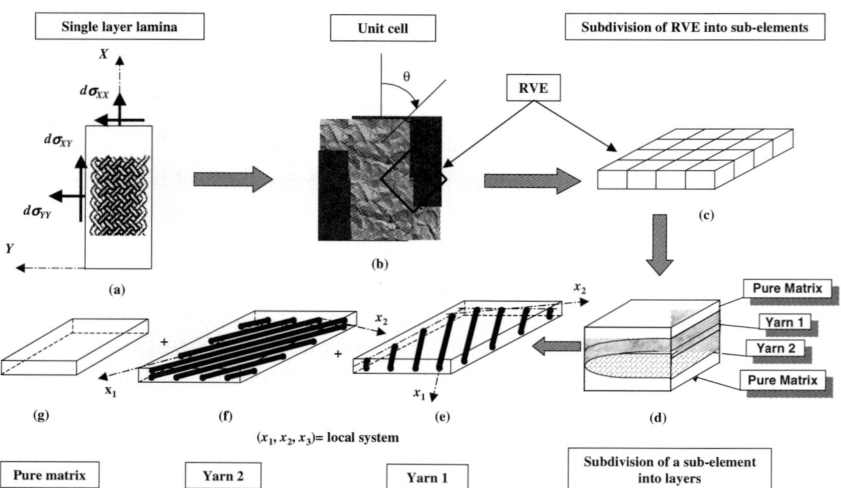

Figure 9–22 Subdivision of a braided fabric composite into UD laminae

9.4.5.5 *Analysis outline for a knitted fabric composite*

Figure 9–23 shows the analysis steps for a laminate reinforced with multi-layers of knitted fabric composite lamina. Several single-layer resin-impregnated knitted fabrics (Figure 9–23(a)) are stacked together (Figure 9–23(b)) to make a laminate panel, which is subjected to an arbitrary load condition as indicated in Figure 9–23(c). An incremental solution is applied. The load components sustained by each layer of the laminate in the global coordinate system (Figure 9–23(d)) is determined by using a laminate analysis procedure [88]. Before proceeding to the analysis for a single layer of the knitted fabric composite, a coordinate transformation is necessary to transform the stress state in the global coordinate system into the ply system (Figure 9–23(e)).

The analysis steps for a single layer of the knitted fabric composite are schematically shown in Figure 9–24, with respect to the ply coordinate system. Figure 9–24(a) shows that the entire fabric can be constructed using a repeating unit cell (Figure 9–24(b)), which can be further divided into four symmetrical or identical sub-cells. One such sub-cell is taken as the RVE for the knitted fabric composite, as indicated in Figure 9–24(c).

There are two yarns in the RVE, whose geometric positions are critical. Fortunately, for the present plain weft-knitted fabric structure, the Leaf and Glaskin model can be employed to specify its geometry [89]. For the geometrical descriptions of some other fabric structures, please refer to Huang and Ramakrishna (2000) [90].

The RVE in Figure 9–24(c) is subdivided into even smaller elements along the *x*-direction. Due to the small element size after subdivision, the yarn segment together with its surrounding matrix can be regarded as a UD composite which has an inclined angle with the *x*-direction (Figure 9–24(d)). The response of the UD composite in its local coordinate system is determined through the bridging model. Then, the RVE properties can be obtained by assembling the contributions of all the sub-elements. More details can be found in Huang *et al.* (1999) [89], Huang and Ramakrishna (2000) [90], and Huang *et al.* (2001) [88].

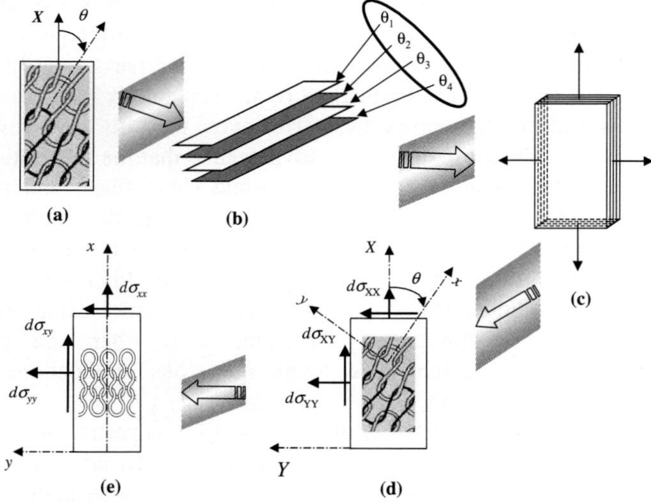

Figure 9–23 Analysis of a knitted fabric reinforced laminate

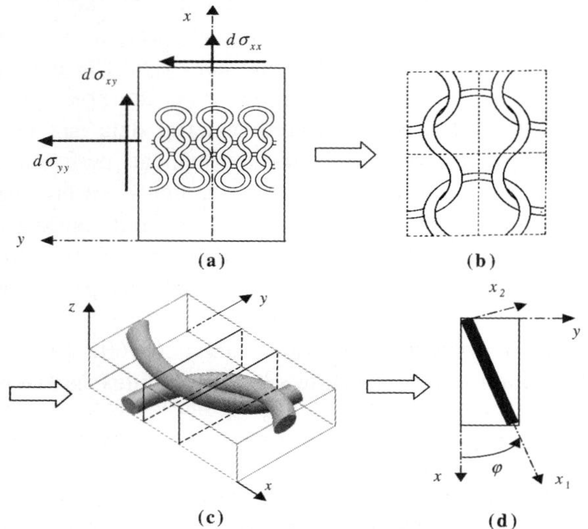

Figure 9–24 Analysis steps for a single layer of knitted fabric reinforced composite

9.4.6 *Mechanical Properties of Short Fiber and Particulate Composites*

Composites reinforced with short (chopped or whisker) fibers and particulates constitute another class of composite materials for bioengineering applications. For short fiber composites, three types of reinforcements can occur: uniaxially aligned short fibers, off-axially aligned short fibers, and randomly oriented short fibers. The first two types have their fiber orientations in the same direction — they are hence rarely found in reality, whereas the third type is the most common. Compared with continuous fiber counterparts, the mechanical performance of short fiber and particulate reinforcements is inferior: they have lower stiffness and strength properties. However, they do have several very attractive features. The most significant advantage is that the fabrication cost of short fiber (especially that of randomly oriented short fiber) and particulate reinforced composites is low. Another advantage is that these composites can assume very complicated contour geometry. Short fibers and particulates can be easily mixed with liquid polymer resin, and the resin-fiber mixture can be fabricated in large volumes into complex component shapes using injection or compression molding technique. Therefore, short fiber and particulate reinforced polymer composites have found numerous applications in areas where a secondary load is applied.

Randomly oriented short fiber composites as well as particulate composites display isotropic characteristics when subjected to an external load. For these composites, perhaps the simplest as well as the best way to understand their mechanical response is through an experiment. However, the experimental measurement can be performed only after composite fabrication has been accomplished. This is not convenient for composite design. Although randomly oriented short fiber and particulate composites are essentially isotropic, they are basically different from conventionally homogeneous isotropic materials such as metals. For the latter materials, measured material data can be used in the design. However for a composite, its mechanical performance depends significantly on fillers (reinforcements) — the contents, arrangements, shapes, and properties of these fillers. Knowledge of the relationship between the mechanical performance of the resulting composite and the properties and geometric information of its constituent materials brings great benefit to composite design.

For particulate reinforced composites, Paul (1960) [91] obtained an approximation equation for the composite's elastic modulus, as given below:

$$E = E_m \frac{E_m + (E_d - E_m)V_d^{2/3}}{E_m + (E_d - E_m)V_d^{2/3}(1 - V_d^{1/3})} \qquad (25)$$

where E_m is the matrix modulus, E_d the particulate (dispersion) modulus, and V_d the volume fraction of the particulate (dispersion). Using this formula, Paul calculated the moduli of tungsten carbide particulate reinforced cobalt matrix composites and compared with his measurements. Good correlation was reported.

As for short fiber composites, Cox (1952) [92] using a RVE shown in Figure 9–25 derived a formula for the longitudinal modulus of a uniaxially aligned short fiber composite, as shown below:

$$E_{11} = \left[1 - \frac{\sinh(\beta L/2)}{(\beta L/2)\cosh(\beta L/2)} \right] V_f E_{11}^f + V_m E_m \tag{26a}$$

$$\beta^2 = \frac{2\pi G_m}{A_f E_{11}^f \ln(D/d)} \tag{26b}$$

where x_1 is along the fiber axial direction, L is the fiber length, d is the fiber diameter, $A_f = 0.25\pi d^2$ is the fiber cross-sectional area, G_m is the shear modulus of the matrix, and D is the outer diameter of the RVE (Figure 9–25). Suppose the distance between the two adjacent fiber ends is e (Figure 9–25) and the fiber volume fraction is V_f, the following formula is derived:

$$\ln(D/d) = \frac{L}{2V_f(L+e)} \tag{26c}$$

Halpin and Tsai proposed a set of empirical formulae, known as Halpin–Tsai equations, which can also be used to estimate the engineering moduli of a uniaxially aligned short fiber composite. The Halpin–Tsai equations read as follows:

$$E_{11} = E_m \frac{1+\xi\eta V_f}{1-\eta V_f} \tag{27a}$$

$$E_{22} = E_m \frac{1+\varsigma\lambda_1 V_f}{1-\lambda_1 V_f} \tag{27b}$$

$$G_{12} = G_m \frac{1+\varsigma\lambda_2 V_f}{1-\lambda_2 V_f} \tag{27c}$$

$$\eta = \frac{E_{11}^f/E_m - 1}{E_{11}^f/E_m + \xi}, \quad \xi = 2L/d, \quad \lambda_1 = \frac{E_{22}^f/E_m - 1}{E_{22}^f/E_m + \varsigma}, \quad \lambda_2 = \frac{G_{12}^f/E_m - 1}{G_{12}^f/E_m + \varsigma} \tag{27d}$$

In the above equations, ζ is a "curve-fitting" parameter which can be taken as '2' for E_{22} and '1' for G_{12} if no other information is available [93]. Halpin (1969) [94] also concluded that v_{12} is not significantly affected by fiber length. Therefore, equation (7b) can be used to calculate v_{12}.

The elastic properties of an off-axially aligned short fiber composite can be obtained through a coordinate transformation, which is derived as follows:

$$[S_{ij}^G] = [T_{ij}]_s [S_{ij}] [T_{ij}]_s^T \tag{28}$$

where $[T_{ij}]_s$ is given by equation (23). Note that the compliance matrix, $[S_{ij}]$, of the uniaxially aligned short fiber composite used in equation (28) needs to be defined using the Halpin–Tsai equations, as the Cox equations are not adequate for this purpose.

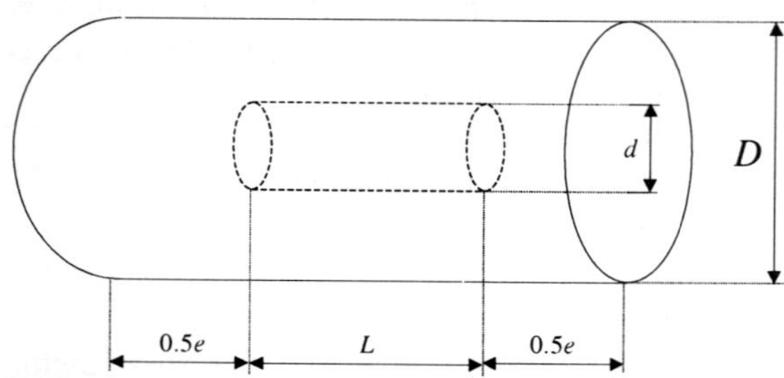

Figure 9–25 A RVE for uniaxial aligned short fiber composite

As mentioned before, randomly oriented short fiber composites display isotropic behaviors. If the fiber length is significantly larger than the composite's thickness, which may occur in composite panels made from sheet-molding compounds or resin transfer moldings, then composite isotropy occurs in the composite plane. In such a case, the Cox model gives the following approximation to the composite's Young's modulus and Poisson's ratio [95]:

$$E = E_{11}^{f} V_f /3, \quad \nu = 1/3 \tag{29a}$$

If, however, the composite is truly three-dimensional, *i.e.*, the fiber length is significantly smaller than the composite's thickness, the Cox model gives another pair of formulae for the composite's Young's modulus and Poisson's ratio — as shown below:

$$E = E_{11}^{f} V_f /6, \quad \nu = 1/4 \tag{29b}$$

The development of strength theories for short fiber or particulate composites is far behind that of continuous fiber composites. Only several attempts have been made to provide theoretical analysis of the tensile strength of short fiber reinforced polymer matrix composites [96]. For a reasonable engineering estimation, a modification to the rule of mixture formula has been effectively used as follows [96]:

$$\sigma_c = \sigma_p V_p + \sigma_f V_f \varepsilon_1 \varepsilon_0 \tag{30}$$

where σ_c is the tensile strength of the composite;

$\quad$ σ_p is the tensile strength of the polymer;

$\quad$ σ_f is the tensile strength of reinforcing fibers;

$\quad$ V is the volume fraction;

$\quad$ ε_0 is an efficiency factor related to the orientation of fibers in the composite;

$\quad$ ε_1 is an efficiency factor related to the effectiveness of load transfer between the fiber and matrix.

According to Bigg (1990) [96], if the fibers are uniaxially oriented, ε_0 is 1.0. When they are randomly dispersed in a plane, the value of ε_0 is 0.33. For very small reinforcing fibers, three-dimensional random isotropy is possible, in which case ε_0 is approximately 0.162. In a complex part, ε_0 can have different localized values. In such cases, a finite element analysis for that part can be made, taking the localized fiber orientation into account. One of the primary problems associated with designing short fiber reinforced composites is their anisotropy. Different regions of a molded part will have not only different fiber orientations but also different fiber concentrations. Moreover, fiber orientations may be varied not only in the in-plane dimension but also within the thickness of the part.

Besides the problems associated with ε_0 determination, the value of ε_1 is even more difficult to determine because it is different for each polymer-fiber combination. For example, the value of ε_1 is strongly affected by the effectiveness of coupling agents. ε_1 is equal to 1.0 for continuous fibers. For discontinuous fibers, ε_1 is related to the critical aspect ratio for the fiber-matrix combination. The equation used to establish the critical fiber aspect ratio is as follows [96]:

$$(L/D)_c = \sigma_f/(2\tau_1) \tag{31}$$

where σ_f is the tensile strength of the fiber, and τ_1 is the interfacial strength between the fiber and the matrix.

The shear strength of the polymer is often used as an estimate for τ_1 [97]. In most cases, however, τ_1 is determined from fiber pull-out experiments [98]. Typical values of $\varepsilon_0\varepsilon_1$ for short glass fiber reinforced injection molded materials range between 0.10 and 0.18. For carbon fiber reinforced compounds, they can be as high as 0.25; while for less well bonded fibers such as aramid, $\varepsilon_0\varepsilon_1$ can be as low as 0.07.

9.5   Future Advances

It is a relatively recent clinical practice where composite materials are used in biomedical applications. For implants which have been developed based on composite technology, many are still at laboratory-development stage. One major flaw is the lack of proper design theory with composite materials [99]. Many researchers used directly the design standards which were originally developed for isotropic materials to produce polymer composite implants. However, composite materials are distinctly different from homogenous materials in terms of anisotropy, fracture behavior, and environmental sensitivity. As such, polymer composite implants must be designed using criteria separate from those intended for isotropic material-based implants. Innovations — such as spatially-varying fiber contents and reinforcing structures — are adding new types of functionally graded composite materials to implant applications. New design criteria need to be developed to explore the potential of this new class of materials and to design implants with improved performance.

The success of polymer composites as biomaterials also relies substantially on implants quality — which is determined by the reproducibility of the fabrication process. Current practices use a trial-and-error approach, resulting in limited success in clinical applications. The composite fabrication methods employed in engineering applications have been directly adopted for producing implants. It is important to realize that the requirements for the two applications are different. Hence the composite fabrication methods for biomedical applications must be modified to meet the specific needs of each application. For example, in a hip joint replacement application, the composite material surface should be completely covered with a continuous matrix layer to prevent any potential release of fiber particle debris during implantation. Moreover, the fabrication method needs to be optimized such that it enables desired local and global arrangements of reinforcement phase so as to make the composite implant structurally compatible with the host tissues. Thus far, polymer composite biomaterials are mainly reinforced with particulates, short fibers, and unidirectional fiber prepregs — very few reports on woven fabric composites are available. The many advantages offered by textile composite materials have not been well exploited in the biomedical field. Efforts should be made to harness the potential of textile composite materials in designing implants with improved performance.

It is now clear that for greater success, implants should be surface compatible as well as structurally compatible with the host tissues. In this regard, polymer composite biomaterials are particularly attractive because of their tailorable manufacturing processes, as well as properties that are comparable to those of the host tissues. In addition, other factors help to heighten the appeal of polymer composite biomaterials. Innovations in composite material design, improvements in polymer matrices and fabrication processes — all these raise the possibility of achieving implants with improved performance. However, for successful application, surgeons must be convinced with the long-term durability and reliability of polymer composite biomaterials. Monolithic materials have long been used and there are considerable experimental and clinical data supporting their continued usage. Such data in terms of polymer composite biomaterials are relatively scarce. Considerable research efforts are required to elucidate the long-term durability of composite biomaterials in the human body conditions. Nevertheless, in view of their promising potential of high performance, composite materials are likely to be increasingly utilized as biomaterials in the future.

Appendix

Acronym	Meaning
BIS–GMA	bis-phenol A glycidyl methacrylate
C	Carbon
CF	Carbon fibers
GF	Glass fibers
HA	Hydroxyapatite
HDPE	High density polyethylene
KF	Kevlar fiber
LCP	Liquid crystalline polymer
LDPE	Low density polyethylene
MMA	Methylmethacrylate
PA	Polyacetal
PBT	Polybutylene terephthalate
PC	Polycarbonate
PCL	Polycaprolactone
PE	Polyethylene
PEA	Polyethylacrylate
PEEK	Polyetheretherketone
PEG	Polyethylene glycol
PELA	Block copolymer of lactic acid and polyethylene glycol
PET	Polyethylene terepthalate
PGA	Polyglycolic acid
PHB	Polyhydroxybutyrate
PHEMA	Poly(HEMA) or Poly(2–hydroxyethyl methacrylate)
PLA	Polylactic acid
PLDLA	Poly L–DL–lactide
PLLA	Poly(L–lactic acid)
PMA	Polymethylacrylate
PMMA	Polymethylmethacrylate
Polyglactin	Copolymer of PLA and PGA
PP	Polypropylene
PS	Polysulfone
PTFE	Polytetrafluroethylene
PU	Polyurethane
PVC	Polyvinylchloride
SR	Silicone rubber
THFM	Tetrahydrofurfuryl methacrylate
UHMWPE	Ultra-high molecular weight polyethylene

References

1. G. O. Hofmann, Biodegradable implants in orthopedic surgery — A review on the state-of-the-art, Clinical Materials, 1992, 10:75–80.
2. K. P. Baidya, S. Ramakrishna, M. Rahman, A. Ritchie, and Z. M. Huang, An investigation on the polymer composite medical device — external fixator, Journal of Reinforced Plastics & Composites, 2003, 22(6):563–590.
3. P. Tormala, J. Vasenius, S. Vainionpaa, J. Laiho, T. Pohjonen, and P. Rokkanen, Ultra-high-strength absorbable self-reinforced polyglycolide (SR–PGA) composite rods for internal fixation of bone fractures: *In vitro* and *in vivo* study, J. Biomedical Materials Research, 1991, 25:1–22.
4. K. B. Chandran and S. W. Shalaby, Soft tissue replacements, in The Biomedical Engineering Handbook, ed. J. D. Bronzino, (CRC Press, 1995) pp:648–665.
5. B. J-L. Moyen, P. J. Lahey, E. H. Weinberg, and W. H. Harris, Effects on intact femora of dogs of the application and removal of metal plates, J. Bone and Joint Surgery, 1978, 60A(7):940–947.
6. H. K. Uhthoff and M. Finnegan, The effects of metal plates on post-traumatic remodeling and bone mass, J Bone and Joint Surgery, 1983, 65B(1):66–71.
7. P. Christel, L. Claes, and S. A. Brown, Carbon reinforced composites in orthopedic surgery, in High Performance Biomaterials: A Comprehensive Guide to Medical and Pharmaceutical Applications, ed. M. Szycher, (Technomic Publishing Co., Inc., Lancaster, USA, 1991) pp:499–518.
8. J. S. Bradley, G. W. Hastings, and C. Johnson-Nurse, Carbon fiber reinforced epoxy as a high strength, low modulus material for internal fixation plates, Biomaterials, 1980, 1:38–40.
9. G. B. McKenna, G. W. Bradley, H. K. Dunn, and W. O. Statton, Mechanical properties of some fiber reinforced polymer composites after implantation as fracture fixation plates, Biomaterials, 1980, 1:189–192.
10. K. Tayton, C. Johnson-Nurse, B. Mckibbin, J. Bradleym, and G. W. Hastings, The use of semi-rigid carbon fiber reinforced plastic plates for fixation of human fractures, J. Bone and Joint Surgery, 1982, 64B(1):105–111.
11. G. Peluso, L. Ambrosio, M. Cinquegrani, L. Nicolis, S. Saiello, and G. Tajana, Rat peritoneal immune response to carbon fiber reinforced epoxy composite implants, Biomaterials, 1991, 12:231–235.
12. C. Morrison, R. Macnair, C. MacDonald, A. Wykman, I. Goldie, and M. H. Grant, *In vitro* biocompatibility testing of polymers for orthopedic implants using cultured fibroblasts and osteoblasts, Biomaterials, 1995, 16(13):987–992.
13. S. Ramakrishna, J. Mayer, E. Wintermantel, and K. W. Leong, Biomedical applications of polymer-composite materials: a review, Comp. Sci. & Tech., 2001, 61(9):1189–1224.
14. K. Fujihara, Z. M. Huang, S. Ramakrishna, K. Satkunananntham, and H. Hamada, Development of braided carbon/PEEK composite bone plates, Advanced Composite Letters, 2001, 10(1):13–20.
15. J. Choueka, J. L. Charvet, H. Alexander, Y. H. Oh, G. Joseph, N. C. Blumenthal, and W. C. LaCourse, Effect of annealing temperature on the degradation of reinforcing fibers for absorbable implants, J. Biomedical Materials Research, 1995, 29:1309–1315.

16. M. Zimmerman, J. R. Parsons, and H. Alexander, The design and analysis of a laminated partially degradable composite bone plate for fracture fixation, J. Biomedical Materials Research: Applied Biomaterials, 1987, 21(A3):345–361.

17. P. Tormala, S. Vainionpaa, J. Kilpikari, and P. Rokkanen, The effects of fiber reinforcement and gold plating on the flexural and tensile strength of PGA/PLA copolymer materials *in vitro*, Biomaterials, 1987, 8:42–45.

18. A. Nazre and S. Lin, Theoretical strength comparison of bioabsorbable (PLLA) plates and conventional stainless steel and titanium plates used in internal fracture fixation, in Clinical and Laboratory Performance of Bone Plates, eds. J. P. Harvey Jr. and F. Games, 1994, pp:53–64.

19. T. W. Lin, A. A. Corvelli, C. G. Frondoza, J. C. Roberts, and D. S. Hungerford, Glass peek composite promotes proliferation and osteocalcin production of human osteoblastic cells, J. Biomedical Materials Research, 1997, 36(2):137–144.

20. J. Kettunen, A. Makela, H. Miettinen, T. Nevalainen, M. Heikkila, P. Tormala, and P. Rokkanen, Fixation of femoral shaft osteotomy with an intramedullary composite rod: An experimental study on dogs with a two-year follow-up, J. Biomaterials Science Polymer Edition, 1999, 10(1):33–45.

21. M. van der Elst, C. P. A. T. Klein, P. Patka, and H. J. T. M. Haarman, Biodegradable fracture fixation devices, in Biomaterials and Bioengineering Handbook, ed. D. L. Wise, (Marcel Dekker, Inc., New York, 2000), pp:509–524.

22. N. Ashammakhi and P. Rokkanen, Absorbable polyglycolide devices in trauma and bone surgery, Biomaterials, 1997, 18:3–9.

23. P. Tormala, P. Rokkanen, J. Laiho, *et al.*, Material for osteosynthesis devices, US Patent 4,743,257, 1988.

24. S. Ramakrishna and Z. M. Huang, Biocomposite materials, in Comprehensive Structural Integrity, Vol. 9: Bioengineering, eds. S. H. Teoh and Y. W. Mai, (Elsevier Science Publisher, UK, 2003) (in press).

25. S. Santavirta, Y. T. Konttinen, T. Saito, *et al.*, Immune response to polyglycolide acid implants, J. Bone and Joint Surgery, 1990, 72(B):597–600.

26. O. Bostman, E. K. Partio, E. Hirvensalo, *et al.*, Foreign-body reactions to polyglycolide screws, Acta Ortop Scand, 1992, 63:173–176.

27. A. Ignatius, K. Unterricker, K. Wenger, M. Richter, and L. Claes, A new composite made of polyurethane and glass ceramic in a loaded implant model: a biomechanical and histological analysis, J. Materials Science: Materials in Medicine, 1997, 8:753–756.

28. L. Claes, M. Schultheiss, S. Wolf, H. J. Wilke, M. Arand, and L. Kinzl, A new radiolucent system for vertebral body replacement: Its stability in comparison to other systems, J. Biomedical Materials Research — Applied Biomaterials, 1999, 48(1):82–89.

29. M. Marcolongo, P. Ducheyne, J. Garino, and E. Schepers, Bioactive glass fiber/polymeric composites bond to bone tissue, J. Biomedical Materials Research, 1998, 9(1):161–170.

30. J. W. Brantigan, A. D. Steffee, and J. M. Geiger, A carbon fiber implant to aid interbody lumbar fusion mechanical testing, Spine, 1991, 16(6S):S277–S282.

31. P. Ciappetta, S. Boriani, and G. P. Fava, A carbon fiber reinforced polymer cage for vertebral body replacement: A technical note, Neurosurgery, 1997, 41(5):1203–1206.

32. Q. B. Bao, G. M. McCullen, P. A. Higham, J. H. Dumbleton, and H. A. Yuan, The artificial disc: theory, design and materials, Biomaterials, 1996, 17:1157–1167.

33. J. R. Urbaniak, D. S. Bright, and J. E. Hopkins, Replacement of intervertebral discs in chimpanzees by silicone–Dacron implants: A preliminary report, J. Biomedical Materials Research Symposium, 1973, 4:165–186.

34. S. Ramakrishna, S. Ramaswamy, S. H. Teoh, and C. T. Tan, Development of a knitted fabric reinforced elastomeric composite intervertebral disc prosthesis, Proc. ICCM–11, Vol. 1, (Conard Jupiters–Golad Coast, Australia, 1997) pp:458–466.

35. L. Ambrosio, P. A. Netti, S. Iannace, S. J. Huang, and L. Nicolais, Composite hydrogels for intervertebral disc prostheses, J. Materials Science: Materials in medicine, 1996, 7:251–254.

36. K. H. Bridwell, R. L. DeWald, J. P. Lubicky, D. L. Spencer, K. W. Hammerberg, D. R. Benson, and M. G. Neuwirth, The textbook of spinal surgery, (J. B. Lippincott Company, Philadelphia, USA, 1991).

37. K. H. G. Schmitt-Thomas, Z. G. Yang, and T. Hiermer, Performace characterization of polymeric composite implant rod subjected to torsion, Proceedings of ICCM–11, (Gold Coast, Australia, 1997) pp:V277–V286.

38. N. Rushton and T. Rae, The intra-articular response to particulate carbon fiber reinforced high density polyethylene and its constituents: an experimental study in mice, Biomaterials, 1984, 5:352–356.

39. M. Deng and S. W. Shalaby, Properties of self-reinforced ultra-high-molecular weight polyethylene composites, Biomaterials, 1997, 18:645–655.

40. H. Gese, *et al.*, Relativbewegungen und stress-shielding bei zementfreien Hüftendoprothesen - eine Analyse mit der Methode der Finiten Elemente, in Die zementlose Hüftprothese, (Demeter Verlag, Gräfelfing, 1992), pp:75–80.

41. K. R. John St., in Applications of Advanced Composites in Orthopedic Implants. Biocompatible Polymers, Metals, and Composites, ed. M. Szycher, (Technomic Publishing Co., Inc., Lancaster, USA, 1983) pp:861–871.

42. P. Christel, A. Meunier, and S. Leclercq, Development of a carbon-carbon hip prosthesis, J. Biomedical Materials Research, 1987, 21:191–218.

43. F. K. Chang, J. L. Perez, and J. A. Davidson, Stiffness and strength tailoring of a hip prosthesis made of advanced composite materials, J. Biomedical Materials Research, 1990, 24:873–899.

44. J. A. Simoes, A. T. Marques, and G. Jeronimidis, Design of a controlled-stiffness composite proximal femoral prosthesis, Comp. Sci. & Tech., 1999, 60:559–567.

45. E. Wintermantel and J. Mayer, Anisotropic biomaterials strategies and developments for bone implants, in Encyclopedic Handbook of Biomaterials and Bioengineering, Part B–1, eds. D. L. Wise, D. J. Trantolo, D. E. Altobelli, J. D. Yaszemiski, J. D. Gresser, and E. R. Schwartz, (Marcel Dekker, New York, 1995) pp:3–42.

46. E. Wintermantel, A. Bruinink, K. Eckert, K. Ruffiex, M. Petitmermet, and J. Mayer, Tissue engineering supported with structured biocompatible materials: goals and achievements, in Materials in Medicine, ed. M. O. Speidel, (ETH Zurich, Switzerland, 1998) pp:1–136.

47. M. Akay and N. Aslan, Numerical and experimental stress analysis of a polymeric composite hip joint prostheses, J. Biomedical Materials Research, 1996, 31:167–182.

48. S. Saha and S. Pal, Mechanical properties of bone cement: a review, J. Biomedical Materials Research, 1984, 18:435–462.

49. H. D. Wagner and D. Cohn, Use of high-performance polyethylene fibers as a reinforcing phase in poly(methylmethacrylate) bone cement, Biomaterials, 1989, 10:139–141.

50. J. M. Yang, P. Y. Huang, M. C. Yang, and S. K. Lo, Effect of MMA–g–UHMWPE grafted fiber on mechanical properties of acrylic bone cement, J. Biomedical Materials Research, 1997, 38(4):361–369.

51. R. M. Pilliar, R. Blackwell, I. Macnab, and H. U. Cameron, Carbon fiber reinforced bone cement in orthopedic surgery, J. Biomedical Materials Research, 1976, 10:893–906.

52. J. L. Gilbert, D. S. Ney, and E. P. Lautenschlager, Self-reinforced composite poly(methyl methacrylate): static and fatigue properties, Biomaterials, 1995, 16(14):1043–1055.

53. L. D. T. Topoleski, P. Ducheyne, and J. M. Cuckler, The fracture toughness of titanium-fiber-reinforced bone cement, J. Biomedical Materials Research, 1992, 26:1599–1617.

54. J. B. Park and R. S. Lakes, Biomaterials: An introduction, (Plenum Press, New York, 1992) pp:169–183.

55. J. Tamura, K. Kawanabe, T. Yamamuro, T. Nakamura, T. Kokubo, S. Yoshihara, and T. Shibuya, Bioactive bone cement: The effect of amounts of glass powder and histologic changes with time, J. Biomedical Materials Research, 1995, 29:551–559.

56. T. N. Gerhart, R. L. Miller, S. J. Kleshinski, and W. C. Hayes, *In vitro* characterization and biomechanical optimization of a biodegradable particulate composite bone cement, J. Biomedical Materials Research, 1988, 22:1071–1082.

57. Q. Liu, J. R. de Wijn, and C. A. van Blitterwijk, Composite biomaterials with chemical bonding between hydroxyapatite filler particles and PEG/PBT copolymer matrix, J. Biomedical Materials Research, 1998, 40(3):490–497.

58. S. Higashi, T. Yamamuro, T. Nakamura, Y. Ikada, S. H. Hyon, and K. Jamshidi, Polymer-hydroxyapatite composites for biodegradable bone fillers, Biomaterials, 1986, 7:183–187.

59. W. Bonfield, M. D. Grynpas, A. E. Tully, J. Bowman, and J. Abram, Hydroxyapatite reinforced polyethylene — a mechanically compatible implant material for bone replacement, Biomaterials, 1981, 2:185–186.

60. C. P. A. T. Klein, H. B. M. van der Lubbe, and K. de Groot, A plastic composite of alginate with calcium phosphate granules as implant material: an *in vivo* study, Biomaterials, 1987, 8:308–310.

61. W. R. Krause, S. H. Park, and R. A. Straup, Mechanical properties of BIS–GMA resin short glass fiber composites, J. Biomedical Materials Research, 1989, 23:1195–1211.

62. F. Issidor, P. Odman, and K. Brondum, Intermittent loading of teeth restored using prefabricated carbon fiber posts, Int. J. Prosthodontics, 1996, 9(2):131–136.

63. S. Ramakrishna, V. K. Ganesh, S. H. Teoh, P. L. Loh, and C. L. Chew, Fiber reinforced composite product with graded stiffness, Singapore Patent Application No. 9800874–1, 1998.

64. R. P. Kusy, A review of contemporary arch wires: Their properties and characteristics, The Angle Orthodontist, 1997, 67(3):197–207.

65. Z. M. Huang, R. Gopal, K. Fujihara, S. Ramakrishna, P. L. Loh, W. C. Foong, V. K. Ganesh, and C. L. Chew, Fabrication of a new composite orthodontic arch wire and validation by a bridging micromechanics model, Biomaterials, 2003, 24(17):2941–2953.

66. S. W. Zufall, K. C. Kennedy, and R. P. Kusy, Frictional characteristics of composite orthodontic arch wires against stainless steel and ceramic brackets in the passive and active configurations, J Materials Science: Materials in Medicine, 1998, 9:611–620.

67. M. A. Tallent, C. W. Cordova, D. S. Cordova, and D. S. Donnelly, Thermoplastic fibers for composite reinforcement, in International Encyclopedia of Composites, Vol. 2, ed. S. M. Lee, (VCH Publishers, New York, 1990) pp:466–480.

68. Z. M. Huang and S. Ramakrishna, Development of knitted fabric reinforced composite material for prosthetic application, Advanced Composites Letters, 1999, 8(6):289-293.

69. M. N. Pradas and R. D. Calleja, Reproduction in a polymer composite of some mechanical features of tendons and ligaments, in High Performance Biomaterials: A Comprehensive Guide to Medical and Pharmaceutical Applications, ed. M. Szycher, (Technomic Publishing Co., Inc., Lancaster, USA, 1991) pp:519–523.

70. B. B. Seedham, Ligament reconstruction with reference to the anterior cruciate ligament of the knee, in Mechanics of Human Joints: Physiology, Pathophysiology, and Treatment, eds. V. Wright and E. L. Radin, (Marcel Dekker Inc., New York, USA, 1993) pp:163–201.

71. S. Iannace, G. Sabatini, L. Ambrosio, and L. Nicolais, Mechanical behavior of composite artificial tendons and ligaments, Biomaterials, 1995, 16(9):675–680.

72. L. Ambrosio, R. De Santis, S. Iannace, P. A. Netti, and L. Nicolais, Viscoelastic behavior of composite ligament prostheses, J. Biomedical Materials Research, 1998, 42(1):6–12.

73. B. Gershon, D. Cohn, and G. Marom, Utilization of composite laminate theory in the design of synthetic soft tissues for biomedical prostheses, Biomaterials, 1990, 11:548–552.

74. B. Gershon, D. Cohn, and G. Marom, Compliance and ultimate strength of composite arterial prostheses, Biomaterials, 1992, 13:38–43.

75. N. Klein, M. L. Carciente, D. Cohn, G. Marom, G. Uretzky, and H. Peleg, Filament-wound composite soft tissue prostheses: controlling compliance and strength by water absorption and degradation, J. Materials Science: Materials in Medicine, 1993, 4:285–291.

76. B. D. Agarwal and L. J. Broutman, Analysis and performance of fiber composites, (John Wiley & Sons, Inc., New York, 1990).

77. B. T. Astrom, Manufacturing of polymer composites, (Chapman & Hall, London, UK, 1997).

78. K. K. Chawla, Composite materials science and engineering, (Spinger–Verlag, New York, USA, 1998).

79. Z. Maekawa, H. Hamada, A. Yokoyama, and S. Ueda, Tensile behavior of braided flat bar with a circular hole, J. of Japan Society for Comp. Mater., 1988, 14(3):116–123.

80. Z. M. Huang, Micromechanical strength formulae of unidirectional composites, Materials Letters, 1999, 40(4):164–169.

81. D. B. Gundel and F. E. Wawner, Comp. Sci. & Tech., 1997, 57:471.

82. Z. M. Huang, Simulation of the mechanical properties of fibrous composites by the bridging micromechanics model, Composites Part A, 2001a, 32(2):143–172.
83. Z. M. Huang, Modeling strength of multidirectional laminates under thermo-mechanical loads, J. Comp. Mater., 2001b, 35(4):281–315.
84. R. F. Gibson, Principles of composite material mechanics, (McGraw–Hill, Inc., New York, 1994) pp:201–207.
85. Z. M. Huang, K. Fujihara, and S. Ramakrishna, Bending failure characterization of laminated beams with braided fabric reinforcement, Advanced Composites Letters, 2003, 12(3):85–96.
86. Z. M. Huang, The mechanical properties of composites reinforced with woven and braided fabrics, Comp. Sci. & Tech., 2000, 60(4):479–498.
87. Z. M. Huang and S. Ramakrishna, Towards automatic designing of 2D biaxial woven and braided fabric reinforced composites, J. Comp. Mater., 2002, 36(13):1541–1579.
88. Z. M. Huang, Y. Z. Zhang, and S. Ramakrishna, Modeling progressive failure process of multilayer knitted fabric reinforced composite laminates, Comp. Sci. & Tech., 2001, 61(14):2033–2046.
89. Z. M. Huang, S. Ramakrishna, and A. A. O. Tay, A micromechanical approach to the tensile strength of a knitted fabric composite, J. of Comp. Maters., 1999, 33(19):1758–1791.
90. Z. M. Huang and S. Ramakrishna, Micromechanical modeling approaches for the stiffness and strength of knitted fabric composites: A review & comparative study, Composites A, 2000, 31(5):479–501.
91. B. Paul, Prediction of elastic constants of multiphase materials, Trans. Metallurgical Society of AIME, 1960, pp:36–41.
92. H. L. Cox, The elasticity and strength of paper and other fibrous materials, British Journal of Applied Physics, 1952, 3:72–79.
93. S. R. Swanson, Introduction to design and analysis with advanced composite materials, (Prentice–Hall International, Inc., New Jersey, USA, 1997).
94. J. C. Halpin, Stiffness and expansion estimates for oriented short fiber composites, J. Comp. Mater., 1969, 3:732–734.
95. T. W. Chou, Micromechanical design of fiber composites, (Cambridge University Press, Cambridge, UK, 1992).
96. D. M. Bigg, in International Encyclopedia of Composites, Vol. 2, ed. S. M. Lee, (VCH, New York, 1990) pp:10–34.
97. J. V. Milewski, Plst. Comp., 1982, 5(3):71.
98. Y. W. Mai and J. K. Kim, Composite interfaces, (Elsevier Science Publishers, UK, 1998).
99. T. E. Matikas and N. J. Pagano, Recent advances in composite science (editorial), Composites Part B, 1998, 29B:91–92.

CHAPTER 10

NEW METHODS AND MATERIALS IN PROSTHETICS FOR REHABILITATION OF LOWER LIMB AMPUTEES

Peter V. S. Lee

Division of Bioengineering
National University of Singapore
E-mail: bieplvs@nus.edu.sg

Restoration of gait in lower limb amputees requires the aid of an artificial limb or prosthesis. This chapter discusses the methods and materials related to lower limb prosthetics. Attention is paid particularly to the interface between the amputee's stump and the prosthesis, *i.e.*, the prosthetic socket, where man interfaces with machine. The basic considerations, background, and constraints of various state-of-the-art techniques applied to prosthetics are discussed. These include the function and safety of prostheses, computer-aided design and fabrication methods, prosthetic socket and foot designs. The field of prosthetics relies heavily on innovative use of existing materials often found in other industries. The choice of materials is primarily derived from novel methods used in prostheses fabrication or components design, in order to achieve both function and safety for the amputee.

10.1 Introduction

Rehabilitation can be broadly defined as practices that lead to functional physical recovery. It encompasses a wide variety of professionals that can include counselor therapist, doctor, and engineer, all working towards a similar goal. Rehabilitation engineering as Reswick [1] described is the application of science and technology to ameliorate the handicaps of individuals with disabilities. It applies methods and materials to design and manufacture devices suited to individuals in order to recover physical capabilities. A prosthesis or artificial limb is one such device that aims to substitute the loss of a limb with cosmetic and functional desirability to the amputee. Lower extremities amputation continues to be a major problem due to motor vehicle and landmine accidents, and vascular related diseases.

A lower limb prosthesis can consist of an assembly of several component parts such as socket, knee, shank, ankle, and foot as shown in Figure 10–1. It is no surprise that modern engineering methods and materials applicable to other industries, e.g., aerospace, have been used in the field of prosthetics. New technology has undoubtedly brought upon many accomplishments. How the wooden artificial limb of the 1950s is being transformed to a leg with flexible plastic socket, computer controlled knee, carbon-fiber shank, and energy storing foot is certainly commendable. In the 1996 Paralympics in Atlanta, Tony Volpentest of USA, a double-leg amputee set an athletic 100-meter record of 11.36 seconds — about two seconds behind the world record for able-bodied athletes — using modern prostheses.

This chapter focuses on the latest methods and materials that have impacted the field of prosthetics for rehabilitation of lower limb amputees. Prosthetics is only one of the many areas in rehabilitation. The other specialties would require chapters in their own rights.

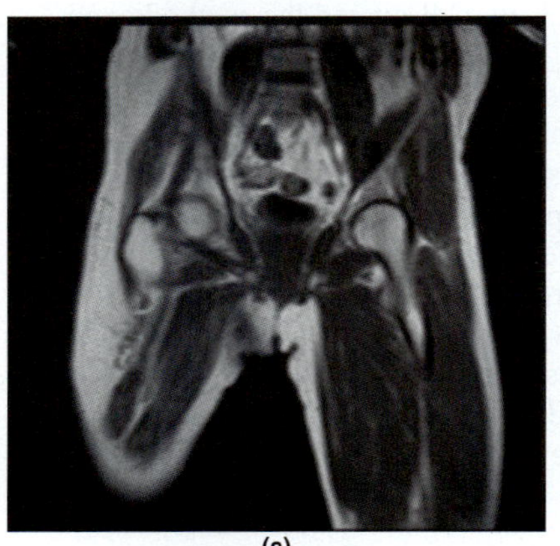

(a)

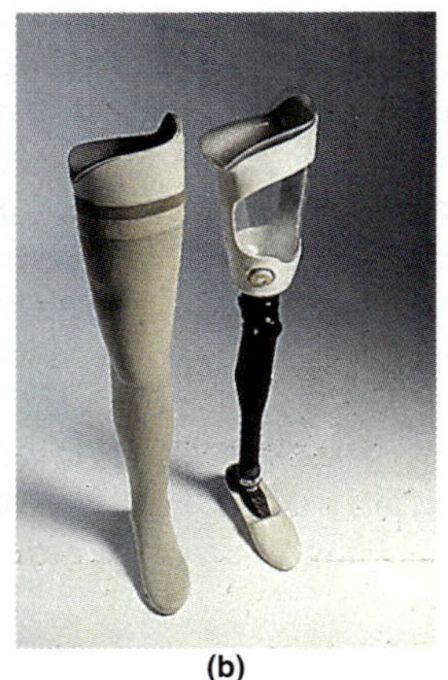

(b)

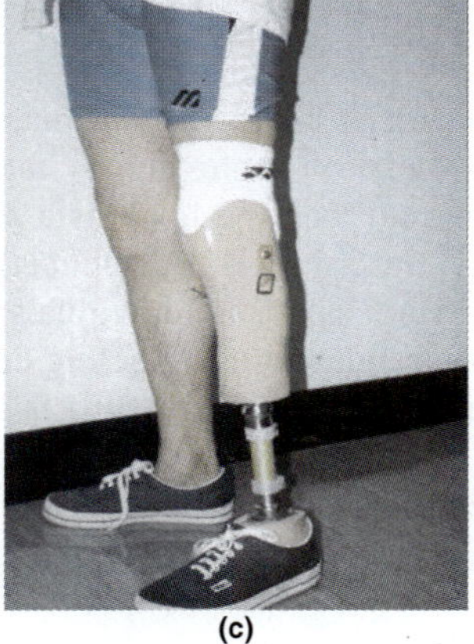

(c)

Figure 10–1 (a) MRI of trans-femoral (above-knee) amputation stump; (b) trans-femoral prostheses; (c) trans-tibial (below-knee) amputee wearing prosthesis

10.2 Function and Safety

The motivation to introduce new methods and materials is to improve function and safety for the amputee during walking. When a human walks, the position of the leg can be broken down into repetitive cycles consisting of swing and stance phases. At swing phase, the foot moves through the air; during stance or support phase, the foot is in contact with the ground. The stance phase can then be further divided into heel contact, mid stance and toe off or push off phases (Figure 10–2).

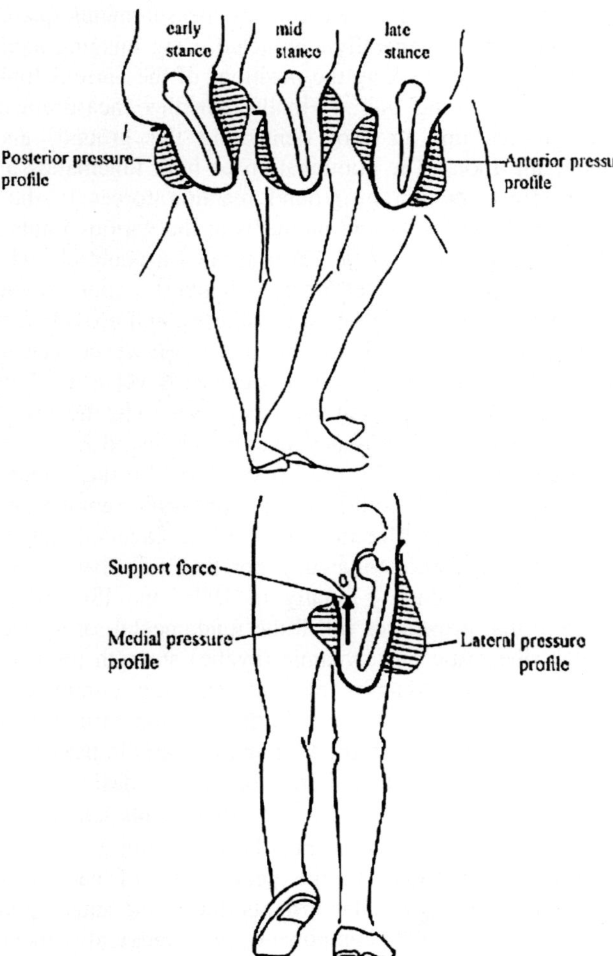

Figure 10–2 Amputee's stump/prosthesis interaction during stance phase of the gait cycle

Prosthetic components therefore have to be optimized for all phases of gait — for example, lightweight for swing phase and high strength for stance phase. To this end, amputee's gait has been analyzed extensively to help design and evaluate prosthetic components. A complete gait analysis includes the study of temporal-distance measurements, kinematics and kinetics analyses, energy factors, and muscular activities. Temporal-distance parameters include walking speed, stride length, step length, cadence, and gait cycle. A trans-femoral amputee (above-knee) walks about 40 percent slower than normal, increasing the duration of the gait cycle by an average of 0.36 seconds and reducing the stride length by about 20 percent. Kinematics measurements quantify motion with respect to time and are generally conducted using imaging methods in the form of video photography, tracking the positions of the various limb segments relative to each other during gait. Finally, kinetics measurements include ground reaction forces due to foot contacting the ground, and pressure distribution under the foot. The combination of both kinematics and kinetics data enables the transformation of ground reaction forces to the respective anatomical joints, defining forces and moments at the various joints. Applying gait analysis techniques, Linden *et al.* [2] described a comprehensive study of four different types of prosthetic feet for trans-femoral amputees. Such studies contribute to the design and evaluation of prostheses, and provide a quantitative measurement on gait restoration for the amputees. However, gait analysis for individual patient prescription of prosthetic devices is yet to be fully explored [3]. The high cost of performing a gait analysis proves to be the key obstacle.

In addition to function, safety issues must be addressed for any new design or material introduced to prosthetics. Safety concerns for the amputee have led to major research efforts and meetings by international communities, the most notable being the 'Philadelphia Meeting' in 1978 [4]. Detailed gait analysis data of normal and amputee gait were collated, generating a database to help develop an international safety standard. Finally in 1996, the ISO 10328 [5] was developed to ensure that prostheses fulfill the fundamental safety requirements. The standards describe static and dynamic (cyclic) strength tests that evaluate the structural and design strengths of load carrying components of both trans-femoral and trans-tibial prostheses. In the principal structure test, the test prosthesis can consist of the socket, the foot and all parts in between, or just the individual components. The principal structure test is designed such that the desired loading at both the knee and ankle components can be achieved by applying only a single test load to the prosthesis (Figure 10–3). The desired loads generated then correspond to the peak value of each load carrying component, occurring at the particular instants during the stance phase of gait. To achieve accurate loading to the components, the relative alignment of the test components to each other is therefore very crucial [6]. The test is configured into the two major phases of gait, heel strike and toe off. Both these events produce complex loading in the prosthesis, which can principally be divided into the following components: axial load, anterior-posterior and medial-lateral bending moments, and torsional moment.

The prosthetic ankle/foot devices present an interesting challenge in strength testing. The ISO 10328 requires the heel and forefoot to be loaded alternately in both static and dynamic (cyclic) conditions. It must be noted that the ISO 10328 focuses on the structural integrity of prosthetic devices. However, it is becoming difficult to delineate structural and functional integrity for prosthetic components. Recent attempts have therefore been made to apply physiological testing conditions, using six-degree-of-freedom gait simulator that 'walks' the foot to study both structure and function [7].

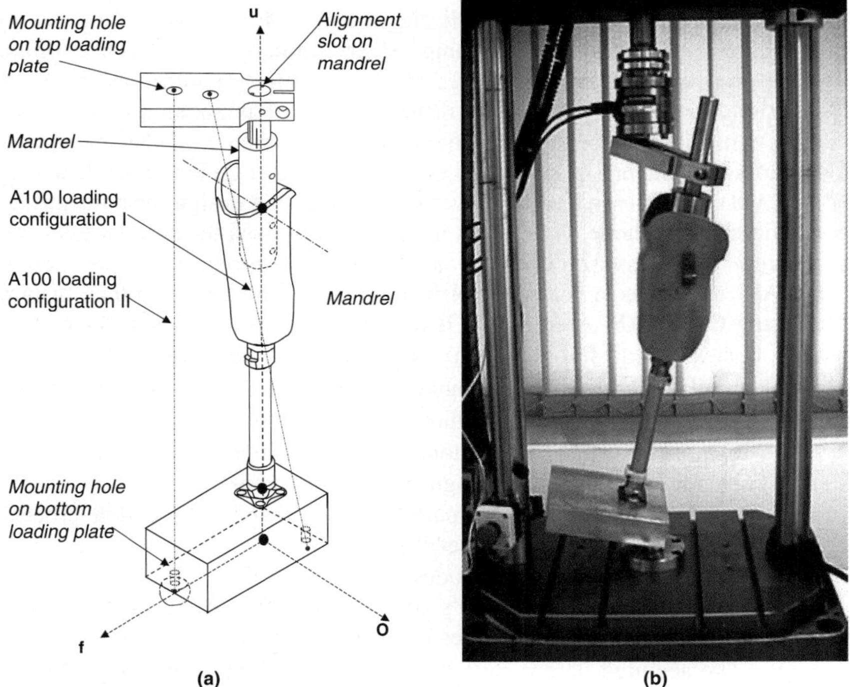

Figure 10–3 (a) Principal structure test setup; (b) heel strike setup for static and cyclic test conditions

10.3 Methods and Materials

The process of implementing new methods and materials is slow due to the complexity at the man and machine interface, *i.e.*, amputee-prosthesis interaction. In addition, the rehabilitation industry relies heavily on prosthetists' expertise and skills — which are derived from artisan methods, and which cannot be easily replaced with technology. New methods and materials — in terms of safety and function — are primary guided by ISO safety standards and driven by patients' needs. Successful methods and component designs demonstrate excellence in balancing the two. The following sections thus discuss state-of-the-art techniques applicable to artificial limb components.

10.3.1 Prosthetic Socket

10.3.1.1 Computer-aided Design and Manufacturing (CAD/CAM)

The most important aspect of the artificial limb is the socket — which constitutes the critical interface between the amputee's stump and prosthesis. The design and fitting of the socket is also the most difficult procedure due to the uniqueness of each amputee's stump. Every fitting requires much attention from the prosthetist. Although at present, there exists systemization of artisan practices to design and fit sockets for different levels of amputation, a successful fitting is still highly dependent on the skill and experience of the prosthetist. Nevertheless, Computer-Aided Design and Computer-Aided Manufacturing (CAD/CAM) has emerged as methods that influence the design, manufacturing, and services of prosthetic sockets. Its initiation arises from the need to automate procedures to increase productivity and quality of products. The present CAD/CAM system is a much simplified process compared to other mature engineering CAD/CAM operations. It basically comprises a computer (which controls a shape acquisition system) and a carving machine. The system processes closely copy the artisan techniques (Figure 10–4) of making prosthetic sockets. A similar three-phase procedure is as follows (Figure 10–5):

1) Measurement of body contours where analogue measurements are converted to digital data recognized by computers;
2) Shape generation and manipulation — a shape rectification process controlled by the software user; and
3) Physical realization of socket design.

The initial shape of the amputee's stump is first recognized through shape measurement or acquisition techniques using non-contact laser scanner (Figure 10–5(a)). The acquired data is further interpreted by CAD software packages, which enable the stump shape to be displayed as computer graphics. The rectification phase of the software allows the acquired shape to be manipulated by decreasing or adding volume to it, moving and slicing it to any desired field of view (Figure 10–5(b)). Finally, a replica of the final socket shape is manufactured through computer codes sent to a numerically controlled milling machine which carves on plaster, foam, or wax (Figure 10–5(c)). Depending on the final material of the socket, it can be vacuum formed by draping heated thermoplastics or by applying layers of woven material with acrylic resin over the carved model. The latter is a time consuming process and may require several days for the resin to cure — which severely hampers CAD/CAM's productivity. However, recent studies have shown that it is feasible to produce sockets directly without the need of any positive model. This is done by dispensing semi-molten polypropylene onto a machine table to form a prosthetic socket. Rovick *et al.* [8] and Ng *et al.* [9,10] described the process using SQUIRT and RMM machines, which are capable of fabricating sockets within 30 minutes and three hours respectively. The Rapid Manufacturing Machine (RMM) consists of two main components: the robotic system and the dispenser. Polypropylene filaments are fed into the heated dispenser and extruded in a semi-molten state. A filament is then dispensed onto the machine table according to the cross-sectional contour of the socket. The second layer is laid in a similar manner on top of the first. The process continues until the whole socket is built (Figure 10–6).

Due to the layering process, concerns arose over the delamination of socket material. The socket materials were then tested using ASTM material test standards. Test results showed that they compared well with polypropylene sheets used typically for socket fabrication. Moreover, the results indicated minimal strength loss [8,9]. Ng *et al.* [9,10] went on further to perform successfully the ISO 10328 principal structure test on the socket.

10.3.1.2 Intelligent CAD/CAM system

The introduction of CAD/CAM system for prosthetics has generated much debate. Pritham [11] suggested that until CAD/CAM reaches a product standard equivalent to that of the manual method, its application could not be justified. There are numerous studies comparing the outcome of CAD/CAM and manual sockets [12]. Nevertheless, it is clear the major technical disadvantage of the CAD/CAM system is that no new principles are introduced to optimize socket fit. The system offers only a controlled socket reproduction technique based on conventional principles. The system is still highly dependent on the skill of the prosthetist to produce a good fitting socket. As described by Klasson [13], "a good fit is primarily not defined by a particular shape of socket, but by the accommodation of forces or pressure between the stump and the socket, to provide for comfortable and harmless weight bearing, stabilization and suspension". In line with this definition, stump/socket interface pressure is widely accepted as a quantitative way of evaluating socket fit.

As early as the 1960s, experimental studies on stump/socket interface pressure measurement were attempted [14]. Only recently, the Finite Element (FE) method — a computation technique that enables the prediction of soft tissue displacement from input forces/pressures and vice-versa — was recognized to be of great potential in the field of lower limb prosthetics. Combining CAD/CAM with FE analysis, ideal pressure distribution over the stump/socket interface can be achieved and evaluation of different types of socket design can be made quantitatively. This could lead to a new generation of CAD/CAM systems — the intelligent CAD/CAM. A review of the use of FE method for sockets design can be found in the survey by Zhang *et al.* [15].

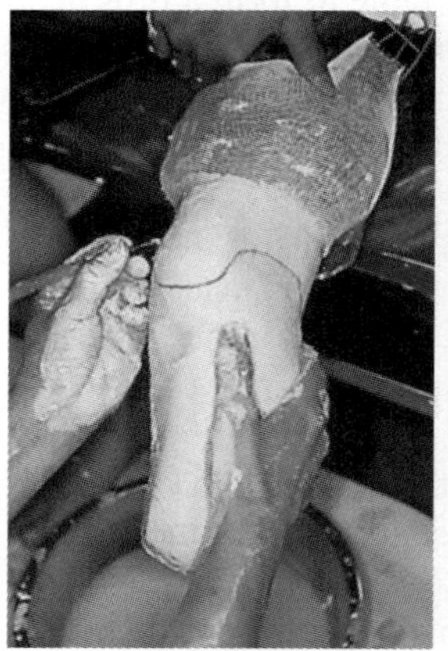 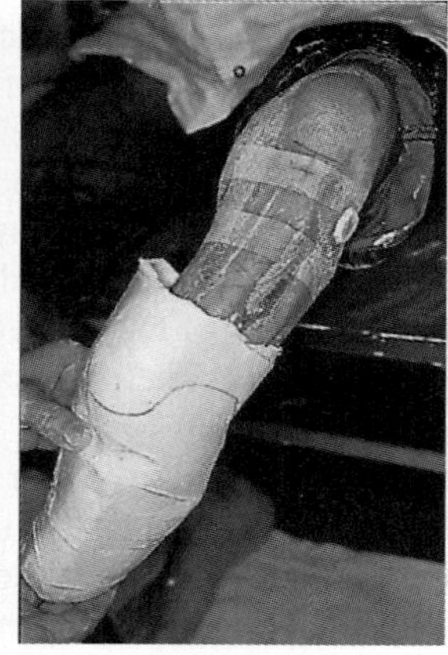 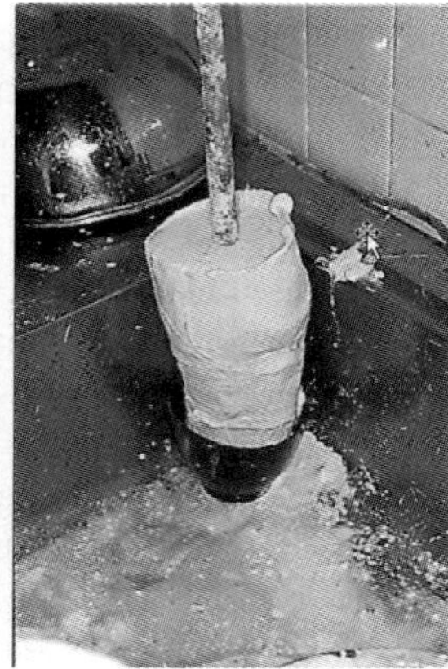

(a) Shape acquisition using plaster cast

(b) Plaster of paris to create positive model

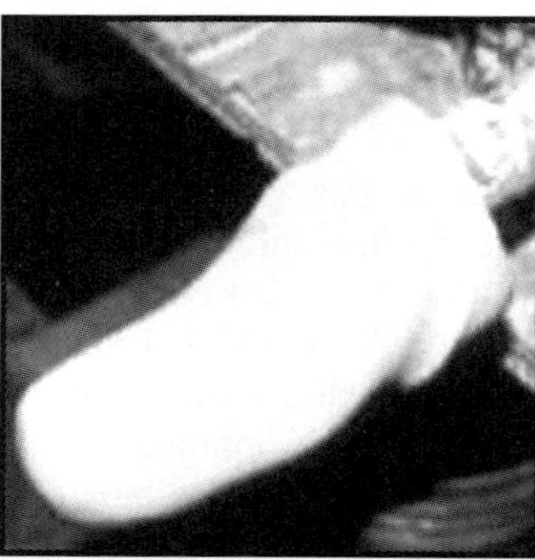

(c) Shaping the positive model to form the socket shape; socket fabricated by draping plastic or laminating woven fabrics with resin over positive model

Figure 10–4 Artisan techniques and stages of trans-tibial prosthetic socket fabrication

Figure 10–7 describes the concept of an intelligent CAD/CAM process:
1) Acquire stump shape.
2) Input shape acquisition data to the CAD software so that an initial socket shape can be defined.
3) Transfer socket geometry data and other parameters required for a FE model to the FE analysis (FEA) program.
4) Calculate stump/socket interface pressure. (At this stage, an iterative loop can be formed — each time the CAD software re-creates a new socket shape, the system re-calculates the new pressure until a satisfactory pressure distribution over the stump is obtained.)

5)　An alternative approach to step (4) is to define the desired pressure distribution as loading conditions for the FE model, and thereby solve for a new socket shape.

The system described above can provide quantitative feedback information to the prosthetist recommending rectification in the CAD software, or even better, create a new socket shape with known and desired pressure distribution. In this manner, the CAD/CAM system can move on from being just a socket reproduction system to a genuine socket design and optimization technology.

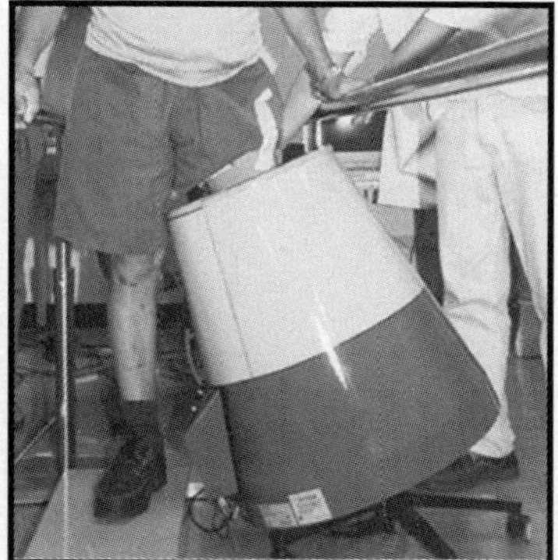

(a) Shape acquisition using stump laser scanner

(b) Rectify scanned model to socket shape

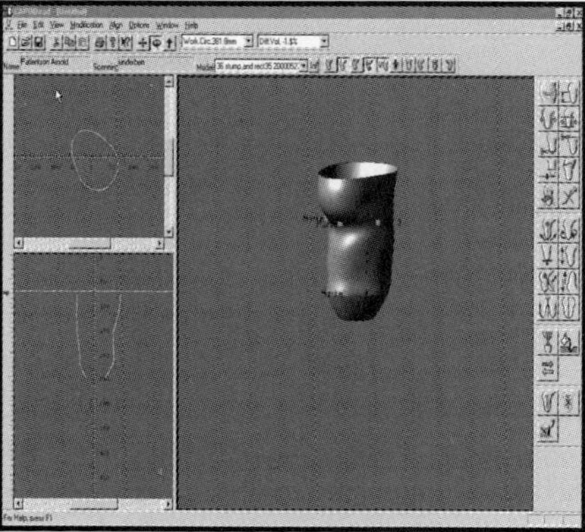

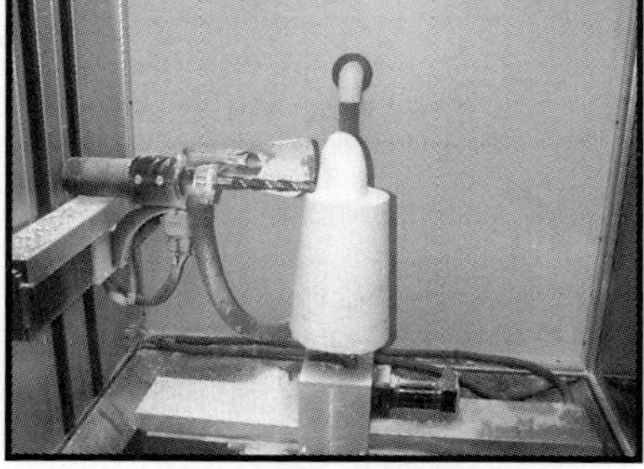

(c) Milling machine fabricates rectified positive model

Figure 10–5　CAD/CAM process of socket design and fabrication

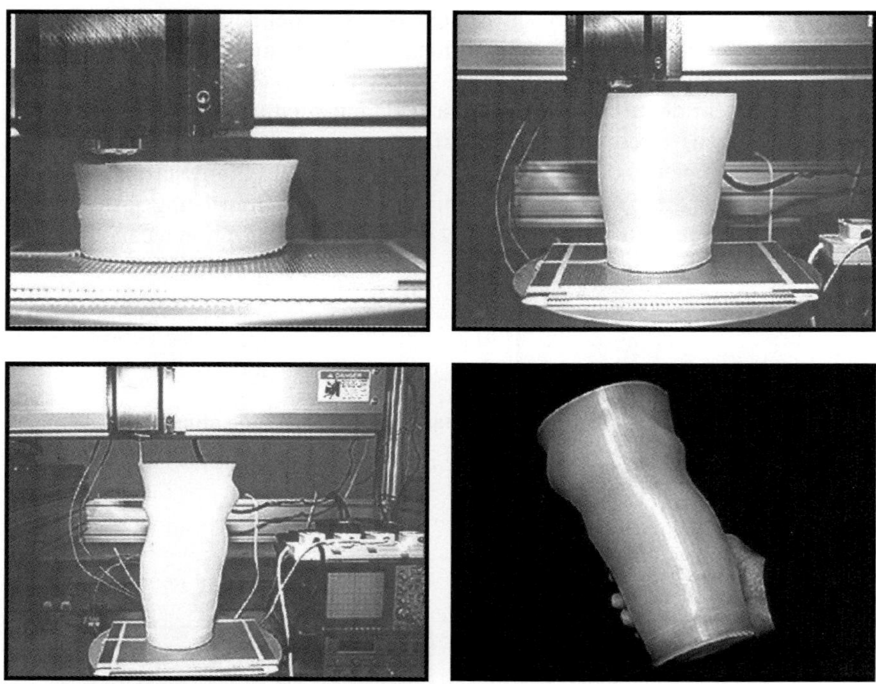

Figure 10–6 Rapid Manufacturing Machine (RMM), where socket is fabricated by controlled layering of molten polypropylene

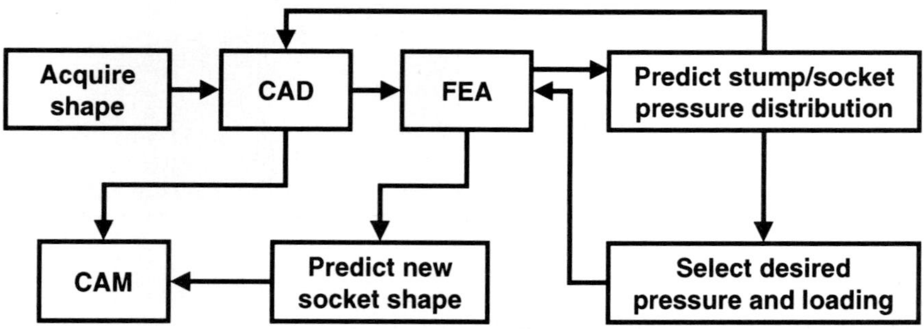

Figure 10–7 Concept of an intelligent CAD/CAM system for prosthetic socket fabrication

Lee *et al.* [16] reported integrating a CAD system (CAPODCad, CAPOD Systems) with a FE software (ANSYS, SAS IP Inc.). A volunteer trans-tibial amputee and an experienced prosthetist tested the integrated CAD–FE system. The amputee's stump geometry was captured using a non-contact optical scanner from CAPOD Systems. The stump's shape was further rectified using CAD–FE process by the prosthetist to create a definitive socket shape. A customized program converted the CAD information to FE codes that automatically performed meshing of the stump geometry, followed by assigning suitable material properties, loading and boundary conditions to create the FE model (Figure 10–8).

10.3.1.3 Prosthetic socket design

The above sections described state-of-the-art technologies in prosthetic socket fabrications. With the advent of high-speed computers, SQUIRT, and RMM, productivity in sockets fabrication would become less of a problem. However, what remains lacking are technologies that can provide the best or optimal socket fit for an individual patient, according to his unique biomechanical properties. What is the optimal fit for a patient is an arresting research question. Mak *et al.* [17] discussed various techniques that have been attempted to elucidate the biomechanics at the stump/socket interface. Factors affecting the acceptability of a socket fit can include stump's external and internal geometry, tissue viability (pain, vascular response, lymphatic supply, skin temperature, and abrasion), tissue's mechanical properties, socket-liner's geometrical and mechanical properties, and finally stump/socket interface mechanics generated via external loading (walking, running, and standing). These parameters are highly dependent on each other. For example, different socket materials would produce different stump/socket pressure patterns, resulting in different comfort levels and varying gait patterns.

A 'good fit' is highly dependent on the skill of the prosthetist, his/her knowledge and experience. He/she must create a socket that will encourage muscles usage, relieve pressure at pressure intolerant areas, distribute pressure around the stump to tolerant areas, and maintain suspension of the prosthesis throughout the gait cycle. All these are achieved through geometrical changes of the socket. Socket shapes or designs and their complementary materials have therefore evolved as one of the more controversial topics in prosthetics. The following sections illustrate some of their key developments.

Trans-femoral prosthetic socket

Currently, two main types of trans-femoral prosthetic socket are in use: the quadrilateral (quad) socket developed in the 1950s [18] and the ischial containment (IC) socket developed in the 1980s [19]. The quad socket (Figure 10–9) takes its name from its shape when viewed in a transverse plane at the ischial tuberosity level. Four distinct walls make up the quad socket. At proximal brim level of the posterior wall, there is a wide (25 mm) seat parallel to the ground, known as the ischial seat. A large percentage of body weight is directed to this ischial seat via the ischial tuberosity. The gluteal musculature also transmits vertical force onto this shelf. The newer socket design possesses an elliptical rather than a quadrilateral shaped brim (Figure 10–9). The IC socket was initiated when Long [20] investigated the femoral angle of 100 trans-femoral amputees prescribed with the quad socket. By using X-rays, he found 92 to have a difference in angle compared to the sound limb. But the more significant revelation was that 91 of the amputees experienced femoral abduction. Following this finding, new socket designs were attempted to maintain the femur in adduction. Instead of providing an ischial seat, the configuration encloses the ischial tuberosity and ramus within the socket. Hence, this design is generally termed ischial containment socket or quite often ischial ramal weight bearing socket.

Clinical and laboratory evaluations of the IC socket have been carried out by various independent researchers. Gailey *et al.* [21] studied 10 unilateral amputee subjects, each fitted alternately with quad and IC sockets. Oxygen consumption and heart rate were measured for two speeds of ambulation. The results showed a reduction in the oxygen intake when the amputees used the IC sockets, resulting in about 20 percent less energy. Lee *et al.* [22] measured the pressure profile of two volunteer trans-femoral amputees fitted with both types of socket. Comparison made between the two sockets indicated that higher pressures were recorded at the proximal brim of the quad socket whereas the IC socket produced a more evenly distributed pressure profile. The pressure distributions on the medial and lateral walls of both types of socket were similar but in the anterior and posterior walls, significant differences were noted.

Trans-tibial prosthetic socket

The current trans-tibial socket of choice is the Patellar Tendon Bearing (PTB) socket that was developed in the late 1950s at the University of California [23]. The socket design leverages on the pressure tolerant areas in the trans-tibial stump, especially that of the patellar tendon and the posterior aspect of the stump. PTB socket advocates so determined that the patellar tendon area could carry a substantial amount of the total load, therefore the patellar tendon bar was introduced to help relieve loading at other regions of the socket. However, considerable skill is required to generate a good PTB socket fit. Many prosthetists faced difficulties in consistently producing satisfactory socket fits. As early as the 1960s, a technique known as pressure casting was introduced to address these inconsistency problems. Gardner [24] introduced a pneumatic pressure sleeve that wrapped the entire stump during cast taking. Murdoch [25] described another pressure casting concept where fluid was used as a medium to apply uniform pressure around the stump. The aim of these experiments was to eliminate some factors related to manual dexterity during the casting process, hence addressing the inconsistency problems.

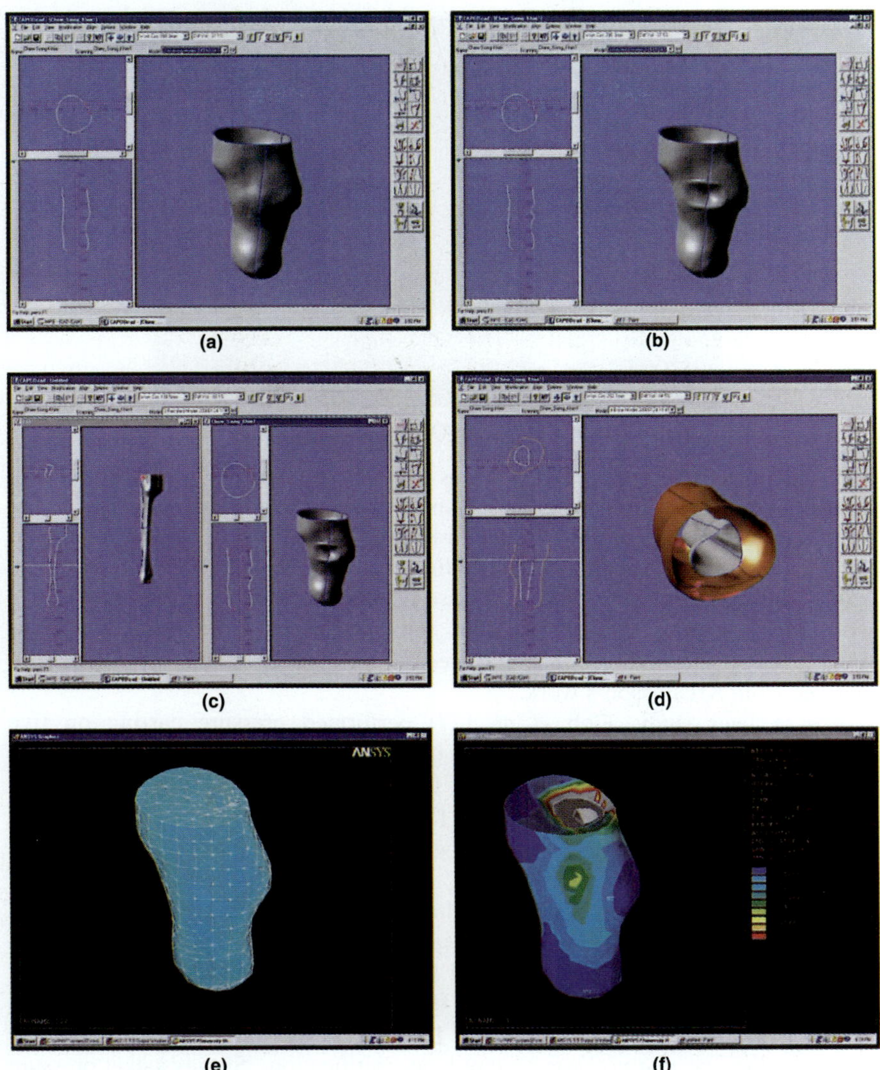

Figure 10–8 Example showing FE stress prediction on stump due to a localized compression introduced at the rectification stage: (a) original scanning obtained from AK/BK scanner; (b) prosthetist performed rectification to obtain rectified model; (c) imported a generic bone scaled to the amputee's anatomical landmarks; (d) positioned bone in stump to form bone model; (e) transformed and combined data from stump, and rectified bone model to create FE final model; (f) predicted stump/socket interface pressure, providing quantitative feedback to prosthetist

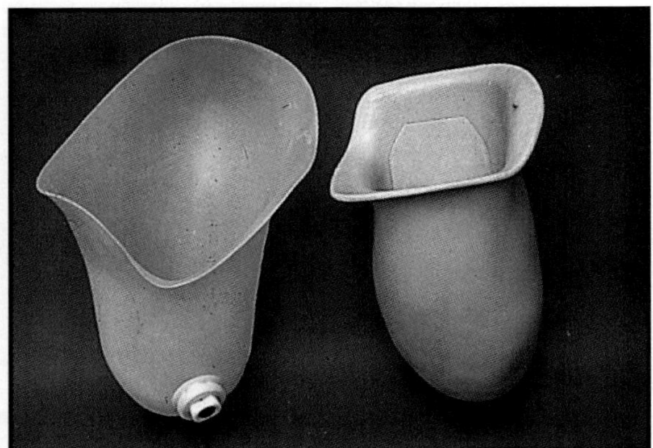

Figure 10–9 Comparing Quad and IC socket designs

The pressure casting concept was recently revived by Kristinsson [26], where air was used as a medium. Using an air pressure chamber, the socket shape was defined by casting plaster wrap over the stump wearing silicone liner. In addition to the silicone liner, padding was placed over bony areas of the stump during the casting process. Casting was performed on the patient in a non-weight bearing fashion (*i.e.*, not standing) in an air pressure chamber. Figure 10–10 shows the commercial Icecast® air bladder system from Ossur hf., derived from Kristinsson's work.

In a later study, Goh *et al.* [27] performed pressure casting on five trans-tibial amputee subjects. Instead of using air as a medium, pressure was applied to each amputee's stump in a tank separated from the hydraulic fluid medium by a diaphragm (Figure 10–11). Prior to the amputee placing his/her stump in the tank, a plaster wrap cast was applied over the stump. The patient was requested to stand without any aid, *i.e.*, in a normal standing position under weight bearing situation, applying almost half of his body weight on the pressurized medium. Once the plaster wrap hardened, the system was depressurized and the plaster removed from the stump. A positive model was generated from the wrap cast and finally, a socket was fabricated using traditional lamination methods (Figure 10–12). A very important aspect of this investigation was that no casts required any rectification. Stump/socket pressure was measured for the five subjects, and socket fits were found acceptable by the subjects.

The impact in generating an acceptable fit using pressure casting methods is tremendous and worth investigating. The hypothesis in pressure casting is "let nature dictate the most realistic and achievable pressure distribution". Such a method will remove all manual dexterity and inter-prosthetist variances. In addition, innovative use of prosthetic socket materials could be derived. The commercial Icex® system developed by Ossur hf. takes advantage of pressure casting where there is no need for socket rectification, thus no need for a positive model. Lee *et al.* [28] similarly reported the use of braided carbon fiber sock impregnated with quick curing resin prior to casting. The sock was donned directly on the stump, instead of a plaster cast. The sock hardened within minutes to form the final socket when pressure casting was completed (Figure 10–13).

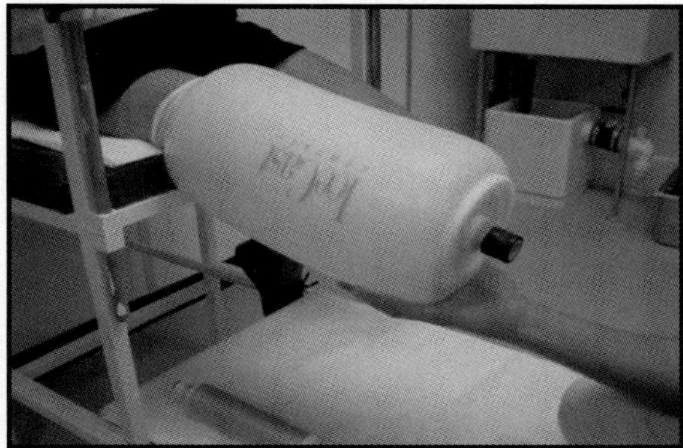

Figure 10–10 Icecast® pneumatic casting system for trans-tibial amputee

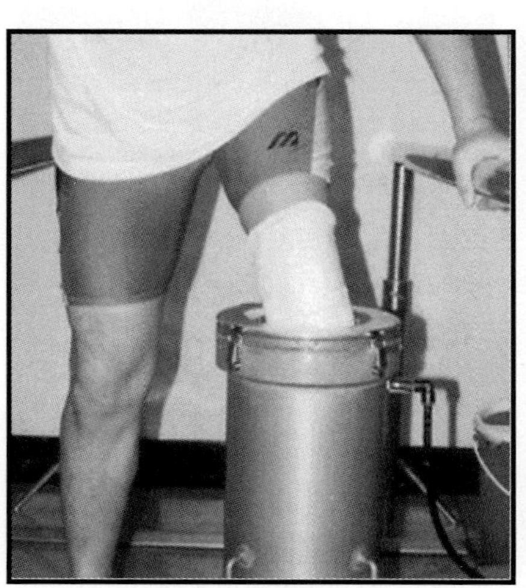

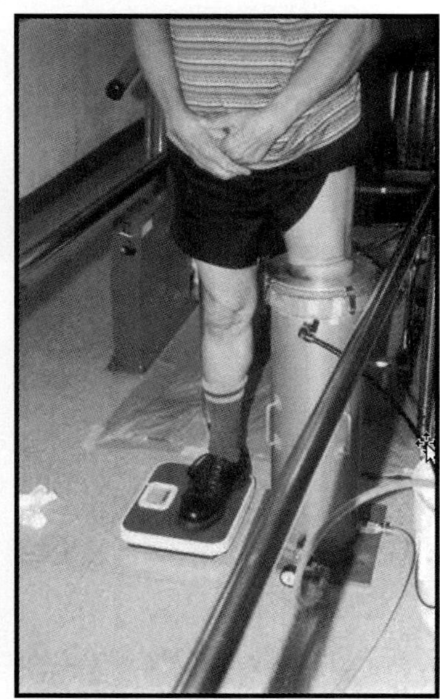

Figure 10–11 Pressure casting using hydraulic medium

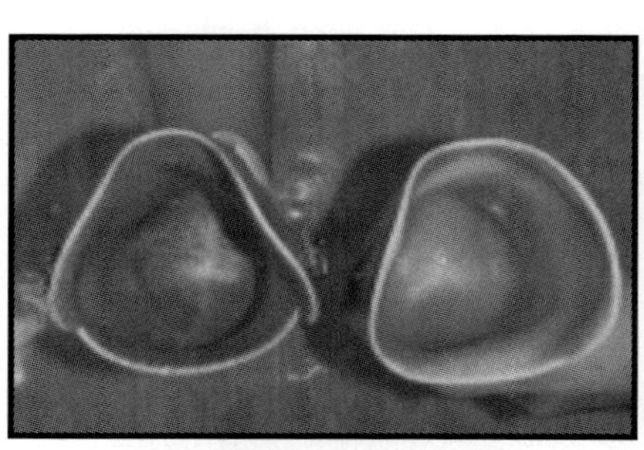

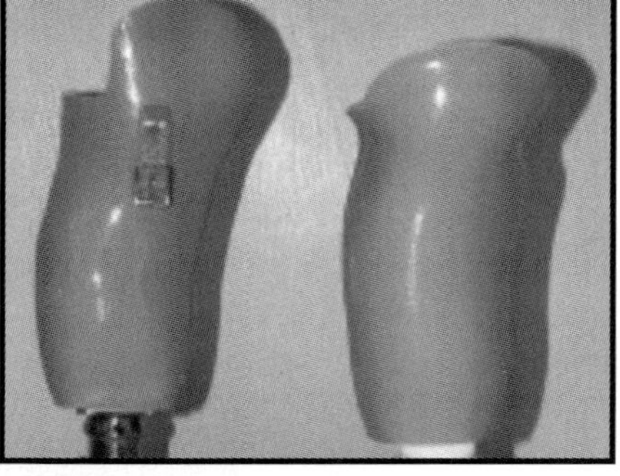

Pressure Cast   **PTB**   **Pressure Cast**   **PTB**

Figure 10–12 Comparing PTB socket and pressure cast socket

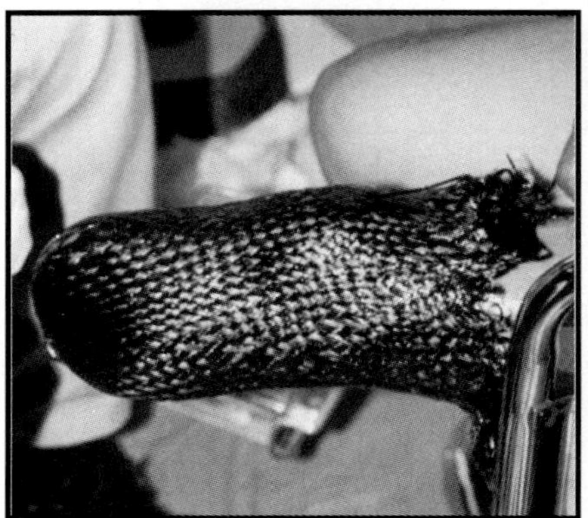

(a) Resin-impregnated carbon fiber sock draped over stump

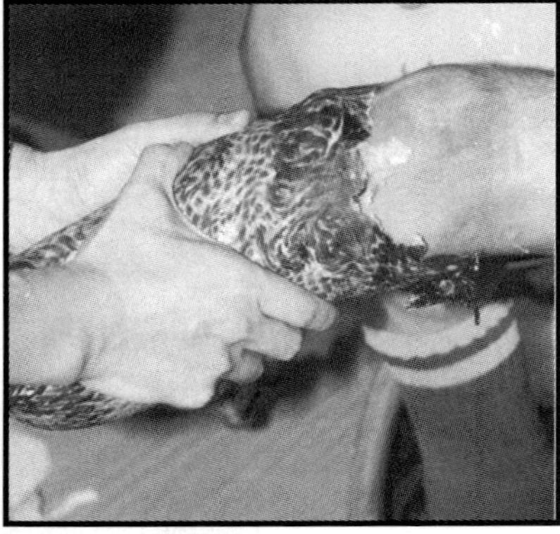

(b) Sock hardened to form socket after pressure casting

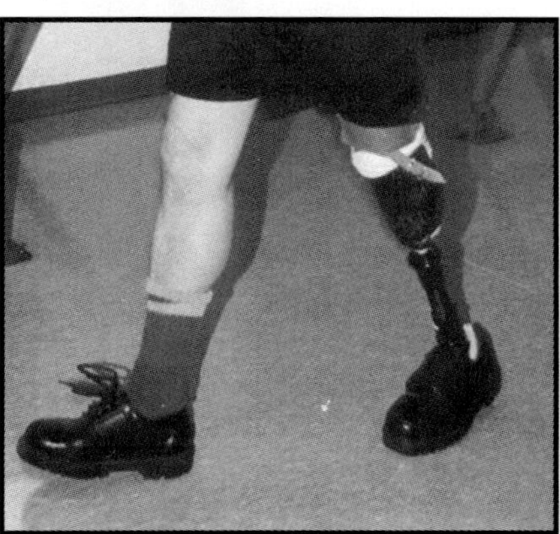

(c) Socket fitted with the rest of the modular components

Figure 10–13 Direct socket casting used with pressure casting system

10.3.2 Prosthetic Foot

In recent years much emphasis has been placed on improving the lifestyle of active amputees. There was thus an explosion of high-end prosthetics componentry in the market that caused much confusion to both providers and patients. The prosthetic foot has seen so many changes that the old designs are now known simply as the conventional foot. The newer designs are called energy storing prosthetic foot (ESPF), or more recently energy storage and return (ESAR) [29]. As the name suggests, ESAR is designed to store energy during stance and release energy during the push off phase to help propel the body, hence reducing fatigue and improving comfort to the amputee. The materials of ESAR foot are high in strength while the design or geometry of the foot gives it flexibility or the spring-like effect. Materials used include carbon fiber and Kevlar®. In addition, most designs allow 'stiffness tuning' to suit the patient's body weight and choice of activities. Stiffness tuning methodology can include attaching additional vertical shock pylon to the foot or simply choosing a desired foot stiffness provided by the manufacturer. The latest foot designs have built-in shock pylons (Figure 10–14).

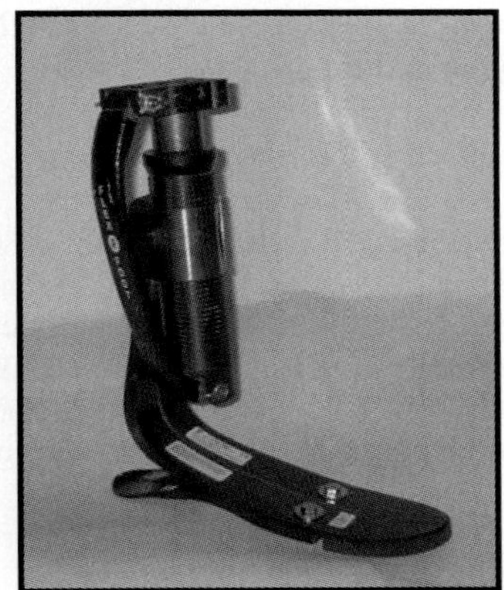

Figure 10–14 ESAR prosthetic foot with built-in shock absorbers

With growing parameters arising from new components, it becomes adversely difficult to optimize an amputee's gait. In addition, gait itself is a continuous process with an infinite number of variables. For example, an incorrect or correct foot stiffness could have an exponential effect to the overall prosthetic fit and rehabilitation outcome. This has led to numerous biomechanical studies quantifying the energy storage and release effects with respect to improving a patient's gait efficiency [2]. Other groups of studies are qualitative evaluations to elucidate patients' preference between the conventional foot and the varieties of ESAR foot [30]. However, it is interesting to note that Hafner *et al.* [31] indicated that biomechanical studies of ESAR foot often do not commensurate those of patients' perceptive findings. The authors provided a comprehensive review of previous studies and suggested that the link between biomechanical and clinical studies is still unclear.

10.3 Conclusion

Highlighted in this chapter are current research issues that face the prosthetic community on the utilization of novel methods and new materials. CAD/CAM has helped to increase productivity in sockets fabrication, but currently faces new challenges to quantify socket fits and to better socket designs. However, the topic of designing an optimal socket fit is still being deliberated relentlessly. Simple pressure casting methods that aim to provide a consistent 'perfect design' for every individual confront traditional concepts. Nevertheless, new quick-curing direct socket materials have emerged and are capable of achieving same-day prosthesis delivery. Prosthetic feet have also seen significant changes over the years — revolutionized by innovative designs and high-strength materials. New socket fitting methods and components have indeed improved the lifestyle and capabilities of amputees. Nevertheless, their introduction will always be greeted with both excitement and skepticism.

References

1. J. B. Reswick, Rehabilitation engineering, Annu. Rev. Rehabil., 1980, 1:55–79.
2. M. L. van der Linden, S. E. Solomonidis, W. D. Spence, N. Li, and J. P. Paul, A methodology for studying the effects of various types of prosthetic feet on the biomechanics of trans-femoral amputee gait, J. Biomech., 1999, 32:877–889.
3. J. M. Czerniecki and A. J. Gitter, Gait analysis in amputee: Has it helped the amputee or contributed to the development of improved prosthetic components?, Gait Posture, 1996, 4:258–268.
4. ISO Standards for lower limb prostheses, The Philadelphia Report, International Society of Prosthetics and Orthotics, Copenhagen, 1978.
5. ISO10328, Prosthetics — structural testing of lower limb prostheses, International Standards Organization, Geneva, 1996.
6. L. D. Neo, V. S. P. Lee, and J. C. H. Goh, Specimen preparation and principal structural testing of trans-tibial prosthetic assemblies, Prosthet. Orthot. Int., 2000, 24:241–45.
7. Six DOF Gait Simulator, www.mts.com.
8. S. Rovick, D. S. Childress, and R. Chan, An additive fabrication technique for the CAM of prosthetic sockets, J. Rehab. Res. Dev., Progress Reports, 1996, 33:1.
9. P. Ng, P. S. V. Lee, and J. C. H. Goh, Prosthetic socket fabrication using rapid prototyping technology, Rapid Prototyping J., 2002, 8(1):53–59.
10. J. C. Goh, P. V. Lee, and P. Ng, Structural integrity of polypropylene prosthetic sockets manufactured using the polymer deposition technique, Proc. Inst. Mech. Eng. H., 2002, 216(6):359–368.

11. C. H. Pritham, The application of advanced technology to the production of positive models: A sceptic's point of view, Report, ISPO workshop on CAD/CAM in prosthetics and orthotics, USA, 1988, 8–12th June.

12. B. Klasson, Computer-aided design, computer-aided manufacture and other computer aids in prosthetics and orthotics, Prosthet. Orthot. Int., 1985, 9(1):3–11.

13. B. Klasson, Evaluation of CASD CAM, Report, ISPO workshop on CAD/CAM in prosthetics and orthotics, USA, 1988, 8-12th June.

14. F. A. Appoldt and L. Bennett, Preliminary report on dynamic socket pressure, Bull. Prosthet. Res., 1967, 10(8):20–55.

15. M. Zhang, A. F. T. Mak, and V. C. Roberts, Finite element modeling of residual lower limb in prosthetic socket: a survey of the development in the first decade, Med. Eng. Phys., 1998, 20:360–373.

16. V. S. P. Lee, S. K. Cheung, S. K. Pan, J. C. H. Goh, and S. DasDe, Computer Aided Design (CAD)-Finite Element Analysis (FEA) integration for prosthetic socket design, 10th Int. Conf. Biomed. Eng., Singapore, 2000, 415–416.

17. A. F. T. Mak, M. Zhang, and D. A. Boone, State-of-the-art research in lower limb prosthetic biomechanics-socket interface, J. Rehab. Res. Dev., 2001, 38(2):161–174.

18. C. W. Radcliffe, Functional considerations in the fitting of above-knee prostheses, Artificial Limbs, 1955, 2(1):35–60.

19. J. Sabolich, Contoured Adducted Trochanteric-Controlled Alignment Method (CAT-CAM): Introduction and basic principles, Clin. Prosthet. Orthot., 1985, 9(4):15–26.

20. I. A. Long, Allowing normal adduction of femur in above-knee amputations, J. Orthot. Prosthet., 1975, 8(1):6–8.

21. R. S. Gailey, D. Lawrence, H. C. Burdi, P. Spyropoulos, C. Newell, and M. S. Nash, The CAT-CAM socket and quadrilateral socket: A comparison of energy cost during ambulation, Prosthet. Orthot. Int., 1993, 17:95–100.

22. V. S. P. Lee, W. D. Spence, and S. E. Solomonidis, Stump/socket interface pressure as an aid to socket design in prostheses for trans-femoral amputees — A preliminary study, Proc. Inst. Mech. Eng. H., 1997, 211:167–180.

23. C. W. Radcliffe, The biomechanics of below-knee prostheses in normal level, bipedal walking, Artificial Limbs, 1961, 6:16–24.

24. H. Gardner, A pneumatic system for below-knee casting, Prosthetic International, 1968, 3(4/5):12–14.

25. G. Murdoch, The Dundee socket for below-knee amputation, Prosthetic International, 1965, 3(4/5):15–21.

26. O. Kristinsson, Pressurized casting instruments, 7th World Congress ISPO, Chicago, 1992, 43.

27. J. C. H. Goh, P. V. S. Lee, and S. Y. Chong, Stump/socket pressure profile of the pressure cast (PCast) prosthetic socket, Clin. Biomech., 2003, 18(3):237–243.

28. P. Lee, J. Goh, and V. Tong (2000), Biomechanical evaluation of the pressure cast (PCast) prosthetic socket for trans-tibial amputee, World Congress on Medical Physics and Biomedical Eng., Chicago, 2000, 23rd July.

29. J. E. Sanders, S. G. Zachariah, A. B. Baker, J. M. Greve, and C. Clinton, Effects of changes in cadence, prosthetic componentry, and time on interface pressures and shear stresses of three trans-tibial amputees, Clin. Biomech., 2000, 15:684–694.

30. R. C. Crandall, T. F. Anderson, B. Backus, and T. Frucci, Clinical evaluation of an articulated dynamic-response prosthetic foot in teenage trans-tibial and syme-level amputee, J. Prosthet. Orthot., 1999, 11(4):185–192.
31. B. J. Hafner, J. E. Sanders, J. Czerniecki, and J. Fergason, Energy storage and return prostheses: does patient perception correlate with biomechanical analysis?, Clin. Biomech., 2002, 17:325–344.

CHAPTER 11

CHITIN-BASED BIOMATERIALS

Eugene Khor

Department of Chemistry, National University of Singapore
E-mail: chmkhore@nus.edu.sg

Chitin is a unique biopolymer based on the N–acetyl–glucosamine monomer. Over the years, there has been much interest in exploiting this biopolymer and its variants for a myriad of biomedical applications. Chitin and its derivatives have been shown to be useful as wound dressing materials, drug delivery vehicles, and increasingly a candidate for tissue engineering. The potential for this biomaterial is immense and will continue to increase: studies are underway to explore its utilization in new biomedical applications as well as to investigate the chemistry of extending its capability.

11.1 Introduction

Traditionally, implants or "body part" replacements were fabricated from inert biomaterials such as metals, ceramics, and synthetic polymers. In recent years, science and technology trends of medical devices have been directed at more "temporal" tissue-engineered implants, which are fabricated using a combination of cells and biodegradable biomaterials. These implants are expected to perform transient roles without upsetting the body's functions and eventually be replaced by the body's own cells with the biodegradable property (which permits the biomaterial to be removed in a non-toxic manner). The use of biopolymers as biomaterials for such purposes is becoming increasingly popular as materials derived from nature are expected to exhibit greater compatibility with humans, and may be bioactive and biodegradable. Among the candidate biopolymers for this purpose is chitin.

11.2 Chitin Occurrence and Isolation

Chitin is a co-polymer of N–acetyl–glucosamine and N–glucosamine units (Figure 11–1) randomly or block distributed throughout the biopolymer chain — depending on the processing method used to derive the biopolymer. When the number of N–acetyl–glucosamine units is higher than 50 percent, the biopolymer is termed chitin. Conversely, when the number of N–glucosamine units is higher, the term chitosan is used. Chitin chains are strongly hydrogen bonded, making the biopolymer insoluble in common solvents. Chitosan is the deacetylated chemical derivative of chitin and has been the more prevalent version of the biopolymer because of its ready solubility in dilute acids — rendering chitosan more accessible for chemical reactions and a preferred choice for utilization.

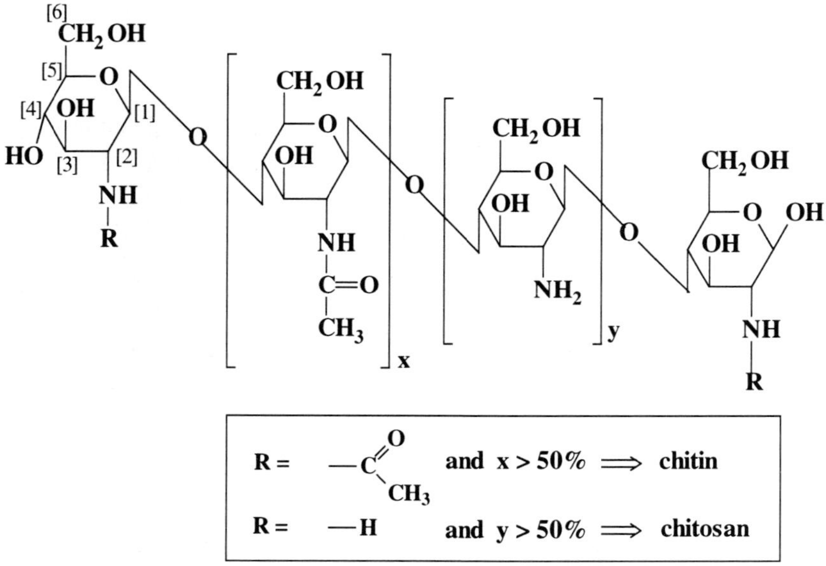

Figure 11–1 Chemical structure of the biopolymer chitin and its derivative, chitosan (Reprinted from "E. Khor, Chitin: Fulfilling a biomaterial's promise, ISBN 008 04410185" with permission from Elsevier)

Chitin is a biopolymer found in nature — primarily in the shells of crustaceans and mollusks, in the backbone of squids and the cuticle of insects [1]. Chitin is also present in the algae commonly known as marine diatoms, in protozoa and the cell wall of several fungal species [2]. Chitin from the diatom spines — such as *Cyclotella cryptica* and *Thalassiosira fluviatilis* — is the only form reported to be 100% poly-N–acetyl–glucosamine; that is, it is not associated with proteins and is termed chitan [3]. A small number of fungal strains are known to produce chitosan in preference to chitin [4]. Chitosan is not native to animal sources and is normally obtained by the deacetylation of shellfish-derived chitin using sodium hydroxide [5].

The primary biological function of crustacean chitin and fungal chitin is to provide a structural scaffold to support the animal exoskeleton or fungal cell wall. While this is achieved differently in animals and plants, the common feature is an intimate link between the biopolymer with the biological system in which it is found. Isolation of the biopolymer involves a systematic destruction of its links with the biological system, as well as removal of components such as proteins, calcium carbonate, and β-glucans. Efficiency of the methods used to remove these components has significant bearing on the final quality of chitin and chitosan materials [6]. Presently, the chemical method using hydrochloric acid for decalcification and sodium hydroxide for deproteination is practiced on shellfish, although milder enzymatic methods are beginning to make inroads.

11.3 Chitin as a Biomaterial

The potential for chitin as a biomaterial has been reported in scientific literature for more than 40 years. Chitin and chitosan have been shown to be useful materials in biomedical applications such as wound dressings, hemocompatible coatings, drug delivery, tissue engineering, and cell encapsulation. Wound dressings and hemocompatibility coatings are normally external device applications, while tissue engineering and drug delivery are intended for internal use that requires biodegradability — except possibly when drug delivery is *per os*. In this chapter, chitin as a biomaterial in wound dressings, tissue engineering, and drug delivery will be discussed to illustrate its huge potential in biomedical applications.

11.3.1 Wound Healing

Prudden *et al.* were the first to use chitin as a wound dressing material. Chitin obtained from shrimp and fungal sources was ground into topical powders and applied to wounds. It was found to accelerate wound healing. The rationale was such that the lysozyme enzyme — which is abundantly present in fresh and healing wounds — acted to break down the chitin powder to release N–acetyl–glucosamine required for wound healing [7]. Soon after, reports followed in which chitin was cited to be used as a wound dressing material in more conventional ways like as a film or in a woven form. For example, in a report published in the 1980s, chitosan films of differing molecular weights were assessed in wound model studies in which animal models were used. In some instances, the films were even coated with a silver antibiotic. It was demonstrated that animals covered with the chitosan films had a better chance of survival [8].

As for non-woven, fabric-type chitin dressing, the first step in its preparation was to make the chitin fiber. The fiber was then cut into segments of desired length, followed by dispersing the cut segments in water and binders, thereby giving rise to non-woven sheets. These non-woven chitin sheets have

been shown to be effective in treating burns, skin ulcers, and skin-graft areas —
where wounds were kept dry and that the dressing adhered to the wounds well
[9]. Another chitin source for this dressing method is from fungal mycelia,
which when applied directly as a wound dressing led to favorable results in rat
model studies [10].

Fluid absorbing chitin beads and a bi-layered chitosan membrane obtained
by "immersion-precipitation phase inversion" have also been proposed as a
wound dressing material [11,12,13]. In the fluid absorbing chitin bead, the
primary feature was an external layer of carboxymethyl–chitin (CM–chitin)
with a chitin core (Figure 11–2). The bi-layered membrane was a thin
layer of chitosan which acted as antibacterial and moisture control barrier,
and which was affixed to a sponge layer to absorb wound exudates.
N–carboxybutyl–chitosan has also been developed as a wound dressing. The
water-soluble, gel-forming ability and ease of sterilization are advantages of this
chitosan derivative. Favorable wound healing observations, such as formation
of repair tissue and the absence of scar formation and contraction, were noted in
animal model studies and human patients [14,15,16].

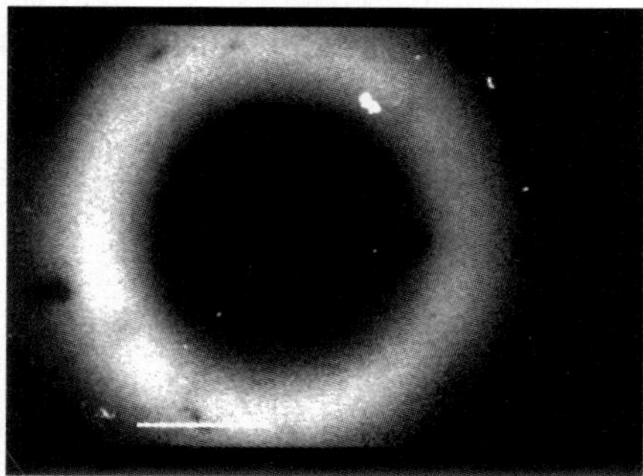

Figure 11–2 Confocal microscope image of chitin bead showing outer core of
CM–chitin (light ring) and inner core of chitin (dark circle) (Reprinted from "Journal of
Biomedical Materials Research©, 2001" with permission from John Wiley & Sons, Inc.)

Instead of being the only material in wound dressing applications, chitosan
materials have been combined with other materials such as collagen and
glycosaminoglycans (GAG). Under such compositions, wound healing was
found to be comparable, if not better, than with only single materials [17,18].
The inclusion of anti-microbial agents (such as silver sulfadiazine and
chlorhexidine) into wound dressings has also been shown to be promising
[19,20]. Both instances exhibited favorable infection control or antibacterial
activity.

Today, chitosan gauze is widely used in wound dressing applications.
However, given the extensive scientific studies devoted to investigating the
candidacy of chitin and chitosan as wound dressings, the full potential of these
biopolymers is just waiting to be tapped.

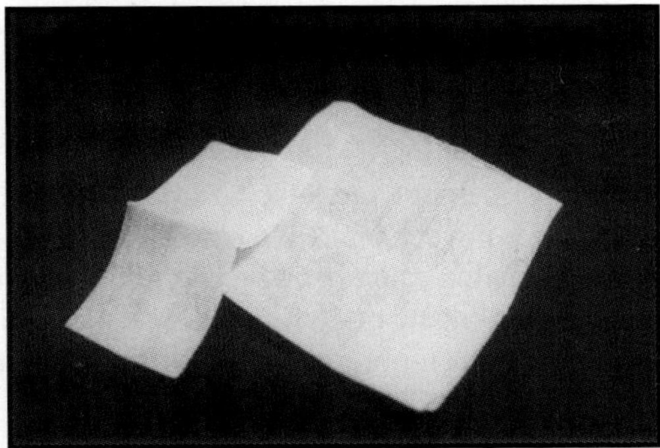

Figure 11–3 Chitosan gauze

11.3.2 Tissue Engineering

Tissue Engineering (TE) is defined as "an interdisciplinary field that applies the principles of engineering and life sciences toward the development of biological substitutes that restore, maintain, and improve the function of damaged tissues and organs" [21]. Biomaterials are required in tissue engineering to provide a structure termed "scaffold" onto which cells are seeded and allowed to proliferate to form a "tissue system". Normally, included under the tissue engineering concept is the encapsulation of bioactive substances such as pancreatic β cells that can secrete insulin at a controlled rate. In many instances, biodegradable polymers are used for the scaffolds as they have the advantage of degrading *in vivo* into non-toxic products.

Chitosan is one of the candidates proposed as a suitable polymer to form tissue engineering scaffolds due to the following advantages [22]:

- Chitosan is easily processed as dilute acid solutions into various shapes, films, and fibers. This thus allows scaffolds to be prefabricated in all forms and sizes, including three-dimensional assemblies.
- Since chitosan is insoluble at the physiological pH of 7, the structure once formed is maintained. Moreover its monomeric unit N–glucosamine that is found in human extracellular matrices gives non-toxic residues upon biodegradation.
- Chitosan can be chemically modified at its C–6 and N–2 positions to give new derivatives, hence extending its versatility.

Porous chitosan scaffolds are commonly prepared in two steps. First, controlled freezing of chitosan solutions and gels to yield pore sizes ranging from 1 μm to 250 μm. Subsequently, it is lyophilization that produces the freeze-dried construct. From this simple two-step process, variously shaped scaffolds that fit the desired applications can be fabricated. The porous nature of the scaffolds makes them behave like composite materials where low-modulus and high-modulus regions — which are dependent on pore size and orientation — are present.

Using similar strategies of freezing and lyophilization, chitin scaffolds with pore sizes ranging from <10 μm to 500 μm have been reported (Figures 11–4(a) to 4(d)) [23]. And for any open-pore architecture with pore sizes above 500 μm, it has been prepared using a novel chemical method (Figure 11–4(e)) [24]. This novel chemical method included calcium carbonate in the chitin gel. Depending on the amount of calcium carbonate particles used, reaction with dilute HCl then resulted in a homogeneous open-pore system of 100–500 μm pore size with ~76% porosity and another one of 500–1000 μm pore size with 81% porosity.

Several studies have demonstrated the usefulness of chitosan matrices as tissue engineering scaffolds. For example, Mathew *et al.* reported the use of chitosan in cartilage regeneration [25]. In this study, the cationic character of chitosan enabled the interaction with anionic polymers (such as chondroitin–4–sulfate–A (CSA) basis) to form insoluble complexes for membranes fabrication. The membranes are then used to grow bovine articular chondrocytes with retention of phenotype expression both in morphology and mitosis [26]. Hence this biomaterial could be useful as a carrier for autologous chondrocytes or as a scaffold for generation of cartilage-like "tissue systems". Frondoza *et al.* reported similar observations, however with chitosan only. When in contact with human osteoblasts and chondrocytes, chitosan assisted the continued expression of type I collagen in osteoblasts and type II collagen for chondrocytes, suggesting that chitosan has potential application in bioengineering repair of cartilage and bone defects [27].

Ma *et al.* [28] poured a porogen containing chitosan solution onto a prefabricated chitosan film. The chitosan film was then freeze-dried, and eventually soaked (to dissolve the porogen) in order to produce a bi-layered chitosan film-sponge. Human neofetal dermal fibroblast cells were seeded on this chitosan film-sponge. The growth and proliferation of the cells on the chitosan substrate implied the latter's potential as a tissue-engineered skin substitute.

Using simple methods as described above, chitin and chitosan biomaterials can be manipulated into various shapes to produce scaffolds suitable for tissue engineering. On this note, the potential of chitin and chitosan as biomaterials in tissue engineering is just beginning to be realized.

11.3.3 Drug Delivery

In drug delivery, the drug is normally combined with a polymeric material that serves two purposes: protect the drug from the biological environment prior to its therapeutic action, and make the drug available to the body.

In today's context, the indispensable requirements of controlled release, sustained release and site-specific delivery demand for more sophisticated delivery systems. This is because a regular dosage of drug is delivered for an extended period of time at the target site to attain a specific beneficial, therapeutic effect.

For an intravenous application, the polymer normally deteriorates *in vivo*, preferably at a constant rate, releasing the drug or functioning as a semi-permeable membrane in the release of the drug. The polymeric material has to be compatible with the drug. In other words, the material must be non-toxic, stable, sterilizable, and biodegradable — the very qualities discovered of chitin and chitosan, hence justifying studies of these materials as drug carriers.

Chitosan is an important drug delivery vehicle. It has been shown to enhance drug absorption, controlled release, and bioadhesion [29]. In terms of delivery methods, oral, parenteral, nasal, and ocular routes are available, as well as others such as encapsulation for gene therapy and gel systems. If it is by oral delivery, chitosan can be devised in various forms: microparticulate, liposomal, buccal disk, solution, vesicle, coated film, tablet, or capsule. If it is by parenteral route, chitosan will be delivered in the form of microspheres or solutions.

Early studies utilized gel-based chitin and chitosan for drug delivery applications. For example, the drugs indomethacin and papaverine hydrochloride were included in various chitin or chitosan solutions. Once the solvent evaporated and dried up, the final product was a drug containing chitin or chitosan gel [30]. Steroids, specifically β-oestradiol, progesterone, and testosterone have also been incorporated into chitosan films and beads [31]. Release studies indicated the potential of these chitin and chitosan gels, films, and beads as sustained release agents. Furthermore, dissolution studies on the chitosan films and beads showed no degradation over 30 days, suggesting their usefulness as controlled release systems if degradation of the carrier is not required. Chitosan films containing diazepam have also been prepared for oral administration in rabbit model studies, through which it was shown that film formulations were a suitable alternative to tablet forms [32].

Chitosan and hydroxypropyl–chitosan have been developed for implantable, sustained anticancer drug delivery systems suitable for zero-order drug release [33]. In one preparation the anticancer agent, uracil, was mixed with chitosan and hydroxypropyl–chitosan powders. The mixture was then dissolved using water and acetic acid. The resulting solution was either cast and dried to give a membrane, or extruded through a nozzle into dry air and neutralized with ammonia gas to give stick forms. *In vitro* and *in vivo* studies showed sustained release of uracil.

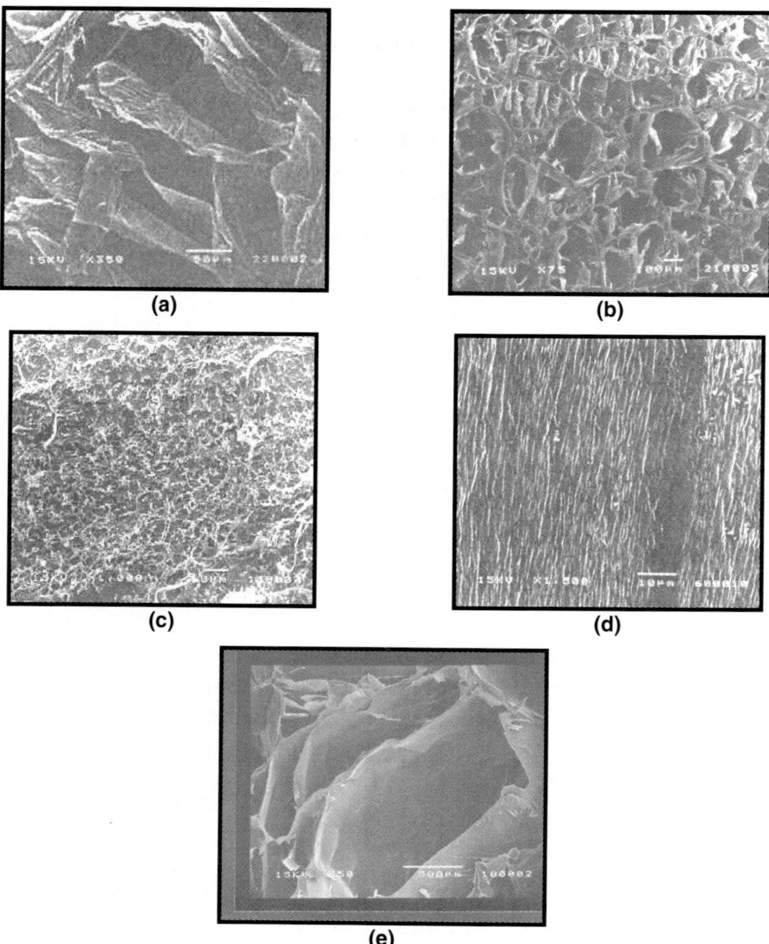

Figure 11–4 Scanning electron photomicrographs showing pore size morphology of variously frozen/lyophilized gels: (a) dry ice/acetone; (b) liquid nitrogen; (c) freezer; (d) Air-dried chitin gel; (e) calcium carbonate-produced matrix (Reprinted from "Journal of Polymer Research, 2001, 8:27–35, f–2" with permission from Kluwer Academic Publishers)

The pro-drug behavior is further demonstrated when the amino functionality of hydroxypropyl–chitosan interacted with the anti-tumor agent cis–diamino–dichloroplatinum (CDDP) [34]. CDDP containing hydroxypropyl–chitosan was prepared as a cotton mesh and implanted onto the tumor surface of mice. The results indicated that this method of drug delivery provided anti-tumor efficacy with no nephrotoxic side effects normally encountered with systemic delivery. In another study, the pro-drug behavior was demonstrated using the carminomycin–chitosan system where a dialdehyde was employed as the linking agent [35]. An aqueous solution of hydroxypropyl–chitosan containing basic fibroblast growth factors (bFGF) was impregnated into Gore Tex® vascular grafts, entrapping the growth factors as they were deposited by the biopolymer in the pores of the graft [36]. The hydroxypropyl–chitosan slowly dissolved, resulting in the sustained release of bFGF.

The anionic carboxymethyl–chitin (CM–chitin) is another chitin-based candidate for drug delivery in pro-drug platforms, in adsorption and entrapment materials or in methods that combine both adsorption and entrapment [36]. Watanabe *et al.* incorporated 30% doxorubicin in a CM–chitin gel and demonstrated the time-dependent release of the drug from the gel as the lysozyme enzyme hydrolyzed the CM–chitin [37].

Combination systems are another popular channel to achieve drug delivery. For example, the simple mixing of chitosan, sodium alginate, and drug powders, followed by compaction into a tablet form gives good bioadhesion to the buccal and sublingual mucosa — justifying this method to be suitable for intraoral drug delivery [39]. Semi-interpenetrating polymer network (semi-IPN) membranes for pH-sensitive drug delivery applications is another demonstration of chitosan as a drug delivery vehicle [40]. *In vitro* results indicated that chitosan gels were sensitive to simulated gastric fluid of low pH, hence swelling significantly; whereas in simulated intestinal fluid at neutral pH, the swelling was nominal.

Other examples include a poly(ethylene–vinylacetate) (PE–VAc) copolymer-chitosan co-matrix developed by Chandy *et al.* [41]. Aspirin was first loaded onto chitosan beads, which were in turn exposed to a PE–VAc solution. The solvent was left to evaporate to generate the co-matrix. Release studies showed a burst effect that could be attenuated by an additional polystyrene butadiene barrier membrane. Chitosan–gelatin sponges are another system that has been shown to give controlled release of prednisolone [42]. Finally, a new pH-sensitive system utilizing an inorganic material tetra-ethyl–orthosilicate (TEOS) with chitosan in a transparent IPN membrane (that swells at low pH and shrinks at physiological pH) can be useful as a delivery system [43].

Microspheres and their more recent descendant nanospheres, well-liked for their better drug release profiles or the ability to protect body tissue from harmful side effects of the drug, are another popular method of effecting drug delivery.

In a series of papers, Nishioka *et al.* described a simple method of preparing CDDP that contains chitosan microspheres. First, the drug cis–diamino–dichloroplatinum (CDDP) was dispersed in chitosan solution to be followed by vortexing until the desired sizes of particles were attained. The particles were cross-linked with glutaraldehyde to derive consolidated microspheres. Finally, lyophilization gave rise to the drug containing chitosan microspheres [44,45,46]. The authors found that increasing the amount of chitosan or adding chitin to the mixture prior to forming the microspheres led to an increase in CDDP incorporation, while at the same time the release rate of CDDP became more regulated with no initial burst effect. The improvement was attributed to better consolidation of the microspheres arising from the higher amount of biopolymers.

In another technique, diclofenac sodium (DS) was dispersed in a chitosan solution followed by dropping via a syringe/needle assembly into a non-solvent tripolyphosphate. This gave rise to microspheres that were roughly 750 μm in diameter with a very narrow size distribution [47]. A slow release of the drug was obtained over six hours *in vitro*, while *in vivo* studies demonstrated effective protection of the gastric mucosa. Other drugs that have been incorporated using similar techniques include 5–fluorouracil, where the drug release characteristics were in turn modified with other substances such as alginic acid, chitin, and agar. Bisphosphonates were used for treating pathological bone conditions, and gadolinium–DTPA for neutron capture cancer therapy [48,49,50]. As for oral vaccination applications, microparticles of chitosan were prepared from a surfactant containing chitosan solution, which was subjected to stirring and sonication. The chitosan microspheres were then loaded with a model antigen, ovalbumin [51]. The experimental results indicated good uptake of ovalbumin, and release studies using Balb/c mice showed good uptake based on Peyer's patches, hence indicating the potential of chitosan microspheres as a vaccine delivery system. The versatility of chitosan microspheres is also extended to nasal administration systems. This application method was exemplified when chitosan containing the luteinizing releasing hormone (LHRH) agonist was used in prostate and advanced breast cancer treatments' preparations [52].

In gene delivery, polycationic systems bound to DNA via ionic interactions have been proposed as one delivery route with chitosan as a convenient candidate biomaterial. Leong *et al.* reported the possible benefits of using chitosan as a delivery system for DNA-polycation nanospheres [53]. Chitosan was found to readily form nanospheres with the possibility of conjugating ligands to the nanospheres for targeting and protecting the DNA during transit and lyophilization for storage.

To enhance recognition of the cellular target, Murata *et al.* have synthesized pendant galactose-containing chitosan [54]. Using N–trimethyl–chitosan (TM–chitosan), galactose units were attached to the C–6 position of the chitosan monomer. The TM–chitosan demonstrated low cytotoxicity while the DNA–galactose conjugate demonstrated receptor recognition. Subsequently, a tetragalactose group was shown to further improve target recognition [55].

Chemical derivatives of chitin have also been used. For example, the complex coacervation of the anionic carboxymethyl–chitin with 6–mercaptopurine (an anticancer agent) in the presence of iron (III) chloride solution produced an ionically cross-linked microsphere system [56]. On the other hand, Genta *et al.* utilized a spray-drying technique to prepare ampicillin containing methylpyrrolidinone–chitosan microspheres [57]. Although release studies have indicated unsatisfactory profiles as a drug release agent, the chitosan microspheres retain their utility in wound treatment [58].

In summary, there are many ways to utilize chitin, chitosan, and their derivatives for drug delivery. Forms such as tablets, films, and gels do not require sophistication in formulation, while microspheres and nanospheres intended for internal use require proper fabrication that takes biodegradability into consideration. The present emphasis is on efforts to better understand the modulating effects of chitosan on drug transport, as well as mechanisms such as muco-adhesion and action at the tight epithelial cells' junction. As these issues get resolved and become better understood, the vast potential for chitin and chitosan in the drug delivery field will increase.

11.4 Processing

When it comes to biomedical applications, it is mandatory that chitin and chitosan be produced under some form of GMP (Good Manufacturing Practice) guidelines. This is because GMP ensures consistency and verifiable characteristics of the chitin-based materials. Some characteristics that must be consistent and verifiable are namely molecular weight and degree of acetylation — a regulatory requirement of the material if it is to be incorporated as a component of a medical device, drug, or other medical products. Several companies have started to actively produce GMP "medical grade" chitosan. Riding on this trend, it is likely that medical grade chitin and other chitin/chitosan derivatives will soon follow in the not-too-distant future [59].

One of the forerunner examples is the process reported by Dornish *et al.* on producing ultra-pure chitosan salts for biomedical and pharmaceutical use [60]. In the Protosan™ process to produce the ultra-pure chitosan salts, the chitin was first isolated from shellfish sources and deacetylated to give crude chitosan. Subsequently, the chitosan was depyrogenized to remove endotoxins, followed by microfiltration and ultrafiltration to remove insoluble materials and low molecular weight compounds respectively.

Several grades of the Protosan™ material were evaluated for oral, intravenous, and intraperitoneal toxicities using a rat model. No observable toxicological effects were found in all the three studies. Several other safety evaluations including hypersensitization studies and the Ames test gave acceptable results.

In summary, the processing of chitin and chitosan has come a long way from the crude treatment with acids and bases to produce chitin and chitosan flakes to refined methods that are more regulatory-compliant for biomedical applications. The proliferation of "medical grade" chitin-based biomaterials in the first decade of the 21st century will certainly springboard these biomaterials as a significant resource for a wide variety of biomedical applications.

11.5 Chitin or Chitosan

Chitosan is the more often cited form of chitin whenever it comes to demonstrating the utility of this biopolymer in biomedical applications. In contrast, the intractability tag has been the cause for the lag in exploiting chitin although the advent of the solvent system N, N′, dimethylacetamide/5% lithium chloride is changing this trend. The importance of chitin should be underscored — chitin is the first isolate while chitosan is chemically derived from chitin. This suggests that chitin is more natural, a fact that may be significant where biomedical applications are concerned.

The utilization of chitin or chitosan — as noted in the survey of biomedical applications — is likely to proliferate, in particular with applications that require the biodegradability property. Increasingly, there will be a need to look at this property more thoroughly. The true biodegradability or bioassimilation of chitin, chitosan, and their derivatives over a defined time period, as well as the consequences of bioaccumulation must be fully addressed before chitin-based biomaterials receive general acceptability for biomedical applications.

11.6 Future Outlook

Chitin-based biomaterials have been poised to be an important biopolymer for the present and future needs of biomaterials. The survey in this chapter gives a flavor of the wide-ranging application potential of this biopolymer and its variants. The eventual realization of biomedical products from this biomaterial will vindicate the foresight and hopes currently pinned on this biomaterial, based on its potential and versatility in utilization.

References

1. G. A. F. Roberts, Chitin Chemistry, (Macmillan Press Ltd., UK, 1992) Ch. 1.
2. E. P. Feofilova, D. V. Nemtsev, V. M. Tereshina, and V. P. Kozlov, Polyaminosaccharides of mycelial fungi: New biotechnological use and practical implications (review), Appl. Biochem. Microbio., 1996, 32:437–445.
3. J. McLachlan, A. G. McInnes, and M. Falk, Studies on the chitan (Chitin: Poly-N–acetylglucosamine) fibers of the diatom *thalassiosira fluviatilis hustedt*, 1. Production and isolation of chitin fibers, Can. J. Botany, 1965, 43:707–713.
4. S. Arcidiacono, S. J. Lombardi, and D. L. Kaplan, Fermentation, processing and enzyme characterization for chitosan biosynthesis by *Mucor Rouxii*, in Chitin and chitosan: Sources, chemistry, biochemistry, physical properties and applications, eds. G. Skjåk-Bræk, T. Anthonsen, and P. Sanford, (Elsevier Appl. Sci., UK, 1989) pp:319–332.
5. H. K. No and S. P. Meyers, Preparation of chitin and chitosan, Chitin Handbook, eds. R. A. A. Muzzarelli and M. G. Peters, (Atec Edizioni, Italy, 1997) pp:475–489.
6. E. Khor, Chitin: Fulfilling a biomaterial's promise, (Elsevier Sci. Pub., UK, 2001) Ch. 5.
7. J. F. Prudden, P. Migel, P. Hanson, L. Freidrich, and L. Balassa, The discovery of a potent pure chemical wound-healing accelerator, Amer. J. Surg., 1970, 119:560–564.
8. G. G. Allan, L. C. Altman, R. E. Bensinger, D. K. Ghosh, Y. Hirabayashi, A. N. Neogi, and S. Neogi, Biomedical applications of chitin and chitosan, in Chitin, Chitosan and Related Enzymes, ed. J. P. Zikakis, (Academic Press Inc., Orlando, FL, USA, 1984) pp:119–133.
9. Y. Oshshima, K. Nishino, Y. Yonekura, S. Kishimoto, and S. Wakabayashi, Clinical applications of chitin non-woven fabric as wound dressing, Europ. J. Plast. Surg., 1987, 10:66–69.
10. C. H. Su, C. S. Sun, S. W. Juan, C. H. Hu, W. T. Ke, and M. T. Sheu, Fungal mycelia as the source of chitin and polysaccharides and their applications as skin substitutes, Biomaterials, 1997, 18:1169–1174.
11. Y. W. Cho, Y. N. Cho, S. H. Chung, G. Yoo, and S. W. Ko, Water-soluble chitin as a wound healing accelerator, Biomaterials, 1999, 20:2139–2145.
12. N. L. B. M. Yusof, L. Y. Lim, and E. Khor, Preparation and characterization of chitin beads as a wound dressing precursor, J. Biomed. Matls. Res., 2001, 54:59–68.
13. F. L. Mi, S. S. Shyu, Y. B. Wu, S. T. Lee, J. Y. Shyong, and R. N. Huang, Fabrication and characterization of a sponge-like asymmetric chitosan membrane as a wound dressing, Biomaterials, 2001, 22:165–173.
14. G. Biagini, A. Pugnaloni, A. Damadei, A. Bertani, A. Belligolli, V. Bicchiega, and R. Muzzarelli, Morphological study of the capsular organization around tissue expanders coated with N–carboxybutyl chitosan, Biomaterials, 1991, 12:287–291.
15. G. Biagini, A. Bertani, R. Muzzarelli, A. Damadei, G. Dibenedetto, A. Belligolli, and G. Riccotti, Wound management with N–carboxybutyl chitosan, Biomaterials, 1991, 12:281–286.

16. G. Biagini, R. A. A. Muzzarelli, R. Giardino, and C. Castaldini, Biological materials for wound healing, Advances in Chitin and Chitosan, eds. C. J. Brine, P. A. Sandford, and J. P. Zikakis, (Elsevier Appl. Sci, New York, 1992) pp:16–24.

17. O. Damour, P. Y. Gueugniaud, M. Berthin-Maghit, P. Rousselle, F. Berthod, F. Sahuc, and C. Colombel, A dermal substrate made of collagen–GAG–chitosan for deep burn coverage: First clinical uses, Clin. Matls., 1994, 15:273–276.

18. G. Kratz, C. Arnander, J. Swedenborg, M. Back, C. Falk, I. Gouda, and O. Larm, Heparin–chitosan complexes stimulate wound healing in human skin, Scand. J. Plast. Recon. Hand Surg., 1997, 31:119–123.

19. Y. M. Lee, S. S. Kim, M. H. Park, K. W. Song, Y. K. Sung, and I. K. Kang, β-Chitin-based wound dressing containing sulfurdiazine, J. Matls. Sci.: Mats. Med., 2000, 11:817–823.

20. W. K. Loke, S. K. Lau, L. Y. Lim, E. Khor, and K. S. Chow, Wound dressing with sustained anti-microbial capability, J. Biomed. Matls. Res., 2000, 53:8–17.

21. B. E. Chaignaud, R. Langer, and J. P. Vacanti, The history of tissue engineering using synthetic biodegradable polymer scaffolds and cells, in Synthetic Biodegradable Polymer Scaffolds, eds. A. Atala, D. Mooney, R. Langer, and J. P. Vacanti, (Birkhauser, Boston, USA, 1997) pp.1.

22. S. V. Madihally and H. W. T. Matthew, Porous chitosan scaffolds for tissue engineering, Biomaterials, 1999, 20:1133–1142.

23. K. S. Chow, E. Khor, and A. C. A. Wan, Porous chitin matrices for tissue engineering: Fabrication and *in vitro* cytotoxic assessment, J. Polym. Res., 2001, 8:27–35.

24. K. S. Chow and E. Khor, Novel fabrication of open-pore chitin matrixes, Biomacromol., 2000, 1:61–67.

25. J. K F. Suh and H. W. T. Matthew, Application of chitosan-based polysaccharide biomaterials in cartilage tissue engineering: a review, Biomaterials, 2000, 21:2589–2598.

26. V. F. Sechriest, Y. J. Miao, C. Niyibizi, A. Westerhausen-Larson, H. W. Matthew, C. H. Evans, F. H. Fu, and J. K. Suh, GAG-augmented polysaccharide hydrogel: A novel biocompatible and biodegradable material to support chondrogenesis, J. Biomed. Matls. Res., 2000, 49:534–541.

27. A. Lahiji, A. Sohrabi, D. S. Hungerford, and C. G. Frondoza, Chitosan supports the expression of extracellular matrix proteins in human osteoblasts and chondrocytes, J. Biomed. Matls. Res., 2000, 51:586–595.

28. J. Ma, H. Wang, B. He, and J. Chen, A preliminary *in vitro* study on the fabrication and tissue engineering applications of a novel chitosan bi-layer material as a scaffold of human neofetal dermal fibroblasts, Biomaterials, 2001, 22:331–336.

29. V. Dodane and V. D. Vilivalam, Pharmaceutical applications of chitosan, Pharm. Sci. Tech. Today, 1998, 1:246–253.

30. S. Miyazaki, K. Ishii, and T. Nadai, The use of chitin and chitosan as drug carriers, Chem. Pharm. Bull., 1983, 31:2507–2509.

31. T. Chandy and C. P. Sharma, Biodegradable chitosan matrix for the controlled release of steroids, Biomat. Artif. Cells Imm. Biotech., 1991, 19:745–760.

32. S. Miyazaki, H. Yamaguchi, M. Takada, W. M. Hou, Y. Takeichi, and H. Yasubuchi, Pharmaceutical application of biomedical polymers XXIX, Preliminary

study of film dosage form prepared from chitosan for oral drug delivery, Acta Pharm. Nordica, 1990, 2:401–406.

33. Y. Machida, T. Nagai, M. Abe, and T. Sannan, Use of chitosan and hydroxypropylchitosan in drug formulations to effect sustained release, Drug Design Del., 1986, 1:119–130.

34. K. Suzuki, T. Nakamura, H. Matsuura, K. Kifune, and R. Tsurutani, A new drug delivery system for local cancer chemotherapy using cisplatin and chitin, Anticancer Res., 1995, 15:423–426.

35. N. Todorova, M. Krysteva, K. Maneva, and D. Todorov, Carminomycin–chitosan: A conjugated antitumor antibiotic, J. Bioact. Compat. Polym., 1999, 14:178–184.

36. K. Yamamura, T. Sakurai, K. Yano, T. Nabeshima, and T. Yotsuyanagi, Sustained release of basic fibroblast growth factor from the synthetic vascular prosthesis using hydroxypropylchitosan acetate, J. Biomed. Matls. Res., 1995, 29:203–206.

37. S. Tokura, Y. Miura, Y. Kaneda, and Y. Uraki, Drug delivery system using biodegradable carrier, in Polymeric Delivery Systems: Properties and Applications, eds. M. A. El-Nokaly, D. M. Platt, and B. A. Charpentier, (ACS Symposium Series 520, 1993) pp:351–361.

38. K. Watanabe, I. Saiki, Y. Uraki, S. Tokura, and I Azuma, 6–O–Carboxymethyl–chitin (CM–chitin) as a drug carrier, Chem. Pharm. Bull., 1990, 38:506–509.

39. S. Miyazaki, A. Nakayama, M. Oda, M. Takada, and D. Attwood, Chitosan and sodium alginate based bioadhesive tablets for intraoral drug delivery, Bio. Pharm. Bull., 1994, 17:745–747.

40. V. R. Patel and M. M. Amiji, pH-sensitive swelling and drug-release properties of chitosan-poly(ethylene oxide) semi-interpenetrating polymer network, eds. Raphael M. Ottenbrite, Samuel J. Huang, and Kinam Park, (ACS Symposium Series 627, 1996) pp:209–220.

41. S. C. Vasudev, T. Chandy, and C. P. Sharma, Development of chitosan/ polyethylene vinyl acetate co-matrix: controlled release of aspirin–heparin for preventing cardiovascular thrombosis, Biomaterials, 1997, 18:375–381.

42. C. C. Leffler and B. U. W. Müller, Chitosan–gelatin sponges for controlled drug delivery: the use of ionic and non-ionic plasticizers, S. T. P. Pharma Sci., 2000, 10:105–111.

43. S. B. Park, J. O. You, H. Y. Park, S. J. Haam, and W. S. Kim, A novel pH-sensitive membrane from chitosan–TEOS IPN: preparation and its drug permeation characteristics, Biomaterials, 2001, 22:323–330.

44. Y. Nishioka, S. Kyotani, M. Okamura, Y. Mori, M. Miyazaki, K. Okazaki, S. Ohnishi, Y. Yamamoto, and K. Ito, Preparation and evaluation of albumin microspheres and microcapsules containing cisplatin, Chem. Pharm. Bull., 1989, 37:1399–1400.

45. Y. Nishioka, S. Kyotani, H. Masui, M. Okamura, M. Miyazaki, K. Okazaki, S. Ohnishi, Y. Yamamoto, and K. Ito, Preparation and release characteristics of cisplatin albumin microspheres containing chitin and treated with chitosan, Chem. Pharm. Bull., 1989, 37:3074–3077.

46. Y. Nishioka, S. Kyotani, M. Okamura, M. Miyazaki, K. Okazaki, S. Ohnishi, Y. Yamamoto, and K. Ito, Release characteristics of cisplatin chitosan microspheres and effect of containing chitin, Chem. Pharm. Bull., 1990, 38:2871–2873.

47. M. Açikgöz, H. S. Kaş, Z. Hasçelik, Ü. Milli, and A. A. Hincal, Chitosan microspheres of diclofenac sodium, II: *In vitro* and *in vivo* evaluation, Pharmazie, 1995, 50:275–277.

48. J. Akbuğa and N. Bergişadi, 5–Fluorouracil-loaded chitosan microspheres: preparation and release characteristics, J. Microencap., 1996, 13:161–168.

49. S. Patashnik, L. Rabinovich, and G. Golomb, Preparation and evaluation of chitosan microspheres containing bisphosphonates, J. Drug Targeting, 1997, 4:371–380.

50. H. Tokimitsu, H. Ichikawa, T. K. Saha, Y. Fukumori, and L. H. Block, Design and preparation of gadolinium-loaded chitosan particles for cancer neutron capture therapy, S. T. P. Pharma Sci., 2000, 10:39–49.

51. I. M. van der Lubben, J. C. Verhoef, A. C. can Aelst, G. Borchard, and H. E. Junginger, Chitosan microparticles for oral vaccination: preparation, characterization and preliminary *in vivo* uptake studies in murine Peyer's patches, Biomaterials, 2001, 22:687–694.

52. L. Illum, P. Watts, A. N. Fischer, I. Jabba Gill, and S. S. Davis, Novel chitosan-based delivery systems for the nasal administration of a LHRH-analog, S. T. P. Pharma Sci., 2000, 10:89–94.

53. K. W. Leong, H. Q. Mao, V. L. Troung-Le, K. Roy, S. M. Walsh, and J. T. August, DNA-polycation nanospheres as non-viral gene delivery vehicles, J. Cont. Rel., 1998, 53:183–193.

54. J. Murata, Y. Ohya, and T. Ouchi, Possibility of application of quaternary chitosan having pendant galactose residues as a gene delivery system, Carbohydrate Polym., 1996, 29:69–74.

55. J. Murata, Y. Ohya, and T. Ouchi, Design of quaternary chitosan conjugate having antennary galactose residues as a gene delivery tool, Carbohydrate Polym., 1997, 32:105–109.

56. F. L. Mi, C. T. Chen, Y. C. Tseng, C. Y. Kuan, and S. S. Shyu, Iron(III)–carboxymethylchitin microsphere for the pH-sensitive release of 6–mercaptopurine, J. Control. Rel., 1997, 44:19–32.

57. P. Giunchedi, I. Genta, B. Conti, R. A. A. Muzzarelli, and U. Conte, Preparation and characterization of ampicillin loaded methyl–pyrrolidinone chitosan and chitosan microspheres, Biomaterials, 1998, 19:157–161.

58. B. Conti, P. Giunchedi, I. Genta, and U. Conte, The preparation and *in vivo* evaluation of the wound-healing properties of chitosan microspheres, S. T. P. Pharma Sci., 2000, 10:101–104.

59. E. Khor, Chitin: a biomaterial in waiting, Current Opinion in Solid State & Materials Science, 2002, 6:313–317.

60. M. Dornish, A. Hagen, E. Hansson, C. Pecheur, F. Verdier, and Ø. Skaugrud, Safety of Protosan™: Ultrapure chitosan salts for biomedical and pharmaceutical use, Advances in Chitin Science, Volume II, eds. A. Domard, G. A. F. Roberts, and K. M. Vårum, (Jacques Andre Publisher, Lyon, 1997) pp:664–670.

SUBJECT INDEX